Aging and
Communication

FOR CLINICIANS BY CLINICIANS

Michael P. Cannito and Deannie Vogel, Series Editors

This book, *Aging and Communication,* is the ninth volume in the For Clinicians by Clinicians series of texts on the diagnosis and clinical management of speech, language, and voice disorders. Each text provides a contemporary perspective on one major disorder or clinical area and is designed for use in clinical methodology courses and continuing education programs. Authors have been selected who represent a broad spectrum of clinical interests and theoretical positions and who hold the common belief that their viewpoints, experiences, and successes should be shared in order to provide a forum for clinicians by clinicians.

Volumes already published in this series are *Treating Language Disorders, Treating Articulation Disorders, Case Studies in Aphasia Rehabilitation, Treating Cerebral Palsy, Alaryngeal Speech Rehabilitation, Treating Disordered Speech Motor Control, Cleft Palate,* and *Language Intervention: Beyond the Primary Grades.*

Dedication

Audrey L. Holland, PhD
University of Arizona

Aging and Communication is dedicated to Dr. Audrey L. Holland, whose pioneering work in functional aspects of communication in adults with aphasia refocused our attention on the client as a whole person, and whose contributions to research and clinical practice in normal aging, dementia, and aphasia are immeasurable. Although well known as an educator and scientist, Dr. Holland's priorities are in and greatest satisfaction have come from her clinical work. Her career exemplifies the clinician orientation of the *For Clinicians by Clinicians* series.

Aging and Communication

For Clinicians by Clinicians

Edited by

Barbara B. Shadden
Mary Ann Toner

pro·ed

8700 Shoal Creek Boulevard
Austin, Texas 78757-6897

pro·ed

© 1997 by PRO-ED, Inc.
8700 Shoal Creek Boulevard
Austin, Texas 78757-6897

Library of Congress Cataloging-in-Publication Data

Aging and communication / edited by Barbara B. Shadden, Mary Ann
  Toner.
    p.   cm.—(For clinicians by clinicians)
   Includes bibliographical references and index.
   ISBN 0-89079-711-0 (alk. paper)
   1. Communicative disorders in old age—Treatment.   2. Aged-
-Communication.   I. Shadden, Barbara B. (Barbara Bennett).
II. Toner, Mary Ann, 1954-   . III. Series.
RC429.A35   1997
618.97′6855—dc20   96-38710
                                                          CIP

This book is designed in Eras and Palatino.

Production Manager: Alan Grimes
Production Coordinator: Karen Swain
Managing Editor: Tracy Sergo
Designer: Thomas Barkley
Reprints Buyer: Alicia Woods
Editor: Sue Motzer
Production Assistant: Claudette Landry
Editorial Assistant: Suzi Hunn

Printed in the United States of America

1 2 3 4 5 6 7 8 9 10   01 00 99 98 97

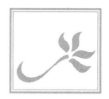

Contents

Contributors

Jane A. Barr, MSW, PhD
University of Arkansas
Department of Sociology
Old Main 211
Fayetteville, AR 72701

Faerella Boczko, MS
The Jewish Home and Hospital
    for the Aged
100 West Kingsbridge Road
Bronx, NY 10468

Michelle S. Bourgeois, PhD
The Florida State University
412 Regional Rehabilitation
    Center
Tallahassee, FL 32306-2007

Anthony J. Caruso, PhD
School of Speech Pathology and
    Audiology
PO Box 5190
Kent State University
Kent, OH 44242-0001

Lynne W. Clark, PhD
Hunter/Mt. Sinai Geriatric
    Education Center
Communication Sciences
    Program
Hunter College, City University
    of New York
425 East 25th Street
Nyack, NY 10010

Carol S. Crichley, PhD
Department of Audiology and
    Speech Pathology
Ithaca College
304 Smiddy Hall
Ithaca, NY 14850

Patricia Duckworth, MSN
Area Health Education
    Cooperative
Pea Ridge Medical Office
801 N. Curtis Avenue
Pea Ridge, AR 72751

Patricia J. Dukes, PhD
Speech and Hearing Clinic
1410 Lower Campus Drive
University of Hawaii
Honolulu, HI 96822

Susan E. Durnford, MA
Department of Audiology and
    Speech Pathology
304 Smiddy Hall
Ithaca College
Ithaca, NY 14850

Holly H. Elliott, MS, MFCC
1300 NE 16th Avenue
#1408
Portland, OR 97232-1454

Susan F. Erler, PhD
Communication Sciences and
    Disorders
Frances Searle Building
2299 North Campus Drive
Northwestern University
Evanston, IL 60208-3550

Dean C. Garstecki, PhD
Audiology and Hearing Sciences
    Program
Frances Searle Building
2299 North Campus Drive
Northwestern University
Evanston, IL 60208-3550

Laurel E. Glass, MD, PhD
1300 NE 16th Avenue
#1408
Portland, OR 97232-1454

Joan K. Glickstein, PhD
Glickstein-Neustadt, Inc.
321 Challen Drive
Pittsburgh, PA 15236

Daniel J. Johnson, PhD
Health South Rehabilitation
    Hospital of Fort Smith
1401 South "J" Street
Fort Smith, AR 72901

John A. Krout, PhD
Gerontology Institute
Ithaca College
170 Dillingham Center
Ithaca, NY 14850

Jon Lyon, PhD
Center for Living with
    Aphasia, Inc.
6344 Hillsandwood Road
Mazomanie, WI 53560

Peter B. Mueller, PhD
School of Speech Pathology and
    Audiology
PO Box 5190
Kent State University
Kent, OH 44242-0001

Gail K. Neustadt, MA
Glickstein-Neustadt, Inc.
516 Harrogate Road
Pittsburgh, PA 15241

Paul R. Rao, PhD
Clinical Services Department
Quality Improvement and
    Customer Service
Stroke Recovery Program
National Rehabilitation Hospital
102 Irving Street NW
Washington, DC 20010

Mary Jo Santo Pietro, PhD
Speech–Language Pathology
Kean College of New Jersey
1000 Morris Avenue
Union, NJ 07083

Barbara B. Shadden, PhD
University of Arkansas Speech
    and Hearing Clinic
410 Arkansas Avenue
Fayetteville, AR 72701

Sheela Stuart, PhD
New Mexico State University
Special Education/Communi-
    cation Disorders
Department 3SPE, Box 30001
Las Cruces, NM 88003-0001

Mary Ann Toner, PhD
University of Arkansas Speech
    and Hearing Clinic
410 Arkansas Avenue
Fayetteville, AR 72701

Larry D. Wright, MD
Bates Medical Center
602 N. Walton Boulevard
Bentonville, AR 72714

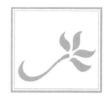

Preface

The For Clinicians by Clinicians series has become synonymous with relevant, clinician-oriented information about assessment and intervention approaches for specific communication disorders. When we were first approached about the prospect of editing a text on aging for the series, we were delighted by the opportunity to create a publication on aging and communication that would emphasize model clinical practices founded on sound theoretical and informational bases. At the same time, we recognized that such a text would represent a radical departure from the rest of the For Clinicians by Clinicians series, because aging itself is not a disorder. A significant focus of the text would have to be information about normal aging processes and changes, and about aspects of functioning apart from communication behavior and disorders. *Aging and Communication* is the product of our deliberations about the content needed by practicing and future clinicians in order to work effectively and creatively with older clients.

Aging and Communication makes no attempt to provide a comprehensive description of the characteristics of and/or management approaches for all of the communication disorders found with some frequency in the older population. Information about specific communication disorders is available in many other sources. Instead, the text is divided into two main sections. Section 1 is entitled "Aspects of Aging: A Continuum of Functioning." The purpose of this section is to introduce the reader to information about all aspects of aging and to define characteristics of older adults that may influence responses to communication disorders, performance in assessment and treatment sessions, and communicative effectiveness in real-life situations. Throughout this section, emphasis is placed upon the heterogeneity of the aging experience and of older individuals. The fundamental assumption is that an understanding of life span developmental issues, and of the status of any individual older person, is critical to successful functional interventions.

Section 2 is titled "Intervention Approaches: A Continuum of Care Settings and Service Delivery Models." In this section, some chapters provide the reader with a broad overview of interventions as they are influenced by the realities of working with older adults within existing service delivery environments and constraints. Other chapters address specific clinical populations or needs of older adults and their caregivers, providing innovative models for intervention that represent current practice at its best and that should stimulate practitioners to develop their own creative management approaches.

Section 1 begins with an introductory chapter by Shadden and Toner in which the philosophical framework of the text is outlined. In addition to basic demographics and multicultural considerations, the chapter provides a description of some of the current and projected challenges facing health care practitioners serving older clients. Basic text concepts about the nature and role of communication for older adults are introduced, and a "wish list" for professional preparation and involvement with the elderly is presented. Chapters 2 through 4 examine aging realities in social, physiological–medical, and cognitive–affective domains. Aspects of the aging experience that may influence communicative functioning and/or response to treatment are highlighted. For example, in Chapter 2, Barr focuses on life transitions and role shifts as fundamental to the experience of social aging, closing with a section on personal adaptation and adjustment. Wright and Duckworth emphasize physical and health changes associated with the aging process in Chapter 3 and outline the importance of functional assessment in these domains. In Chapter 4, Johnson summarizes cognitive changes associated with life span development and discusses briefly the nature of depression and dementia in the elderly. Again, functional assessment is described, this time from the perspective of mental status examination.

Chapters 5 through 7 narrow the focus to hearing, speech/voice, and language/communication. In Chapter 5, Garstecki and Erler survey what is known about age-associated hearing loss, acknowledging its unique status as both a normal age change and a disorder. Prevalence and causes of hearing impairment are described. Consequences for speech perception and psychosocial adjustment are discussed. Caruso and Mueller use Chapter 6 to examine the effects of aging on the oral–pharyngeal–laryngeal mechanisms of older adults, exploring the nature and extent of changes in speech, voice, and swallowing behaviors. Finally, Shadden summarizes what is known about language and communication in older adults in Chapter 7. This chapter begins with a brief exploration of the potential indirect and direct effects on communication of aspects of aging described in the previous chapters, followed by a review of current literature on language comprehension and performance in older adults and communicative interactions with the elderly.

Section 2 begins and ends with chapters addressing broad service delivery issues. In Chapter 8, Glickstein identifies the continuum of settings for health care provision. Readers are provided with a detailed description of the many settings in which speech–language pathologists can serve older clients, and models for care delivery within and across settings and professions are presented. Rao's Chapter 9 also explores broad issues of functional assessment as they apply specifically to speech–language pathology. Principles of functional assessment are outlined, followed by a description of some commonly used assessment tools. The need for accommodations to age changes during evaluation is acknowledged.

Chapters 10 through 16 address innovative intervention strategies for communication disorders in the elderly. Chapters with a common focus are placed sequentially to highlight similar themes, populations, and/or settings. For example, in Chapters 10 and 11, caregiver interventions are addressed. In 10, Bourgeois identifies the needs and optimal approaches to caregiver training for coping with Alzheimer's disease. Techniques used in current pilot programs are discussed, and outcomes are described. In Chapter 11, Clark explores the topic of caregiver interventions from the particular perspective of communication strategies. After discussing the nature and causes of communication breakdown, using a family systems approach to explain the impact of the communication disorder, Clark reviews caregiver communication intervention programs.

Chapters 12 through 14 emphasize communication skills training and communication enhancement. In Chapter 12, Dukes provides a unique perspective on the problem-solving role of Quality Assurance Committees in addressing resident communication needs in long-term care (LTC) and retirement facilities. Through a series of problem scenarios, she outlines innovative approaches to a wide range of concerns, from communication maintenance posttreatment to generalization of communication skills, effective management of hearing aids, aural rehabilitation, and monitoring diet levels in dysphagic residents. In Chapter 13, Lyon takes the reader beyond the treatment room and traditional treatment time frame to explore the use of volunteer partners in working with communicatively disordered older adults to maximize their communicative interactions and opportunities in meaningful activities within the community. The chapter traces volunteer training and involvement with one aphasic adult, and proposes applications of the partners program to work with communicatively at-risk older individuals. Finally, in Chapter 14, Stuart addresses augmentative communication interventions with older adults with speech–language disorders from the unique perspective of "playing to the strength" of older persons. The chapter begins with a brief summary of the augmentative and alternative communication (AAC) challenges of different communication disorders. Necessary considerations in designing AAC systems for older adults are outlined, including motivational issues; accommodations to sensory, motor, and cognitive changes; and financial and social/environmental circumstances. The remainder of the chapter focuses on the story-telling abilities of older adults, the communicative functions served by story telling, and the ways that inclusion of story-telling options into AAC systems can maximize communicative interactions and AAC intervention success.

Chapters 15 and 16 explore communication maintenance and enhancement programs from two perspectives. In Chapter 15, Santo Pietro and Boczko outline current communication intervention guidelines for Alzheimer's patients, then describe one innovative program, the Breakfast Club, that has shown measurable success in improving communicative and social adequacy in dementia residents of an LTC facility. Chapter 16 extends the discussion to more general consideration of all kinds of functional maintenance programs in LTC environments, identifying the elements of such programs and mechanisms for reimbursement.

In Chapter 17, Toner considers how primary, secondary, and tertiary aging affect swallowing and eating functions in older adults. A case example illustrates the potential contributions of all three of these aspects of aging on one client's swallowing dysfunction. Assessment approaches that acknowledge the realities of the older individual's circumstances and preferences are identified, as well as management considerations, with the same client being traced throughout her management program. The importance of appropriate inservice and education of caregivers and older adults is stressed. Chapter 18 examines management of hearing impairment in older adults from the perspective of the individual's reaction to and strategies for coping with gradual-onset hearing loss. Authors Glass and Elliot acknowledge the array of technological, medical, and therapeutic interventions possible, but refer the reader elsewhere for commonly available discussions of specific approaches. Instead, they contend that health professionals must understand the experience of adult-onset hearing loss in order to provide maximally effective and holistic services.

Section 2 closes with a final chapter on the aging services network. After the aging services network is defined, the reader is provided with a description of relevant mandates and programs of the Older Americans Act. The need for collaborative interface between communication disorders professionals and this network is emphasized, with barriers to interaction identified and tentative solutions and model programs outlined.

We hope that *Aging and Communication* will serve as a useful resource to professionals seeking to improve the appropriateness, quality, and breadth of interventions with communicatively impaired older adults. Audiologists and speech–language pathologists are already committed to quality of life for persons of all ages and backgrounds. As health care systems and resulting practice patterns continue to evolve, the older segment of the population will require more and more of our clinical focus. Interventions must be grounded in aging realities, while remaining highly individualized. Creativity and innovation are required.

Barbara B. Shadden
Mary Ann Toner

Section 1

Aspects of Aging: A Continuum of Functioning

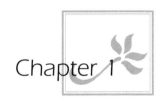

Chapter 1

Introduction: The Continuum of Life Functions

Barbara B. Shadden
Mary Ann Toner

Shadden and Toner provide a philosophical rationale for this text on communication and aging, outlining basic demographic and multicultural considerations and describing challenges facing health care practitioners serving older adults. The importance of communication for older persons is highlighted, and a "wish list" for professional preparation and involvement with the elderly is presented.

1. *What are the demographic trends that suggest that communication disorders professionals will become increasingly involved with older clients? How will the older clients of the future differ from current older individuals? What do we need to learn about communication behavior and disorders in ethnically diverse groups?*

2. *What health care trends are affecting and can be expected to continue to influence communication disorders service delivery to older adults?*

3. *How are our professions preparing for current and future challenges? What needs in professional preparation, research initiatives, and clinical practice still exist?*

4. *What philosophical premises do Shadden and Toner offer for applying gerontological information to clinical management practices? Why should communication be considered a critical element in older adults' adaptation to age changes and life crises?*

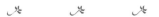

W
ithin recent years, public and professional attention has focused increasingly on a phenomenon known as the "graying of America." By the year 2000, individuals over the age of 65 years will constitute 13% of the country's population, or 35 million adults, more than double the number of children under the age of 5 years (U.S. Department of Commerce, 1992). Soon thereafter, the baby boomers will hit retirement age. By 2020, older persons will constitute 16.9% of our population; by 2030, the number of individuals over 65 will equal the number of individuals under 17 (Brock, Guralnik, & Brody, 1990). Within the older population, the fastest growing segment will be the old-old (over 85 years), a group demonstrating greater frailty and susceptibility to disease processes, as well as greater needs for daily assistance (Holosko & Feit, 1991).

It has been estimated that elderly clients with communication disorders currently constitute 19% of the caseloads of speech–language pathologists and 33% of the caseloads of audiologists (Slater, 1992). These figures suggest that older adults with communicative impairment are already underserved. By the year 2050, it is expected that persons over the age of 65 will constitute 39% of the speech–language impaired population and 59% of the hearing impaired population (Fein, 1983a, 1983b).

Older adults are prone to a wide variety of communication disorders, particularly those that are neurologically based. Duffy (1995) reported that, out of 4,756 clients demonstrating acquired speech–language disorders, neurological impairment accounted for almost 72% of the disorders, with motor speech disorders being most common (36.5%), followed by aphasia (19.5%), other cognitive–linguistic disorders (9.3%), and other neurogenic speech disorders (6.5%). Anatomic deficiency (laryngectomy, glossectomy), nonneurogenic/nonpsychogenic voice disorders (tracheostomy, neoplasms, surgery), idiopathic disorders, and psychogenic disorders completed the caseload. Although this study was not limited to elderly patients, that portion of the population is at greatest risk for most of these acquired disorders. Additionally, dysphagia is often linked to many of the same etiologies. Dysphagia management is the fastest growing area of practice for speech–language pathologists. Although figures may vary, there are more older adults that demonstrate hearing impairment than any other communication disorder. Obviously, as the population ages, clinicians should expect to see ever-expanding numbers of elderly patients who demonstrate some degree of hearing, speech, language, cognitive, or swallowing dysfunction.

Due to the effects of normal aging, elderly persons who experience a communication disorder often demonstrate more severe symptoms and are more likely to experience co-occurring disorders, such as aphasia, dysarthria, and dysphagia. These factors can lead to a poorer prognosis for recovery of skills for the older individual with a communication disorder. It is important, however, that communication disorders specialists do not become comfortable with lower expectations for any group or satisfied with less than optimal recovery. Instead, new methods of prevention and intervention must constantly be sought. Although speech–language pathology and audiology services have demonstrated tremendous change and expansion during the past 20 years, these professions are not ready to meet the demands of the 21st century.

The older adult of the next millennium can be expected to be better educated, more affluent, and generally more sophisticated with respect to rights and needs (Kane, 1994). These "future elderly" come from a generation that has often demanded "more and better" services; they are likely to have higher expectations of health care professionals than the current older generation, demanding greater access to services and better results. There will also be increasing expectations for patient involvement in active decision making. In addition, future professionals need to be prepared for more client variation, allowing for differences in culture and ethnicity.

Ethnicity and Aging

The term *ethnicity* is used here to refer to membership in a group defined or set apart by race, religion, national origin, or a combination of these variables (Stanford, 1990). In the United States, the elderly form a relatively small percentage of non-White ethnic groups at present (e.g., 8.2% of the Black population and 4.9 % of the Hispanic population). However, growth has been and will continue to be most rapid in these groups. For example, it is projected that the Hispanic older population will increase by 76.9% by the year 2000. This trend is already occurring in Native American cultures, where the population over 65 increased by 85% between 1980 and 1990 (U.S. House Committee on Aging, 1988, 1989).

Some facts about multicultural aspects of aging are highlighted here to illustrate the manner in which health care professionals must be sensitive to potential influences of ethnicity on service delivery to and communication in older adults (see references above and Shadden & Warnick, 1994). Clearly, the demographic profile of the elderly varies considerably across ethnic subgroups. For example, non-White older adults have less education and lower median incomes than White older adults. In addition, sources of income differ. Almost 70% of White older adults supplement Social Security income with interest income; in contrast, only 27% of Black and 32% of Hispanic older people have access to similar supplements.

Health profiles and patterns of service utilization also distinguish ethnic groups (Van Nostrand, Furner, & Suzman, 1993). Non-White older adults are more likely to rate their health as fair or poor than White older adults. Non-White elderly persons also experience more days of restricted activity yearly and more difficulty with Activities of Daily Living (ADLs) and Instrumental Activities of Daily Living (IADLs). However, nursing home utilization is lower for the Black older population. Types of health problems also differentiate groups. For example, hearing loss appears to be more prevalent in White older adults than in other ethnic groups. However, Blacks are more susceptible to diabetes, hypertension, and circulatory disorders. Patterns of health service utilization and formal and informal community supports for dependent elders vary widely across cultural boundaries (see Chapter 2).

Clinicians should be sensitive to the fact that ethnic variations may influence the older person's functional and communicative status in a variety of ways. Certainly, the nature of social supports and the degree of real and perceived caregiver burden will vary across ethnic groups. In addition, some individuals may simply lack the necessary resources to access needed services, or may be reluctant to participate in services viewed as dominated by Whites. The effects of age-based stereotypes on communicative interactions may be exacerbated if the communicative exchange involves partners who are not only of different ages, but also from different ethnic and/or cultural backgrounds (Jackson & Ensley, 1995). Finally, little is known about normal speech–language and hearing changes in ethnically diverse older adults and about the prevalence of specific communication disorders in these populations.

Response of the Health Care Industry

The face of the health care industry today has changed radically. Managed care, corporate entrepreneurism, and vertical reorganization of health care sites and services have forced major redefinitions of setting-specific needs and reimbursable services. Further, the enormous escalation of health care costs, particularly for older Americans, has led to public and governmental demands for restraint. In this context, the "graying of America" has profound implications for health care professionals in all settings, for the health care delivery system itself, and for society in general. Resource allocations to older adults are already insufficient. Competition for resources can only increase in the future, particularly in view of health care system mandates emphasizing "more for less." Issues of age-based rationing of services and resources have been raised, kicking up a storm of medical ethics controversies. At the same time, demands are increasing for greater attention to quality-of-life issues, including disease prevention/health promotion programs and maintenance of high levels of functionality in older clients. "Functionality" has become a buzzword linked with personal autonomy and well-being. It would be impossible to address these health care issues in a comprehensive fashion in this chapter. The interested reader is referred to Kane (1994) and Logemann (1994, 1995) for further perspectives on the changing face of health care as it affects our professions.

Where do communication disorders professionals fit within the context of all of these dynamic changes in demographics and associated mandates for system change? As health care delivery systems in our country continue to evolve, communication disorders professionals cannot afford to remain isolated from the critical issues being raised by national changes in service delivery systems, particularly when older adults are considered as a potential client base. The prevailing "more for less" philosophy has led to the search for a "quick fix" in service delivery, with increasing demands for proof of efficacy of services. This has been particularly difficult within the communication disorders professions, because of the complexity and subtlety of many of the behaviors that might be used in establishing efficacy. Some reactions to these expanding needs are already apparent. Communication disorders specialists are providing a greater number of services in more settings than ever before.

However, professional identities inside and outside of the communication disorders discipline are being challenged actively. Individual health care disciplines have increased their advocacy and competition for their particular share of the limited resources available. Speech–language pathology and audiology are struggling with issues of specialization, largely in response to the continually expanding scope of practice. Specialization has significant implications for management of communication disorders in older adults. As noted, many disorders co-occur, and may be overlaid on other aging changes in communicative functioning. Specialists working with geriatric populations must make certain that a holistic approach to assessment and intervention is retained. At the same time, external forces are pushing for more health care generalists, multiskilled practitioners, and lower levels of training for all health care providers. Support personnel have become a reality in speech–language pathology, with few adequate models for the appropriate and creative utilization of such personnel in service delivery to older adults. Some professions are even limiting the number of qualified providers available in the marketplace.

In a 1994 issue of *Asha* focusing on aging, serious questions were raised about the professional preparation of speech–language pathologists and audiologists for work with older clients and for research involving age-related changes in communicative functions. These questions were raised in the context of challenges to practitioners and researchers alike to abandon our professional insularity and our exclusive focus on speech–language and hearing disorders in order to embrace broader, more innovative roles with respect to the spectrum of communication needs of older individuals. As Kane (1994, p. 35) pointed out, it is time for all health care professionals to make "serious efforts to shape rather than prepare to respond to future changes." Passive adaptation to perceived external forces and trends is not sufficient.

There is substantial evidence that the gerontological education of students in speech–language pathology remains insufficient and focused too exclusively on disorders (Clark, Ripich, & Weinstein, 1994; Raiford & Shadden, 1985). Speech–language pathologists and audiologists are most comfortable dealing with aging from the perspective of many of the communication disorders and associated problems found with high prevalence in the older segment of the population, such as aphasia and dysarthria. Less confidence is expressed in the areas of dysphagia, ventilator dependence, and dementia (Shadden & Toner,

1995). In part, the different levels of comfort reflect the availability of both academic coursework and textbooks addressing such disorders, either as separate entities or in the context of geriatric issues and concerns (e.g., Ripich, 1991). Practitioners and administrators in medical speech–language pathology settings also appear most satisfied with the entry-level skills of clinicians as they involve working with traditional speech–language disorders such as aphasia and dysarthria (Shadden & Toner, 1995; Shadden, Toner, & McCarthy, 1995). Because infusion of geriatric information remains the most common method of addressing information on aging in our educational programs, "the philosophy unique to the management of older adults is rarely conveyed to students" (Weinstein & Clark, 1994, p. 36).

Philosophical Premises

Managing the direct consequences of communication disorders might appear to be a sufficient challenge for audiologists and speech–language pathologists working with older adults. However, such management approaches represent the tip of the iceberg of potential service delivery options. In order to understand the broad spectrum of communication needs and intervention strategies and settings presented in this text, it is helpful to keep in mind certain central premises that may provide a clinical framework for applying gerontological information to management practices. The philosophical premises outlined here are those that have shaped the organization and content of this text. They provide a context for understanding aging and the role of the communication disorders professional in working with older adults in this society.

The Importance of Communication for Older Adults

The first, and probably most important, premise is that interpersonal communication is a critical tool in life adjustment for persons of all ages. Kaakinen (1995) identified two critical functions of human communication as part of the adjustment or adaptation process. First, communicative behaviors link the individual with the environment, promoting a sense of well-being and validating self-concept. Second, communication serves as a primary regulator of behavior, both within the individual and in the person-to-person context. In effect, as Lubinski (1991) suggested, communication is "an error-creating and error-correcting mechanism for the establishment of interpersonal relationships" (p. 238).

Successful aging depends, in part, upon being able to use communication resources effectively. Ironically, in the later years, this communication tool is also most vulnerable to a variety of normal and pathological aging processes and changes. Twenty years ago, Oyer and Oyer (1976) listed an extensive number of barriers to communication for the elderly. These barriers are discussed in greater detail in Chapter 7. As our understanding of these barriers and the impact of other aging factors upon communication has increased, it has become clear that both aging and communication are best represented as a continuum of functions.

The Continua of Aging Processes and Communication Behaviors

One of the central tasks facing the clinician is determining the extent to which a given behavior reflects aspects of normal aging, pathological aging, or a specific communication disorder. Implicit in this statement is the concept of aging as occurring on a continuum, from pathological to robust or successful aging (Garfein & Herzog, 1995), with disorders superimposed upon this continuum. Attempts to define clearly what is meant by "normal aging" remain largely unsuccessful, but the term is often used to refer to the expected and unavoidable— the running out of the biological time clock and the readily anticipated responses to the broad spectrum of aging realities. In contrast, "pathological" aging is presumed to refer to some type of premature breakdown of one or more human systems, and is most typically used to describe disease processes leading to dementias or pseudodementias that accelerate signs and products of the normal aging process (Birren, 1986). A similar continuum concept can be applied to communication behaviors across all age groups. A random sampling of older adults will reveal a wide range of interpersonal communication skills, from superior communicators to those at risk for communication breakdown to those with specific communication disorders.

Various factors—genetic, environmental, educational, social, emotional, and financial—influence where each individual will "fall" on these continua. When one considers the interaction of these two continua in the aging adult, it is not surprising that heterogeneity of behavior is the norm.

Aging Is a Life Span Developmental Phenomenon

In the context of the previous statement about the heterogeneity of the aging experience, it may appear odd to assert that aging is a developmental phenomenon. Such a statement implies that there are orderly and sequential changes in attitude, characteristics, and physical status associated with moving through the life span. In reality, these statements are not contradictory. In delivery of services to children, we take for granted that each age and developmental stage has associated with it certain characteristics to which we must accommodate and that we must consider in determining interventions. The stages and effects of developmental changes are more complex and diverse in the older population. To identify older persons in need of intervention, however, we must still be able to recognize deviations from developmental patterns and shifts to the disordered or pathological end of the continuum of aging processes. Further, some aspects of the developmental process of aging allow specific strengths and skills to evolve through experience, strengths that can be harnessed in the managing of life changes and in coping with communication disorders. An understanding of aging as a life span developmental phenomenon also allows us to recognize the central roles of adaptation, and of adaptive strategies, as determinants of communicative behavior and participation in treatment.

Adaptation: A Critical Concept for Understanding the Communication Status of Older Persons

If one views many age-related changes as harbingers of life crises, or more generally as stressors, then one must acknowledge that humans, by nature, are driven to cope or adapt in order to maintain some level of internal equilibrium. There are currently several models reflecting the adaptive nature of communicative behaviors in older adults.

In 1988, Shadden proposed a "communication and aging" model suggesting that, in many domains (including communication), an individual may exist on a continuum of skills or resources, from total deficit/liability at one end to major resource/tool at the other end. The aging individual's status at any point in time can be described in terms of an inventory of personal and situational characteristics that fall either to the debit (risk factor) or credit (resources) side of both the aging and the communication continua. Implicit in the model is the idea that aspects of aging can threaten the older adult's adequacy of communication and thus his or her ability to use communication as a coping strategy or mechanism. The model underscored the fact that older individuals will attempt a variety of coping or adaptive responses to maintain homeostasis in their lives. The more recent Communication Predicament and Enhancement models, proposed by Ryan and colleagues, address similar ideas in a somewhat different format (Orange, Ryan, Meredith, & MacLean, 1995).

Adaptation is also underscored in Trieschman's (1987) model of coping with disability. In this model, Trieschman views the older individual with a disability *in the context* of the total environment, with health or adjustment equated with the interaction among psychosocial, biologic–organic, and environmental influences. Aging itself can be viewed as a change in the balance, often resulting from alteration of biological–organic functions that then modify psychosocial and environmental influences.

A Wish List for the 21st Century

In closing, it seems appropriate to engage in a bit of wishful thinking—for the future of our professions' involvement with older adults and for the achievement of quality of life for older adults through optimal communication. Much of the following wish list evolves logically from the central premises and health care trends identified earlier. All of the items on this list represent challenges to speech–language pathology and audiology today and into the next millennium.

- There is a clear need for improved gerontological preparation related to communication behaviors and disorders in older adults. This preparation must encompass aspects of normal aging, as well as the full continuum of communicative functioning. Students and practitioners need greater understanding of vital issues related to functional status and functional communication assessment, health promotion and prevention of communication breakdown, multidisciplinary service delivery, and setting-specific needs and practices.

- Appropriate accommodations to age-related changes in the individual and the individual's environment must become the norm in assessment and treatment. These accommodations should evolve logically from improved gerontological preparation that emphasizes a developmental approach to aging and acknowledges the vulnerability of the communication continuum to aging forces. We must shift our emphasis to the whole person, and to the environment in which this person exists. As part of these environmental considerations, we must develop systematic methods of promoting family and/or caregiver understanding of and involvement in the intervention process.

- Communication disorders professionals must increase their interprofessional involvement within the aging network to ensure that older adults receive coordinated services and support, and to improve the adequacy, breadth, and comprehensiveness of such services (see Shadden & Barr, 1988; Chapter 19 of this text). As part of this increased involvement, we must begin to see better cross-professional dialogue about ideal service environments and service mechanisms, without petty interdisciplinary squabbles over practice territory.

- Research efforts related to all aspects of aging and the communication continuum must be expanded and refocused (Dancer, 1994) to become (a) more function oriented, (b) more solidly based on interactional aspects of communication, and (c) more interdisciplinary. Research needs include (a) efficacy studies of experimental and innovative programs, including dementia interventions, communication maintenance and enhancement programs for at-risk older adults, and interventions targeting the impairment and disability associated with common communication disorders; (b) further exploration and definition of functional communication baseline and outcome measures; (c) continued attempts to specify the nature of and factors contributing to linguistic and communicative behaviors in older adults; (d) identification of multicultural variations in the prevalence of communication disorders and the impact of normal aging upon language and communication; and (e) further definition of the nature and progression of linguistic and communicative breakdown in individuals with dementia, along with enhanced understanding of dementia subtypes.

It is hoped that if the items on this wish list are realized, communication disorders professionals will become more creative, breaking away from traditional models of intervention and modes of service delivery. We must make a commitment to supporting the role of communication in ensuring quality of life for all older adults. Future interventions should be proactive and preventive in focus, expanding interdisciplinary involvement and broadening outreach to caregivers and significant others (American Speech-Language-Hearing Association Committee on Communication Problems of the Aging, 1988).

Conclusions

Because of the rapidity with which our knowledge base related to aging and to older individuals continues to evolve, it has become virtually impossible for any single text to capture this knowledge base in a readable format that is relevant to practitioners within specific health care disciplines. In the first section of *Communication and Aging,* therefore, contributors have approached the topic of aging from the perspective of what clinicians in speech–language pathology and audiology need to know in order to understand better the complex forces acting upon communication in the older population and to enhance assessment and intervention practices. The second section of the text addresses management issues and approaches specific to the elderly and provides a potpourri of innovative approaches being used with older adults falling at a variety of points along the communication continuum. Although many practitioners will wish to apply one or more of these approaches immediately in clinical practice, it is also hoped that models of creative assessment and intervention will stimulate the development of additional programs and approaches that will benefit future generations of older adults.

References

American Speech-Language-Hearing Association Committee on Communication Problems of the Aging. (1988, March). The roles of speech–language pathologists and audiologists in working with older persons: A position statement. *Asha, 30,* 80–84.

Birren, J. E. (1986). The process of aging: Growing up and growing old. In A. Pifer & L. Bronte (Eds.), *Our aging society* (pp. 259–276). New York: Norton.

Brock, D., Guralnik, J., & Brody, J. (1990). Demography and epidemiology of aging in the United States. In E. Schneider & J. Rowe (Eds.), *Handbook of the biology of aging* (3rd ed., pp. 3–23). San Diego: Academic Press.

Clark, L., Ripich, D., & Weinstein, B. (1994). *Status of geriatric education in the professional education programs of speech–language pathology and audiology.* Unpublished manuscript.

Dancer, J. (1994). Research directions. *Asha, 36,* 37–38.

Duffy, J. R. (1995). *Motor speech disorders: Substrates, differential diagnosis, and management.* St. Louis, MO: Mosby.

Fein, D. J. (1983a). The prevalence of speech and language impairments. *Asha, 25,* 37.

Fein, D. J. (1983b). Projection of speech and hearing impairments to 2050. *Asha, 25,* 31.

Garfein, A. J., & Herzog, A. R. (1995). Robust aging among the young-old, old-old, and oldest old. *Journal of Gerontology, 50B,* 277–287.

Holosko, M., & Feit, M. (1991). *Social work practice with the elderly.* Toronto, Canada: Canadian Scholars Press.

Jackson, J. J., & Ensley, D. E. (1995). Minority elders really ain't all alike. In R. A. Huntley & K. S. Helfer (Eds.), *Communication in later life* (pp. 127–156). Boston: Butterworth-Heinemann.

Kaakinen, J. (1995). Talking among elderly nursing home residents. *Topics in Language Disorders, 15,* 36–46.

Kane, R. L. (1994, April). Looking toward the next millennium. *Asha, 36,* 34–35.

Logemann, J. A. (1994, September). Health care reform: How will it affect you? *Asha, 36,* 3–4.

Logemann, J. A. (1995). The winds of change. In J. Bernthal, E. McNiece, D. Nash, & D. Sorenson (Eds.), *Proceedings of the Sixteenth Annual Conference on Graduate Education* (pp. 17–29). Minneapolis: Council of Graduate Programs in Communication Sciences and Disorders.

Lubinski, R. (1991). Learned helplessness: Application to communication of the elderly. In R. Lubinski (Ed.), *Dementia and communication* (pp. 142–151). New York: Dexter.

Orange, J. B., Ryan, E. B., Meredith, S. D., & MacLean, M. J. (1995). Application of the communication enhancement model for long-term care residents with Alzheimer's disease. *Topics in Language Disorders, 15,* 20–35.

Oyer, H. J., & Oyer, E. J. (1976). Communicating with older people: Basic considerations. In H. J. Oyer & E. J. Oyer (Eds.), *Aging and communication* (pp. 1–16). Baltimore: University Park Press.

Raiford, C. A., & Shadden, B. B. (1985, September). Graduate education in gerontology. *Asha, 27,* 37–43.

Ripich, D. N. (Ed.). (1991). *Handbook of geriatric communication disorders.* Austin, TX: PRO-ED.

Shadden, B. B., & Barr, J. A. (1988). Networking strategies for enhancing interdisciplinary service provision. In B. B. Shadden (Ed.), *Communication behavior and aging: A sourcebook for clinicians* (pp. 360–376). Baltimore: Williams & Wilkins.

Shadden, B. B., & Toner, M. A. (1995, December). *Post-master's education and training needs for adult medical speech–language pathology.* Paper presented at the annual meeting of the American Speech-Language-Hearing Association, Orlando, FL.

Shadden, B. B., Toner, M. A., & McCarthy, S. S. (1995, December). *Administrator perspectives on education for adult medical speech–language pathology practice.* Paper presented at the annual meeting of the American Speech-Language-Hearing Association, Orlando, FL.

Shadden, B. B., & Warnick, P. (1994, April). Multicultural aspects of aging. *Asha, 36,* 45–46.

Slater, S. C. (1992, August). Omnibus survey: Portrait of the professions. *Asha, 34,* 61–65.

Stanford, E. P. (1990). Diverse Black aged. In Z. Harel, E. A. McKinney, & M. Williams (Eds.), *Black aged: Understanding diversity and service needs* (pp. 33–49). Newbury Park, CA: Sage.

Trieschman, R. (1987). *Aging with a disability.* New York: Demos.

U.S. Department of Commerce. (1992). *Statistical abstracts of the United States 1992.* Washington, DC: Author.

U.S. House Committee on Aging. *Demographic characteristics of the older Hispanic population.* 100th Congress, 2nd sess., December 1988. H. Doc. 100-696.

U.S. House Committee on Aging. *Hispanic and Indian elderly: American's failure to care.* 101st Congress, 1st sess., August 7, 1989. H. Doc. 101-730.

Van Nostrand, J. F., Furner, S. E., & Suzman, R., (Eds.). (1993). *Health data on older Americans: United States, 1992* (National Center for Health Statistics Vital Health Statistics Series 2, No. 27). Washington, DC: U.S. Government Printing Service.

Weinstein, B. E., & Clark, L. (1994, April). The educational imperative. *Asha, 36,* 35–36, 47.

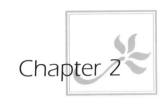

Chapter 2

Continuity and Change: Social Aspects of Aging

Jane A. Barr

Barr explores some of the social aspects of normal aging by focusing on social contacts, social role transitions, financial considerations, and psychological adaptations. Emphasis is placed upon the range of experiences that characterize social aspects of aging and the marked variability in individual coping responses.

1. *Identify some common attitudes and stereotypes about aging and older persons. How does the information in Barr's chapter support or refute such stereotypes?*

2. *What factors influence the nature and frequency of social contacts of older individuals? How do relationships with friends differ from relationships with family in terms of the type of support provided?*

3. *List at least four different role transitions experienced by some older individuals. For each role shift, describe advantages, disadvantages, and potential effects upon communicative interactions.*

4. *Barr suggests that productive aging involves healthy adaptation to age changes. What do we know about the manner in which older adults adapt to such changes, and the factors influencing this adaptation?*

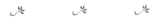

If your ideas about growing old come from the popular press, you are likely to have absorbed two conflicting and polarized images that come to mind when you picture aging in America. On the one hand is the smiling couple, healthy and tan, dressed for golf or tennis. The other image is a frail, shrunken woman, huddled under a tattered blanket in her dingy room, longing for company. Perhaps you envision her as Black, living in a crime-ridden neighborhood and fearful of going out; or, regardless of ethnicity, you imagine her in a nursing home, abandoned by her children and unable to live on her own. The ideal couple, in contrast, retain all their capabilities, live in a retirement community in a sunny climate, and are most certainly White.

As inaccurate as either of these scenarios is as a depiction of normal, or typical, aging, both images do serve to help us identify some of the ways in which the various social "worlds" of older individuals may differ. As for any age group, financial status makes a difference in living conditions and in access to activities and services. The amount of social contact experienced, and with whom, will be influenced by housing arrangements. Physical health may influence the social, work, and leisure roles that are available. All of these aspects of life—social contacts, physical settings, economic conditions, activities, and roles—interact with the personal characteristics of the individual to create his or her unique social world. Communication helps shape the social world, enhancing or limiting encounters and activities; in turn, the social world may have a profound impact upon the communicative functioning of the individual older adult.

The social aspects of a person's life not only influence each other; they come together to form a whole. For example, an older woman who regularly babysits a grandchild while her daughter works is experiencing social contact with the daughter and grandchild. Her day might be described in terms of the particular activities (such as grocery shopping and going to the park) that she does with the grandchild. She is also participating in her family roles of mother and grandmother. At the same time, her experience of all these things depends on the meaning that she attaches to her life and the adaptations that she has made over time. In the following sections, these building blocks of a social world will be discussed under headings such as "social contacts" and "social roles." The categories are a convenience in organizing the information provided, but the reader should remain aware of the overlapping nature of these various life aspects. It is not possible, in one brief chapter, to discuss all the factors that may influence social functioning. The topics that are covered will provide a basic introduction to the range of experiences and issues that are important to understanding the older person's social world.

Social Contacts

One of the most well-researched topics in aging is the nature and impact of social contacts experienced by older adults. Topics related to social contacts include proximity to family, type of residence and relocation, needs for assistance, the positive and negative impact of social supports, and the realities of loneliness and depression among the aged. Each of these will be addressed briefly in following sections.

Physical Proximity to Family

Despite the conflicting popular stereotypes of independent couples in retirement villages and lonely women in single rooms, most older people live near family members and have regular contact with them. This situation has not changed much in the last century. Today, as was the case a hundred years ago, fewer than 5% of people (in all age groups) live alone, and more than 90% live with relatives (Wamboldt & Reiss, 1991). However, when the choice is between living alone and independently, or sharing housing with others who are not immediate family members, even those elderly who are losing their functional abilities tend to prefer to maintain their separate households (Worobey & Angel, 1990).

Data from a national survey indicate that three fourths of people 60 and older, in all racial groups, have a child living less than an hour away. Half have a child living within 5 miles; one fourth have a child living within 1 mile (Lin & Rogerson, 1995). This close proximity has, in some cases, been re-achieved after the adult child moved away in search of jobs or independence and then, at a later life stage, moved back to the original area. In other cases, it was the elderly parent(s) who moved to a retirement area and then moved back to be near the child, possibly after one spouse died or one or both developed some disability that required the assistance of the child (Rossi & Rossi, 1990). Intergenerational proximity is less likely in families with higher income and educational levels than in lower class families (Lin & Rogerson, 1995), but proximity is the most common condition across all groups.

Residence and Relocation

Most older people do not move from the home that they occupied before retirement; many of those who do move subsequently return to their hometowns. Half of those 65 and older who relocate go south and west (Florida, California, Arizona, and Texas are favored), seeking warmer areas where they can avoid snow and ice (Dychtwald & Flower, 1990). For prosperous individuals who want reduced home-care responsibilities, need assistance with some daily activities, and/or want to live among age peers while remaining in their home-town, continuing care retirement facilities are becoming available nationwide (Rector, 1988). Similar services for low-income older people are available at boarding or retirement homes (Down & Schnurr, 1991).

The number of older people who reside in nursing homes at any one time is approximately 1.7 million, less than 5% of the elderly population (Moody, 1994). Some nursing home residents are receiving temporary care following an accident or surgery, and will be returning to their homes in the community, whereas others will require around-the-clock nursing until the end of life. Even among individuals 85 and older, only about one fourth move to a nursing home.

Although it is not the norm, there are some people who do move to the type of large retirement community that constitutes a separate town populated almost entirely by residents of retirement age. Buying property in such a community ensures a large supply of potential same-age friends, as well as recreation areas and activities where it is easy to get acquainted. These communities have been criticized on two grounds. First, some do not live up to their promise of providing an active life, and second, it has been proposed that age segregation of entire communities is not desirable. Regarding the first criticism, Jacobs (1974, 1975) found that only a small percentage of residents actually took part in the touted activities, that the community design (single-family homes on miles of residential streets, with no public transportation and no nearby common areas) encouraged social isolation, and that the geographical isolation discouraged access to cultural events and facilities. Regarding the second criticism, findings about the value of age-segregated living have been mixed (see Kart, 1994, for a discussion). One major study often cited as demonstrating the favorable effects of access to age peers actually found that older residents had the most positive social interactions in apartment buildings that were 50% occupied by elderly residents (Rosow, 1967). Perhaps the older residents were able to form same-age relationships easily, without isolation from younger people or hometown life. Although it is virtually impossible to isolate the effects of age segregation from other factors in research (Kart, 1994), there is an intuitive appeal to the concept that it is more natural for people of varied ages to live near each other, and that interactions across age categories enrich life for all involved.

The stereotypic image of the isolated oldster reflects an expectation that older people lack mobility and must sit passively in their homes, wishing for visitors. In fact, the majority of today's older people are not stranded. Financially well-off retirees who seek access to good weather and recreational activities without moving away from family or hometown roots may choose to travel; 80% of luxury travelers (on cruises or at expensive resorts) are 55 or older (Dychtwald & Flower, 1990). Consistent with other reports, Thorson and Powell (1993) found that, among a large sample of noninstitutionalized older people (ages 60 to 94), more than 85% were able to live their daily lives independently. Among those who require help, many can complete most tasks for themselves.

Issues of Dependence

What about the relatively small numbers who do require regular assistance from someone who can be counted on? Felton and Berry (1992) found that elderly recipients had significantly more positive feelings about their lives when such help was received from kin, rather than from others. Black and White elderly who need assistance are equally likely to have family and close friends available to help them, and to receive social support mainly from relatives (Antonucci & Akiyama, 1987; Chatters, Taylor, & Jackson, 1985), although Blacks are more likely than Whites to receive financial assistance from friends (Ulbrich & Warheit, 1989). Blacks tend to have a larger group of friends, neighbors, and church members providing help than Whites, who tend to rely more heavily on their spouse or one of their children for most assistance (Johnson, Gibson, & Luckey, 1990).

In one study of low-income California elderly, only one in five of those under 80 required any help with daily tasks, but 40% of those over 80 required at least some help. More than 60% of Black and White elderly lived alone, with kin or others coming in to assist when needed. However, Chinese and Mexican households were usually multigenerational, even when both elderly spouses were still alive, meaning that family members were always available and could provide assistance as part of their daily routines (Lubben & Becerra, 1987). Nationally, White older adults are likely to require less help with activities of daily living (such as bathing and dressing) than are members of other groups. In one study, for example, 63% of Whites aged 70 and over maintained their independence in daily tasks over a 2-year period, compared to 54% of Blacks (Van Nostrand, Furner, & Suzman, 1993). Despite their greater need for care, fewer Blacks than Whites utilize nursing homes. Black families' provision of care to elders at home may reflect both the recipients' inability to afford nursing homes and the facilities' history of racial discrimination, as well as ethnic differences in familial expectations (Watson, 1990).

Family and Friendship Social Contacts

It is commonly believed that higher levels of family contact are positive for the elderly, but this is not necessarily true in all cases. Older men have been found to have higher morale when they see their children less often, and receive less aid from them (Lee & Shehan, 1989). Apparently, the effect depends on the meaning of the contact to the individual; those whose values emphasize independence and autonomy prefer less contact, whereas those whose values emphasize family interaction (often women) have higher morale when such interaction is frequent.

Another potential drawback of social support was documented by Wethington and Kessler (1986), who found that those who turn too quickly to others fail to develop their own coping abilities. In addition, Krause (1995) found that overinvolvement of others in the social network increases stress for elders who are already experiencing chronic life strain.

Relationships with spouses, as with any other contacts, may be positive or negative, although there is generally increased satisfaction with marriage in later life (Atchley, 1994). One study of long-married older couples found marital satisfaction to be unrelated to income, education, or number of children. Instead, higher levels of disagreement (e.g., about matters such as recreation and friends) were associated with unhappy marriages, while better physical and psychological health was associated with happy marriages (Levenson, Carstensen, & Gottman, 1993). The authors' interpretation of these results was that unhappy marriages create health problems for women, but not for men, probably because the greater responsibility for the marital relationship's success falls on the woman.

In the last few years, there has been an increasing recognition of the importance of relationships with siblings. There is evidence that siblings experience increased feelings of closeness as they age, valuing their shared memories and mutual life experiences (Gold, 1989). Siblings are likely to help each other in practical ways, particularly in the case of working-class people, who have more limited resources and are more likely to live near each other throughout their lives (Avioli, 1989). In a study of rural elderly, the patterns of sibling contact were virtually identical for Black and White subjects, and were strongly based on mutual helping behavior (Suggs, 1989).

Although family members are generally preferred when help with problems is needed, it is friends who are best at increasing an elder's self-esteem and positive feelings about his or her life because of their reassurance that the person is worthwhile (Felton & Berry, 1992). Possibly, familial attentions can be seen as obligatory. Social contacts with friends are associated with increases in both retirement satisfaction and marital satisfaction (Higginbottom, Barling, & Kelloway, 1993). However, there are marked ethnic variations in the degree to which older adults turn to family versus friends for social support and validation beyond issues of daily assistance (Levitt, Weber, & Guacci, 1993; Lubben & Becerra, 1987).

Limited Social Contacts—Is There a Problem?

It is widely acknowledged that old age is characterized by a reduction in social contacts (Field & Minkler, 1988; Palmore, 1981), but is that reduction a problem? Activity theory suggests that it is. Reduced social contact is conceptualized as resulting from a situational lack of opportunity (due to such changes as health problems or the death of friends) that is negative and should be remedied (Maddox, 1963).

When Lang and Carstensen (1994) compared "old" men and women (70 to 84 years old) with "very old" ones (85 to 104 years old), they found that the social networks of the very old consisted of approximately half as many people as those of the old group. However, the number of very close relationships was the same for both groups, suggesting an active selection process in which individuals had reduced contacts with those who were less important to them. At the same time, there was maintenance of some instrumental relationships with acquaintances and neighbors who could provide assistance. A balanced network of kin and non-kin provides a feeling of emotional belonging and security in having many people to call on, while also allowing some needs to be satisfied without overburdening family and the closest friends (Felton & Berry, 1992; Lang & Carstensen, 1994; Simons, 1983).

The maintenance of close relationships and weeding out of more casual ones was evident among Lang and Carstensen's (1994) very old subjects. Carstensen's (1986) selectivity theory proposes that such choices late in the life cycle are common, reasonable, and adaptive. Furthermore, selectivity in social contacts is congruent with the theory of selective optimization with compensation (Baltes & Baltes, 1990), in which late life adaptation and development are viewed from the perspective of gains and losses (Fredrickson & Carstensen, 1990).

Loneliness and Depression

One stereotype of the elderly is that they are neglected and lonely. Although it is not the norm, there are older people who report that loneliness is a problem for them. In an early national survey by pollsters Louis Harris and Associates (1975), almost one fourth of low-income elderly people said that loneliness was a serious problem in their lives, with the same complaint being voiced by about half as many higher income individuals. The loneliness of the elderly must be taken seriously, because people who are socially isolated are about twice as likely as nonisolated people to get sick, and about twice as likely to die. Loneliness is actually a stronger predictor of death than such widely recognized dangers as smoking and high cholesterol levels (Goleman, 1995). However, loneliness is not particularly a problem of the elderly; in fact, old people may feel less lonely than young and middle-aged adults (Larson, 1978; Revenson & Johnson, 1984).

Similarly, depression and other dysthymic disorders are reported to be no more common among the elderly than in younger populations, affecting approximately 20% of persons 65 and older (Blazer, 1989; Butler, Lewis, & Sunderland, 1991). When depression does occur in older people, there is reason to be concerned, because mood disorders "complicate the treatment of coexisting medical conditions, and increase the risk of death by suicide" (Butler & Lewis, 1995, p. 44). Approximately half of older individuals who experience psychiatric problems do use mental health services, a figure that may be slightly lower than for younger groups because "current cohorts of older adults may have attitudes stressing stoic self-reliance . . . and thus may be less inclined to seek the help of a therapist" (Hooker & Shifren, 1995, p. 115). Diagnosis is complicated by somatic symptoms of the depression itself, its coexistence with other medical problems, and the tendency of older adults to consult their general physician for mental health problems. There are effective treatments available, but primary care physicians fail to identify depression in half of the depressed patients they see (Butler & Lewis, 1995).

Social Role Transition

Disengagement theory, which was very influential when introduced, suggested that it was normal for people to withdraw from social roles as they aged (Cumming & Henry, 1961); that viewpoint has not been supported by research (see Thorson, 1995). Today, it is more common to consider successful aging in terms of adapting to, and compensating for, life changes such as retirement (Baltes & Baltes, 1990). This adaptation is likely to include eliminating some roles and activities, while emphasizing selected others that are more important to the individual.

Marriage and Relationship Roles

People are generally expected to marry in this society, and 95% do marry at least once (Wamboldt & Reiss, 1991), but "spouse" is not always a lifetime role. The chance of divorce for a couple married in 1920 was 18%; this figure rose to 30% for those married in 1950 and to 50% for those married in 1970 (Gottman, 1993). More than 75%

remarry following divorce (Wamboldt & Reiss, 1991), but many of those marriages will also end sooner or later. Marriages may also end in death, and it is largely because of their greater longevity that women are more likely to live alone in old age.

The loss of the role of spouse in old age is considered a life stage marker (George, 1980), which means that it separates clearly distinct phases of life. The scope of adaptation required exceeds that of any other common role change. The remaining spouse must not only develop new daily life habits, but must also develop a new self-iden-tity. The importance of the transition helps to explain the occurrence of extended periods of grief, persisting for as long as 3 years after the spouse's death (Bodnar & Kiecolt-Glaser, 1994; Thompson, Gallagher-Thompson, Futterman, Gilewski, & Peterson, 1991).

It is important, however, to recognize that many widowed elders function well. Some have always preferred a more solitary life, while many have confidants and adequate social contact among friends and relatives (Lowenthal & Haven, 1968). Men are more likely to remarry than women, who are less likely to find an available, appropriate mate. An important consideration about widowhood is the gender disparity, with many more women outliving their spouses. Among those 65 and older, nearly 15% of men are widowed, compared to 42% of women; numbers for those 75 and older are about 25% of men and 66% of women (U. S. Bureau of the Census, 1992). Clearly, at least for women, widowhood must be considered a normal late-life role.

In retirement communities, there are still many peers available after a spouse dies (Dychtwald & Flower, 1990). Because of the greater numbers of women, they commonly develop girlfriend groups, regu-larly scheduling activities with each other. Many come to value their independence and freedom from housekeeping and caregiving roles. They may date; in some cases sex is a part of these relationships but is not necessarily seen as a reason to marry. Although nonmarried sex partner represents a new role for most of these women, those inter-viewed by Dychtwald and Flower (1990) did not seem distressed. Their main concern was that their children might find out about, and be upset by, their activities.

Worker Roles

The role that is most generally abandoned or altered in old age is that of paid worker. In fact, the impression that older people have little social contact may come, in part, from the reality that many of them have retired, thus reducing or eliminating workplace social contacts (Bosse, Aldwin, Levenson, Workman-Daniels, & Ekerdt, 1990). However, the type of social contact provided by co-workers is not usually exclusive to those particular individuals (Felton & Berry, 1992), and their contribution can be replaced (Field & Minkler, 1988). Just as retirement communities offer substitutes for spouses and friends who have been left behind, they also offer substitutes for worker roles. For example, large amounts of the work of the community, including beautification and policing, is done by residents at Sun City. Nationwide, according to a survey sponsored by the American Association of Retired Persons (AARP), more than 30% of older Americans do some kind of volunteer work (Dychtwald & Flower, 1990).

The decision to retire is not generally related to any problem with job performance, which tends to be stable or even improve with age (Waldman & Avolio, 1986). However, to maintain high effectiveness in the face of age-related decline in strength and speed, older workers may have to expend relatively more effort than they did when younger, or may need to adapt in other ways. For example, they may delegate some responsibilities in order to have more time and energy for their most important tasks (Abraham & Hansson, 1995).

It is becoming more common for both famous and ordinary people to follow one career with a completely different kind of work in later life. This represents a societal change from the traditional linear life plan, in which individuals were expected to go through roles in an orderly fashion (child, student, young married, parent, worker, retirement, death), to a cyclic plan in which the order of roles may vary (Dychtwald & Flower, 1990).

Some workers retire from one job, only to take on another immediately (Hayward, Grady, & McLaughlin, 1988). An official of the American Association of Retired Persons estimated that, as of 1995, approximately 35 million experienced people, constituting about one third of retirees over age 65, would like to work, even if they do not require the income (Dychtwald & Flower, 1990). However, they would like to work fewer hours; corporate America is just beginning to develop the flexibility to accommodate them (Fyock, 1990).

The satisfaction of older people with their schedule does not depend on whether they are working or retired, but on the extent to which the amount of work is based on choice rather than necessity. For men and women, in blue collar or professional jobs, "if people work or do not work by their own choice, they . . . report better health and well-being" (Herzog, House, & Morgan, 1991, p. 209). Men who were forced into retirement, as compared to willing retirees, continued to have more depression and lack of adjustment to their status nearly 30 years later (Swan, Dame, & Carmelli, 1991).

For women who did not work outside the home, there is no official retirement and no sudden change in responsibilities. In the future, as more women who have had careers begin to reach retirement age, their experience may more closely resemble that of today's male retirees. Black women are more likely than White women to have worked, and to continue to work past retirement age because the type of employment that was available to them does not lead to pensions and results in only minimal support from Social Security. Black women who continue to work, albeit at a reduced level, tend not to conceptualize themselves as taking on a new identity as retiree (Gibson, 1987).

Caregiver Roles

The caregiver role has received considerable attention because of the stresses that it entails. Ninety percent of caregivers are women, and a third of them are 65 or older (Dychtwald & Flower, 1990). At least for younger caregivers of elderly relatives, there is ample evidence that Black caregivers suffer less stress than White caregivers (Haley et al., 1995). The difference was not explained by the amount of social support extended to them by other relatives.

Caregiving for family members with Alzheimer's disease can be particularly difficult. Hooker, Monahan, Shifrin, and Hutchinson (1992) reported that for caregivers of a spouse with Alzheimer's, the amount of stress experienced by the caregiver was unrelated to the type of care required. Rather, the personality of the caregiver made the most difference. Those who were high in neuroticism or low in dispositional optimism experienced the most depression and other psychological distress (Hooker et al., 1992). This finding is consistent with other studies demonstrating that preexisting caregiver vulnerability, including such characteristics as coping style and attitude, is a major determinant of caregiver distress (see Vitaliano, Russo, Young, Teri, & Maiuro, 1991, for a review).

Grandparent Roles

The role of grandparent is valued in the dominant culture, but the expectation is that grandparents will be allowed to enjoy their grandchildren without having parenting responsibilities. When this expectation is violated, and grandparents take on the major responsibility for raising grandchildren, there are not only direct effects (for example, on the finances and freedom of the grandparent), but also stressful disturbances of the grandparent's overall sense of life course (Jendrek, 1993). According to Saluter (1992), in 1991 approximately 3.3 million children were living in the homes of their grandparents, either without their parents (28%) or with one or more parents (in 50% of cases, the mother) who were also dependent on the grandparent for housing and other assistance. The percentages of children living with grandparents varied by ethnicity, with 3.7% of White children, 5.6% of Hispanic children, and 12.3% of Black children dependent on grandparents.

The violation of expectations regarding grandparent–grandchild relationships also occurs in the opposite direction: Some grandparents may have less involvement than they would wish. Native American (American Indian) grandparents traditionally had a central role in raising their grandchildren. They not only provided daily supervision, but also ensured cultural continuity by teaching traditions to the younger generation. Some grandparents still attempt to fill this role; if they live away from the reservation, however, it becomes very difficult to maintain the culture (Weibel-Orlando, 1990). (For a heartbreaking picture of elders who have lost all of their traditional roles, without hope of replacing them, see Hayes's 1987 account of elderly Hmong immigrants.)

The "Old Person" Role

The role of "old person" is one that calls up societal stereotypes. Thinking of older people as all alike is commonly referred to as "ageism" (Butler, 1975). When Butler coined that word, he described a mostly negative view of old age. In contrast, "New Ageism" (Kalish, 1979) is also an assumption that all old people are alike, but they are assumed to be universally kind, wise, sympathethic, and in need of assistance. Today, stereotypes of the elderly reflect negative characteristics (grouchy, miserly, hard of hearing), but also positive ones (likable, intelligent, experienced). In one survey, respondents indicated that they were aware that these adjectives would correspond with only some, and not all, elders. Older respondents were consistently less willing than younger people to agree with negative stereotypes about their peers (Kite, Deaux, & Miele, 1991). In interviewing people of various ethnic backgrounds, Disman (1987, p. 69) found "few people who, without hesitation, would define them-selves as old. The exceptions were residents of the Chinese [retire-ment] home; an acceptance of old age seems to be embedded in Chinese culture." Matthews (1979) asserted that this denial of being old reflects a healthy coping mechanism involving refusal to accept a stigmatized identity.

Societal attitudes toward the elderly may already be changing, as the average age of the population increases. The "baby boomers," born after World War II, have a strong influence on the nature of the overall population because they form an unusually large cohort, or same-age group. As the baby boomers reach 65, which will begin to happen around the year 2010, the percentage of the population that is elderly will rapidly increase. By 2020, approximately 17% of the pop-ulation (up from about 12% today), or approximately 52 million people, are expected to be 65 or older (Brock, Guralnik, & Brody, 1990).

Money and Social Functioning

According to the 1980 census, about 40% of retired households had incomes that were at least double the poverty level. These households received income from pensions, investments, and/or continued employment, as well as from Social Security (Kart, Longino, & Ullmann, 1989). The majority of households had modest incomes; the typical older person was neither rich nor poor. However, those who have restricted incomes are of the most concern.

A decrease in elderly poverty in the last 15 years is primarily due to rising Social Security benefits, which support recipients at a level barely above poverty (Smeeding, 1990). Inflation can undermine the purchasing power of a fixed income, inexorably shrinking the standard of living of an elderly couple until they can no longer afford medicine, or even adequate food. Across all groups, about 12% of the elderly live below the poverty line—roughly 3.8 million people (Thorson, 1995). Gender differences in income favor men across all ethnic groups. Of those 85 and older (a group including more people who do not qualify for Social Security), 16% of men but 23% of women live at or below poverty level (Barer, 1994). Percentages of elderly living below the poverty level vary substantially by ethnic group. In 1990, they consti-tuted approximately 10% of White, 23% of Hispanic, and 34% of Black elderly (Thorson, 1995). Sixty percent of elderly Black women living alone had incomes below the poverty level (Moody, 1994).

A lack of funds may limit the extent to which elders can compensate for changes associated with aging (for example, by purchasing an effective hearing aid to enable them to continue full social participation). The fact that older Blacks are in poorer health than Whites reflects in part a lifetime of lower income and resultant lack of access to or resources for medical care. Poverty may also limit the ability to relocate if a neighborhood has become dangerous or if additional assistance is needed. The elderly crime victim is more a myth than a common reality, but there are some areas where crime (and realistic fear of crime) does have a serious impact on the older person's social world. Crime rates are high in the inner cities where disproportionately greater numbers of Black, as compared with White, elderly live. Consequently, the percentage of Black older persons who are victims of crimes is almost twice that of White elderly (Johnson et al., 1990).

The importance of financial concerns for the elderly goes beyond actual poverty; it also reflects the experiences of the particular cohort. Those who are 65 and older today grew up with societal fears about money and economic collapse. Those who will be 65 ten years from now grew up in post-World War II prosperity, and can be expected to have different attitudes about money.

There is some evidence that those older individuals who place a higher value on financial success are more likely to experience health problems as a result of financial strain, such as being unable to afford something the family needs. For those individuals, Krause and Baker (1992) found that financial problems produce a sense of loss of personal control, which in turn results in more somatic symptoms of distress, such as headache, difficulty sleeping, a general run-down feeling, nervousness or tenseness, and aches and pains.

Psychological Aspects Help Create the Social World

The Adaptation Process and Stress

Some authors see accommodation to the changes of age as resignation or regression, rather than recognizing the process as constructive. However, Brandtstadter and Rothermund (1994, p. 272) found that "such processes are functional in maintaining a sense of personal efficacy and well-being . . . [in that] older people may adopt a different and more lenient set of standards than younger individuals when describing themselves . . . as healthy." Those people who were able to accommodate changes maintained more of a sense of control and were less vulnerable to depression.

Clearly, productive aging is not a choice between giving up in the face of change, or denying change and insisting on going on as before. To have genuine, healthy adaptation, people must "monitor the important relationships in their lives, anticipate changes that need to be made, and actively take steps to make the necessary adjustments" (Wamboldt & Reiss, 1991, p. 175). Adaptation requires both flexibility and persistence in the face of difficulty, as well as a sense of self-efficacy, defined as a belief in one's ability to do what needs to be done (Bandura, 1986).

Another type of adaptation may explain the ability of older people to cope with major changes when they come on gradually. Rose (1991, p. 64) noted that "one way individuals cope with potentially overwhelming life events is to distance themselves or even to deny the danger or consequences that face them." Such minimalization results in a significant reduction in physiological stress responses and resultant damage to health. Because most of the changes of aging occur gradually, minimalization may occur automatically. The physiological system does not respond to very slow change as novel and threatening, and so there may be habituation to the new functioning level with no conscious awareness and no stress.

Although stress is usually thought of as negative, there is evidence that overcoming difficult experiences can promote self-esteem and self-efficacy in the long run (Moos & Schaefer, 1993). The various challenges of living, which continue into old age, offer opportunities to grow and change. A sense of control and efficacy can be enhanced through accommodation, as described above, but it also can benefit from continued achievement, learning, and change. For example, older men who had low self-efficacy perceptions prior to completing a difficult exercise program showed significantly increased self-efficacy after they succeeded (McAuley, Shaffer, & Rudolph, 1995). Others may challenge themselves mentally, with Elderhostel programs, enrollment in regular colleges, or educational cruises and expeditions (Dychtwald & Flower, 1990).

Personality and Life Stage Development

People develop their own complex combination of personality characteristics, which can be described along three axes: avoiding negative
events, or seeking positive ones; reacting when forced to by circumstances, or proactively controlling; and seeking reinforcement from
others, or from solitary pursuits (Millon, 1991). Jung's view of personality was that, in the second half of life, people develop the characteristics that they downplayed during the first half (Baker & Wheelwright, 1985; Jung, 1930/1976). For example, those who were
outgoing may learn to be more contemplative. There is ample evidence that this switch takes place with regard to gender-identified
personality characteristics. Older women accept and value their own
aggressive and dominant impulses, and older men value their
own nurturant and affiliative impulses, in a reversal of the societal
stereotypes reflected in the responses of younger persons (Neugarten,
1977). Sinnott (1982, 1984) found that older people were more likely
than younger ones to describe themselves on a sex-role inventory as
high in behaviors expressing characteristics commonly associated
both with men (agency, or action) and with women (communion, or
relationship). These changes seem to be internal, rather than clearly
displayed in behavior. That is, older people describe themselves, but
not others, as more androgynous; the characteristics are not observed
by other old people, or by young people (Kite et al., 1991).

At least for some older people, there is an increase in emotional
openness with age. Rather than indicating any "drift toward negative
affect" (Malatesta-Magal, Jonas, Shepard, & Culver, 1992, p. 559), there
is greater honesty and expressiveness regarding anger, sadness, and
interest, and less attempt to conceal emotions. Similarly, young and
old people have been shown to have comparable experiences of emotion and facial expressiveness of emotion, with less physiological indication of inhibition in the older individuals (Levenson, Carstensen,
Friesen, & Ekman, 1991).

One positive characteristic that is popularly associated with aging is
wisdom. Staudinger, Smith, and Baltes (1992) defined *wisdom* as having
good judgment about pragmatic aspects of life and as requiring the following components: factual knowledge, procedural knowledge, knowledge of life span contexts, the recognition of both universal values and
individual differences in goals and priorities, and the acceptance of and

ability to work with uncertainty and ambiguity. There is increasing evidence that social intelligence and professional expertise may show stability or growth throughout the life span (Staudinger et al., 1992). Further, because the general population is now exposed to more information about the life cycle and human behavior, there should be an ongoing increase in this kind of wisdom among the old.

Others would propose that elders also embody a less practical, and more spiritual, kind of wisdom. There is some indication that people may become more religious with age (Koenig, Smiley, & Gonzales, 1988). Aside from organized religion, there are issues of aging that are certainly spiritual or at least philosophical. Peck (1956), for example, proposed that late-life developmental tasks include transcending physical concerns, being less task oriented and guided more by deeper impulses, and being less concerned with one's ego and more concerned with the legacy being left to future generations. This description of later life is reminiscent of Erikson's (1950) familiar designation of later stages as a time of connection with all humanity. Erikson's theory proposes that death will not be feared by people who have accepted the particular life choices they made and experiences they had. In contrast, unsuccessful completion of this last stage consists of despair that it is too late to have a different life.

Jung (1930/1976) believed that the greatest potential for growth is in the latter half of life. He proposed that the tasks of age include acceptance of death, a review of and reflection on one's life, an acceptance that things that have not been accomplished are never to be, a reduction of concern with image or reputation, an opening and increasing receptivity to one's inner life, and the engagement of one's unused potentials in responding freely to whatever possibilities life brings. "Living itself becomes the point. . . . This process is well exemplified by Grandma Moses, whose art originated in her old age" (Baker & Wheelwright, 1985, p. 270). Jung's ideas find a more modern echo in Butler's (1963) concept of life review, and there is experimental support for the similar concept that life satisfaction in later years depends on a sense of meaning or purpose (Zika & Chamberlain, 1992).

Conclusion

This overview of social aspects of aging, although far from complete, is sufficient to illustrate the enormous range of social experiences encountered by older people in America today. Statistics describing people by categories such as ethnicity and age are reported, but should not be allowed to overshadow the fact that no conclusions can be drawn about individuals based solely on their membership in any group. Each person develops his or her own way of coping with aging within the parameters formed by the events of a lifetime. Continuity is evident, for example, in the family ties that tend to be maintained, but it is also clear that people do adjust their social contacts and roles. The importance of personal choice is illustrated in the differing reactions to retirement. Retirement is accompanied by positive feelings among those who freely choose to change their roles, but forced retirement may produce persistent depression.

There is, of course, no justification for social inequalities that leave some elderly without access to adequate housing or medical care. In fact, it seems likely that grinding hardship could undermine self-efficacy and block psychological growth (Maslow, 1970). At the same time, theories of psychological change in old age suggest that a different perspective may develop, in which there is reduced attachment to material goods and other concerns of younger life. For younger people who spend time with the elderly, an appreciation of this possibility can lead to deeper understanding and more productive relationships.

The role of communication in the social world was not directly addressed, but its importance for healthy psychological functioning and for each activity or role discussed can easily be imagined. For example, relationships with family, friends, and co-workers are based on verbal and nonverbal communication. Social roles are constructs that are actually composed of patterns of daily interpersonal interaction. In order to define communicative functioning in the elderly, it is essential to recognize these social aspects of the aging experience.

References

Abraham, J. D., & Hansson, R. O. (1995). Successful aging at work: An applied study of selection, optimization, and compensation through impression management. *Journal of Gerontology, 50B*, P94–103.

Antonucci, T. C., & Akiyama, H. (1987). Social networks in adult life and a preliminary examination of the convoy model. *Journal of Gerontology, 42*, 519–527.

Atchley, R. C. (1994). *Social forces and aging: An introduction to social gerontology* (7th ed.). Belmont, CA: Wadsworth.

Avioli, P. S. (1989). The social support functions of siblings in later life. *American Behavioral Scientist, 33,* 45–57.

Baker, B., & Wheelwright, J. (1985). Analysis with the aged. In M. Stein (Ed.), *Jungian analysis* (pp. 256–274). Boston: Shambhala.

Baltes, P. B., & Baltes, M. M. (1990). Psychological perspectives on successful aging: The model of selective optimization with compensation. In P. B. Baltes & M. M. Baltes (Eds.), *Successful aging: Perspectives from the behavioral sciences* (pp. 1–34). Cambridge, England: Cambridge University Press.

Bandura, A. (1986). *Social foundations of thought and action.* Englewood Cliffs, NJ: Prentice-Hall.

Barer, B. (1994). Men and women aging differently. *International Journal of Aging and Human Development, 38,* 29–40.

Blazer, D. G. (1989). Affective disorders in late life. In E. W. Busse & D. G. Blazer (Eds.), *Geriatric psychiatry* (pp. 369–401). Washington, DC: American Psychiatric Press.

Bodnar, J. C., & Kiecolt-Glaser, J. K. (1994). Caregiver depression after bereavement: Chronic stress isn't over when it's over. *Psychology and Aging, 9,* 372–380.

Bosse, R., Aldwin, C. M., Levenson, M., Workman-Daniels, K., & Ekerdt, D. J. (1990). Differences in social support among retirees and workers: Findings from the Normative Aging Study. *Psychology and Aging, 5,* 41–47.

Brandstadter, J., & Rothermund, K. (1994). Self-percepts of control in middle and later adulthood: Buffering losses by rescaling goals. *Psychology and Aging, 9,* 265–273.

Brock, D., Guralnik, J., & Brody, J. (1990). Demography and epidemiology of aging in the United States. In E. Schneider & J. Rower (Eds.), *Handbook of the biology of aging* (3rd ed., pp. 3–23). San Diego: Academic Press.

Butler, R. N. (1963). The life review: An interpretation of reminiscence in the aged. *Psychiatry, 26,* 65–76.

Butler, R. N. (1975). *Why survive? Being old in America.* New York: Harper & Row.

Butler, R. N., & Lewis, M. I. (1995). Late-life depression: When and how to intervene. *Geriatrics, 50,* 44–55.

Butler, R. N., Lewis, M., & Sunderland, T. (1991). *Aging and mental health.* New York: Mcmillan.

Carstensen, L. L. (1986). Social support among the elderly: Limitations of behavioral interventions. *The Behavior Therapist, 6,* 111–113.

Chatters, L. M., Taylor, R. J., & Jackson, J. S. (1985). Size and composition of the informal helper networks of elderly Blacks. *Journal of Gerontology, 40,* 605–614.

Cumming, E., & Henry, W. E. (1961). *Growing old.* New York: Basic Books.

Disman, M. (1987). Explorations in ethnic identity, oldness, and continuity. In D. E. Gelfand & C. M. Barresi (Eds.), *Ethnic dimensions of aging* (pp. 64–74). New York: Springer.

Down, I. M., & Schnurr, L. (1991). *Between home and nursing home: The board and care alternative.* Buffalo, NY: Prometheus.

Dychtwald, K., & Flower, J. (1990). *Age wave: The challenges and opportunities of an aging America.* New York: Bantam.

Erikson, E. H. (1950). *Childhood and society.* New York: Norton.

Felton, B. J., & Berry, C. A. (1992). Do the sources of the urban elderly's social support determine its psychological consequences? *Psychology and Aging, 7,* 89–97.

Field, D., & Minkler, M. (1988). Continuity and change in social support between young-old and old-old or very-old aged. *Journal of Gerontology, 43,* 100–106.

Fredrickson, B. L., & Carstensen, L. L. (1990). Choosing social partners: How old age and anticipated endings make people more selective. *Psychology and Aging, 5,* 335–347.

Fyock, C. D. (1990). *America's work force is coming of age: What every business needs to know to recruit, train, manage, and retain an aging work force.* Lexington, MA: Lexington Books.

George, L. (1980). *Role transitions in later life.* Monterey, CA: Brooks/Cole.

Gibson, R. C. (1987). Defining retirement for Black Americans. In D. E. Gelfand & C. M. Barresi (Eds.), *Ethnic dimensions of aging* (pp. 224–238). New York: Springer.

Gold, D. T. (1989). Generational solidarity: Conceptual antecedents and consequences. *American Behavioral Scientist, 33,* 19–32.

Goleman, D. (1995). *Emotional intelligence.* New York: Bantam.

Gottman, J. (1993). *What predicts divorce: The relationship between marital processes and marital outcomes.* Hillsdale, NJ: Erlbaum.

Haley, W. E., West, C. A. C., Wadley, V. G., Ford, G. R., White, F. A., Barrett, J. J., Harrell, L. E., & Roth, D. L. (1995). Psychological, social, and health impact of caregiving: A comparison of Black and White dementia family caregivers and noncaregivers. *Psychology and Aging, 10,* 540–552.

Harris, L., & Associates (1975). *The myth and reality of aging in America.* Washington, DC: National Council on Aging.

Hayes, C. L. (1987). Two worlds in conflict: The elderly Hmong in the United States. In D. E. Gelfand & C. M. Barresi (Eds.), *Ethnic dimensions of aging* (pp. 79–95). New York: Springer.

Hayward, M. D., Grady, W. R., & McLaughlin, S. D. (1988). Changes in the retirement process among older men in the United States, 1972–1980. *Demography, 25,* 371–386.

Herzog, A. R., House, J. S., & Morgan, J. N. (1991). Relation of work and retirement to health and well-being in older age. *Psychology and Aging, 6,* 202–211.

Higginbottom, S. F., Barling, J., & Kelloway, K. (1993). Linking retirement experiences and marital satisfaction: A mediational model. *Psychology and Aging, 8,* 508–516.

Hooker, K., Monahan, D., Shifren, K., & Hutchinson, C. (1992). Mental and physical health of spouse caregivers: The role of personality. *Psychology and Aging, 7,* 367–375.

Hooker, K., & Shifren, K. (1995). Psychological aspects of aging. In R. A. Huthley & K. S. Helfer (Eds.), *Communication in later life* (pp. 99–125). Boston: Butterworth-Heinemann.

Jacobs, J. (1974). *Fun city: An ethnographic study of a retirement community.* New York: Holt, Rinehart & Winston.

Jacobs, J. (1975). *Older persons and retirement communities.* Springfield, IL: Thomas.

Jendrek, M. P. (1993). Grandparents who parent their grandchildren: Effects on lifestyle. *Journal of Marriage and the Family, 55,* 609–621.

Johnson, H. R., Gibson, R. C., & Luckey, I. (1990). Health and social characteristics: Implications for services. In Z. Harel, E. A. McKinney, & M. Williams (Eds.), *Black aged: Understanding diversity and service needs* (pp. 69–81). Newbury Park, CA: Sage.

Jung, C. G. (1976). The stages of life (R. F. C. Hull, Trans.). In J. Campbell (Ed.), *The portable Jung* (pp. 3–22). New York: Penguin. (Original work published 1930)

Kalish, R. A. (1979). The New Ageism and the failure models: A polemic. *Gerontologist, 19,* 398–402.

Kart, C. S. (1994). *The realities of aging: An introduction to gerontology* (4th ed.). Boston: Allyn & Bacon.

Kart, C. S., Longino, C. F., & Ullmann, S. G. (1989). Comparing the economically advantaged and the pension elite: 1980 census profiles. *Gerontologist, 29,* 745–749.

Kite, M. E., Deaux, K., & Miele, M. (1991). Stereotypes of young and old: Does age outweigh gender? *Psychology and Aging, 6,* 19–27.

Koenig, H. G., Smiley, M., & Gonzales, J. A. (1988). *Religion, health, and aging.* New York: Greenwood.

Krause, N. (1995). Assessing stress-buffering effects: A cautionary note. *Psychology and Aging, 10,* 518–526.

Krause, N., & Baker, E. (1992). Financial strain, economic values, and somatic symptoms in later life. *Psychology and Aging, 7,* 4–14.

Lang, F. R., & Carstensen, L. L. (1994). Close emotional relationships in late life: Further support for proactive aging in the social domain. *Psychology and Aging, 9,* 315–324.

Larson, R. (1978). Thirty years of research on the subjective well-being of older Americans. *Journal of Gerontology, 33,* 109–125.

Lee, G. R., & Shehan, C. L. (1989). Elderly parents and their children: Normative influences. In J. A. Mancini (Ed.), *Aging parents and adult children.* Lexington, MA: Lexington Books.

Levenson, R. W., Carstensen, L. L., Friesen, W. V., & Ekman, P. (1991). Emotion, physiology, and expression in old age. *Psychology and Aging, 6,* 28–35.

Levenson, R. W., Carstensen, L. L., & Gottman, J. M. (1993). Long-term marriage: Age, gender, and satisfaction. *Psychology and Aging, 8,* 301–313.

Levitt, M. J., Weber, R. A., & Guacci, N. (1993). Convoys of social support: An intergenerational analysis. *Psychology and Aging, 8,* 323–326.

Lin, G., & Rogerson, P. A. (1995). Elderly parents and the geographic availability of their adult children. *Research on Aging, 17,* 303–331.

Lowenthal, M. F., & Haven, C. (1968). Interaction and adaptation: Intimacy as a critical variable. *American Sociological Review, 33,* 93–110.

Lubben, J. E., & Becerra, R. M. (1987). Social support among Black, Mexican, and Chinese elderly. In D. E. Gelfand & C. M. Barresi (Eds.), *Ethnic dimensions of aging* (pp. 130–144). New York: Springer.

Maddox, G. L. (1963). Activity and morale: A longitudinal study of selected elderly subjects. *Social Forces, 42,* 195–204.

Malatesta-Magal, C., Jonas, R., Shepard, B., & Culver, L. C. (1992). Type A behavior pattern and emotion expression in younger and older adults. *Psychology and Aging, 7,* 551–561.

Maslow, A. H. (1970). *Motivation and personality.* New York: Harper & Row.

Matthews, S. H. (1979). *The social world of old women.* Beverly Hills, CA: Sage.

McAuley, E., Shaffer, S. M., & Rudolph, D. (1995). Affective responses to acute exercise in elderly impaired males: The moderating effects of self-efficacy and age. *International Journal of Aging and Human Development, 41,* 13–27.

Millon, T. (1991). Normality: What may we learn from evolutionary theory? In D. Offer & M. Sabshin (Eds.), *The diversity of normal behavior* (pp. 356–404). New York: Basic.

Moody, H. R. (1994). *Aging: Concepts and controversies.* Thousand Oaks, CA: Pine Forge Press.

Moos, R. H., & Schaefer, J. A. (1993). Coping resources and processes: Current concepts and measures. In L. Goldberger & S. Breznitz (Eds.), *Handbook of stress: Theoretical and clinical aspects* (pp. 234–257). New York: Free Press.

Neugarten, B. (1977). Personality and aging. In J. E. Birren & K. W. Shaie (Eds.), *Handbook of the psychology of aging* (pp. 626–649). New York: Van Nostrand Reinhold.

Palmore, E. (1981). *Social patterns in normal aging: Findings from the Duke Longitudinal Study.* Durham, NC: Duke University Press.

Peck, R. (1956). Psychological development in the second half of life. In J. Anderson (Ed.), *Psychological aspects of aging.* Washington, DC: American Psychological Association.

Rector, R. (1988). *Continuing care retirement communities and the life care industry: An annotated bibliography.* Monticello, IL: Vance Bibliographies.

Revenson, T. A., & Johnson, J. L. (1984). Social and demographic correlates of loneliness in late life. *American Journal of Community Psychology, 12,* 71–85.

Rose, R. M. (1991). Normality and stress: Response and adaptation from an endocrine perspective. In D. Offer & M. Sabshin (Eds.), *The diversity of normal behavior* (pp. 60–87). New York: Basic.

Rossi, A., & Rossi, P. (1990). *Of human bonding: Parent–child relations across the life-course.* New York: DeGruyter.

Rosow, I. (1967). *Social integration of the aged.* New York: Free Press.

Saluter, A. F. (1992). Marital status and living arrangement: March 1991. *Current population reports, population characteristics* (Series P-20, No. 461). Washington, DC: U. S. Government Printing Office.

Simons, R. L. (1983). Specificity and substitution in the social networks of the elderly. *International Journal of Aging and Human Development, 18,* 121–139.

Sinnott, J. D. (1982). Correlates of sex roles of older adults. *Journal of Gerontology, 37,* P587–594.

Sinnott, J. D. (1984). Older men, older women: Are their perceived sex roles similar? *Sex Roles, 30,* 847–856.

Smeeding, T. M. (1990). Economic status of the elderly. In R. H. Binstock & L. K. George (Eds.), *Handbook of aging and the social sciences* (3rd ed., pp. 362–381). New York: Academic Press.

Staudinger, U. M., Smith, J., & Baltes, P. B. (1992). Wisdom-related knowledge in a life review task: Age differences and the role of professional specialization. *Psychology and Aging, 7,* 271–281.

Suggs, P. K. (1989). Predictors of asociation among older siblings: A Black/White comparison. *American Behavioral Scientist, 33,* 70–80.

Swan, G. E., Dame, A., & Carmelli, D. (1991). Involuntary retirement, Type A behavior, and current functioning in elderly men: 27-year follow-up of the Western Collaborative Group study. *Psychology and Aging, 6,* 384–391.

Thompson, L. W., Gallagher-Thompson, D. G., Futterman, A., Gilewski, M., & Peterson, J. (1991). The effects of late-life spousal bereavement over a 30-month interval. *Psychology and Aging, 6,* 434–441.

Thorson, J. A. (1995). *Aging in a changing society.* Belmont, CA: Wadsworth.

Thorson, J. A., & Powell, F. C. (1993). The rural aged, social value, and health care. In C. N. Bull (Ed.), *Aging in rural America* (pp. 134–145). Beverly Hills, CA: Sage.

Ulbrich, P. M., & Warheit, G. J. (1989). Social support, stress, and psychological distress among older Black and White adults. *Journal of Aging and Health, 1,* 286–305.

U.S. Bureau of the Census. (1992). *Statistical abstract of the United States: 1992.* Washington, DC: U.S. Government Printing Office.

Van Nostrand, J. F., Furner, S. E., & Suzman, R. (Eds.). (1993). *Health data on older Americans: United States, 1992* (National Center for Health Statistics Vital Health Statistics Series 3, No. 27). Washington, DC: U.S. Government Printing Office.

Vitaliano, P. P., Russo, J., Young, H. M., Teri, L., & Maiuro, R. D. (1991). Predictors of burden in spouse caregivers of individuals with Alzheimer's disease. *Psychology and Aging, 6,* 392–402.

Waldman, D. A., & Avolio, B. J. (1986). A meta-analysis of age differences in job performance. *Journal of Applied Psychology, 71,* 33–38.

Wamboldt, F. S., & Reiss, D. (1991). Task performance and the social construction of meaning: Juxtaposing normality with contemporary family research. In D. Offer & M. Sabshin (Eds.), *The diversity of normal behavior* (pp. 164–206). New York: Basic.

Watson, W. H. (1990). Family care, economics, and health. In Z. Harel, E. A. McKinney, & M. Williams (Eds.), *Black aged: Understanding diversity and service needs* (pp. 50–68). Newbury Park, CA: Sage.

Weibel-Orlando, J. (1990). Grandparenting styles: Native American perspectives. In J. Sokolovsky (Ed.), *The cultural context of aging: Worldview perspectives.* New York: Bergin & Garvey.

Wethington, E., & Kessler, R. C. (1986). Perceived support, received support, and adjustment to stressful events. *Journal of Health and Social Behavior, 27,* 78–89.

Worobey, J. L., & Angel, R. J. (1990). Functional capacity and living arrangements of unmarried elderly persons. *Journal of Gerontology: Social Sciences, 45,* S95–101.

Zika, S., & Chamberlain, K. (1992). On the relation between meaning in life and psychological well-being. *British Journal of Psychology, 83,* 133–145.

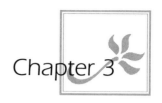

Chapter 3

Physical Aspects of Aging

Larry D. Wright
Patricia Duckworth

Wright and Duckworth approach the topic of physical aspects of aging from the perspective of functional ability as an important indicator of health. Emphasis is placed upon the interplay between normal aging, pathological or disease processes, and extrinsic influences. Structural and functional physical changes associated with aging are discussed, and the importance of functional medical assessment is highlighted.

1. *What are the three factors contributing to functional ability and health, as defined in the model presented in this chapter? In general terms, how does aging influence health by affecting individual responses to physiological and psychological stressors?*

2. *For each of the body systems or aspects addressed in this chapter, list at least three physical changes that accompany normal aging. For each change, identify the functional consequence (if any) for daily activities.*

3. *Functional assessment has become a popular concept in medicine today, particularly as applied to older adults. What are the main elements of a functional geriatric assessment? What are ADLs and IADLs, and how are they evaluated? Should speech–language pathologists and audiologists be concerned with ADL and IADL functioning?*

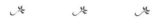

Health-related problems of human aging present formidable challenges to health professionals who work with older adults. The specific insights and approaches that must be developed to address these problems effectively reflect the complexity, frequency, variability, and altered clinical appearance of disease and physiological dysfunction in old age. As a result, clinical geriatric medicine has identified the concept of functional health status as the logical emphasis from which evaluation and treatment of the health problems of older adults can best proceed (Williams, 1994).

This view of functional ability as the most important aspect of health is a departure from the traditional emphasis on medical diagnosis as the goal of clinical assessment and the target of most therapy. The concept of functional health status presents many advantages to the clinician and to the older patient. It acknowledges the multifactorial nature of most health problems of the elderly, as well as the interdisciplinary team approach often required to address them successfully. The health of older adults is understood to be determined by the combined effects of the aging process itself (normal), pathological or disease processes (abnormal), and the interplay of these processes with the extrinsic or environmental influences to which the person is exposed.

Moreover, functional ability or disability presents a common denominator or "bottom line" for practitioners and older patients by emphasizing (a) practical priorities that do not change even when medical problems are incurable, (b) therapeutic goals equally accessible to the patient and to all members of the clinical team, and (c) elimination of false demarcations between the clinical and nonclinical, or among aspects of human performance (e.g., physical, psychological, social). All involved members of the health care team can be enlisted in coordinated efforts designed to promote the optimal level of functional independence. In turn, a target of functional independence may be the most acceptable premise for intervention for some elders whose receptiveness to medical treatments may decline with increasing age.

Health and functional ability can be conceptualized as an optimal balance among the broad dimensions of human life, as illustrated with the interlocking spheres of the physical, psychologic, and socioeconomic domains shown in Figure 3.1. With this concept of health as functional performance, the emphasis becomes restoration and rehabilitation from disability, rather than the false choice of cure versus palliation, which the elderly often assume.

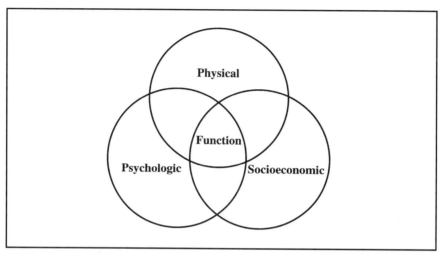

Figure 3.1. Health and functional ability as a balance among overlapping influences from the physical, psychologic, and socioeconomic domains.

It is important for the clinician working with an aging patient to develop an understanding of normal aging changes and their impact on the overall functional and health status of the client. At the most basic level, this understanding is prerequisite to appropriate medical differential diagnosis and selection of treatment options. More broadly, physical changes associated with aging, and general health status, influence an older person's functioning in every arena, including communication. Aspects of functional health and physical aging may require modifications in assessment procedures and/or redirection of management approaches to communication disorders.

This chapter will explore the general nature of the biological aging process, followed by a discussion of normal aging changes within specific systems, common disease processes, and implications for daily performance. Aspects of functional geriatric medical assessment that address the broader concerns shown in Figure 3.1 will be described briefly.

The Aging Process

Aging is an inevitable biological process in all living organisms. The physiological aging process in human beings is a continuum of incremental changes leading to measurable, progressive decreases in basic functions within organ systems. Most organ systems appear to lose function at a rate of about 1% per year beginning at about age 30 (Kane, Ouslander, & Abrass, 1994). Gradually, higher and more integrated functions are affected, resulting in demonstrable impairment of physical, mental, psychological, and social functions. These changes are normal and to be expected. However, for all its normalcy, biological aging has four true characteristics: it is universal, progressive, decremental, and intrinsic (Goldman, 1979).

Observed at the organ system level, these age-related physiological changes can be characterized generally as resulting in the gradual erosion of the *reserve capacity*. This reserve capacity is that part of the functional capability of the organ system that the individual does not use under ordinary circumstances, but that is available on demand. It is this reserve that allows a person to cope with increased performance demands and health challenges and that determines the continuing adaptability and maintenance of homeostasis physiologically as one ages. The physiological decompensation that results when such demands exceed the organ's capacity to increase its performance level typically identifies a threshold of symptoms. In the example of age-related loss of respiratory system reserve, such excessive demand would be manifested in shortness of breath or other symptoms of respiratory distress. This gradual decline in physiologic coping capacity can be viewed as a progressive decrease in the organ systems' ability to maintain homeostasis and an increasing vulnerability to stress. Observed declines vary greatly, not only among older adults but also within the individual. Cells, tissues, organs, and systems age and deteriorate at varying rates. Variation results from, but is not limited to, life-style and/or genetics.

Both childhood/adolescence and old age are times of rapid change and high risk or vulnerability to stress. Thus, change and stress affect optimal functional vitality and independence differentially across the life span (see Figure 3.2). Although *change* and *decline* should not be used synonymously with *disease,* normal aging influences health and the individual's responses to physiological and psychologic stressors. It is the rare older adult who is not affected across many systems and functional planes when change occurs. The older the patient, the greater the impact of normal change and the greater the opportunity for a cumulative negative impact on one or more organ systems. In addition to loss of reserve capacity, decreased

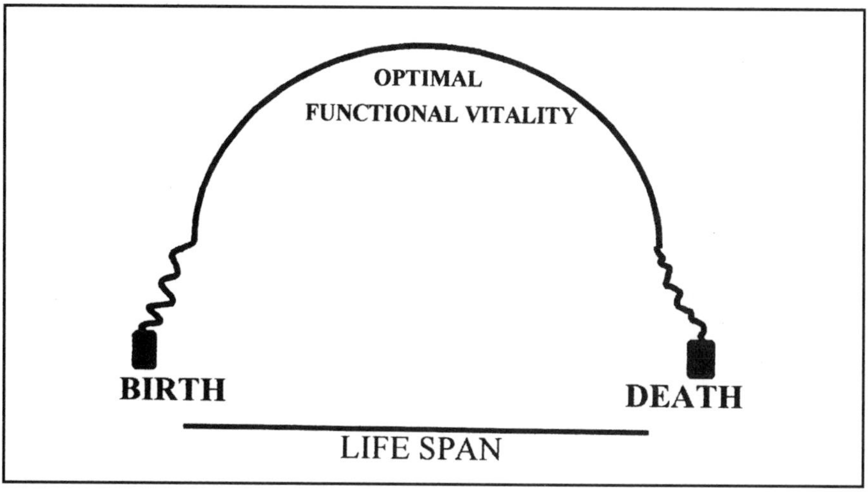

Figure 3.2. Functional independence during the life span. (Jagged lines represent childhood/adolescence and old age, both periods of rapid change and high risk/vulnerability to diverse stressors.)

immune system responsiveness may contribute to the impact of change on health and stress response. One normal aspect of aging is increasing t-cell dysfunction and decreased antibody response. As declines occur in the body's ability to mobilize resources to combat disease processes or increase neurotransmitter production to manage stress, further negative impact on functioning may be observed.

Normal aging changes may actually precipitate an overall decline or an atypical, nonspecific, or obscure presentation of disease. The opposite can also occur: Disease presentation may be interpreted erroneously as a normal change or a consequence of the aging process. For example, constipation and/or fecal impaction, systemic infection without fever, dehydration, drug toxicity, viral infection, and even meningitis may present with general malaise, fatigue, or mental sluggishness, behaviors that may be attributed inappropriately to the normal aging process. Conversely, these signs of normal aging may be interpreted as disease, and aggressive attempts to correct them may be detrimental to the client's overall best health interests.

A logical approach to understanding normal (biological, physical) aging is to examine each body system or aspect separately, then examine their interrelatedness. The social context for aging has already been discussed in Chapter 2. Normal and abnormal changes in cognition, hearing, oropharyngeal and laryngeal structures and functions, and language/communication are addressed in subsequent chapters.

It is important for the clinician working with the aging patient to develop a knowledge base in and awareness of normal aging changes and their impact on the overall functional status of the client. It is also imperative that a thorough health history and health assessment be obtained and medically analyzed prior to the institution of therapy and during the therapy period if unexplained or perplexing signs and symptoms occur. Early intervention in older adults to correct abnormal alterations insures a sustained and optimal level of function for clients. It also insures that clients will receive maximum benefit from all therapeutic interventions. Clinicians can then best adapt their interventions to the individual.

Body Structure and Composition

Kenney (1988) described a number of general aging changes in body structure and composition. One phenomenon noted with increased age is a loss in actual body height, related in part to collapse of the foot arches, narrowing of joint spaces in the legs and spine, and increasing spinal curvature. Decreased body weight is also observed, presumably due to a redistribution of the body elements of water, fat, and nonfat solids. For example, lean body mass decreases. This is related in part to an increase in adipose tissue around and within internal organs, beginning around the age of 40 and progressing until at least age 70 in men and longer in women. Another contributing factor is decreased bone mass, associated with mineral loss, remodeling of bone mass due to physiological stressors, and an erosion of the inner bone core. Loss of muscle tissue also may occur (see later section on musculoskeletal changes).

Changes in Sensory Perception

Sensation is the process by which the mind and body communicate with the external world. The basic senses include taste, smell, hearing, vision, and touch. Additional sensory perceptual information is available through pain, kinesthetic, and proprioceptive receptors, among others. As previously indicated, the sense of hearing is dealt with in depth in Chapter 5 and will not be addressed here.

Taste and Smell

Taste and smell are referred to as *chemosenses;* they rely on chemicals in order to be stimulated and activated. These senses are closely inter-connected. In fact, taste is two thirds dependent on smell (Ebersole & Hess, 1994).

Relevant alterations in taste and smell are discussed in Chapter 6. Changes in both of these senses have profound effects on the maintenance of adequate dietary intake. Foods once enjoyed may become distasteful; foods once disliked may now be eaten with zest. Higher concentrations of the four primary taste perceptions (salt, sweet, bitter, sour) may be required for flavor identification and pleasurable dining. This results in the use of greater amounts of sugar and salt for eating enjoyment. Such use is particularly dangerous when these additives should be restricted, such as in instances of diabetes mellitus, hypertension, and congestive heart failure. Additional discussion of taste and smell in relationship to feeding and swallowing can be found in Chapter 17.

The protective mechanisms of taste and smell may also be lost. For example, the taste or odor of spoiled food or the odor of leaking gas in the home may go undetected. Diminished sense of smell also may result in social alienation if body odors and other offensive household and personal odors cannot be detected.

Vision

Every person will experience changes in sight with age. The impact of the changes may vary in severity. However, diminished sight often is poorly recognized because of the slowness of the onset of most changes and the ability of the older adult to make gradual unnoticed adaptations. Alterations in sight may have serious adverse effects, especially in relation to safety. Of particular concern is the client's ability to drive an automobile safely. Gradual loss of visual acuity, coupled with gradual unconscious adaptation, may result in an unrecognized danger behind the wheel of a vehicle. Loss of vision may also impair social functioning by limiting those activities in which an older adult can comfortably and accurately participate.

Pupil size becomes smaller, limiting the amount of light that can reach the retina. This is the most basic of the mechanisms required for vision. The ability to respond to changes in light and dark, such as when entering a darkened room from a brightly lit area, is impaired. This increases the risk of injury from falls. Three times as much light as that needed by younger persons is required for reading and other close work. It is important to note that, while there is an increased requirement for adequate lighting, there is also an increased sensitivity to glare. Such sensitivity may also impair vision.

Presbyopia, the inability of the eye to accommodate to close and detailed work, begins in the thirties. It also affects the requirement for adequate lighting and may interfere with many social and pleasurable pursuits such as reading, playing cards, sewing, handwork, and other activities and hobbies. Color clarity diminishes by 25% before the age of 60 years is achieved. By the time the 70s are reached, color clarity is diminished by 50%. The blues, violets, and greens are the colors most affected (Ebersole & Hess, 1994). These changes may affect the social acceptability of clothing selection as well as the ability to distinguish identifying colors such as traffic signals.

A milky gray ring around the periphery of the iris is a common age-related change called *arcus senilis* or corneal arcus. Although it occurs in most older individuals at some point, corneal arcus is associated with no significant impairment of vision or other ocular problems. Ptosis, or drooping, of the eyelid occurs commonly with age and may impair vision mechanically if severe. The eyelids may turn outward (eversion) or inward (inversion), resulting in dryness and irritation of the eyeball and its outer layer, the conjunctiva. Tear secretion diminishes. Uncorrected, these changes may result in corneal damage in some cases.

Cataracts, the gradual opacification of the lens, is the most common cause of diminished visual acuity in older persons. This condition apparently results from oxidative damage to the lens, which is, at least partly, due to normal aging. Smoking, poor nutrition, and excessive exposure to ultraviolet light are among the factors that contribute to premature development of cataracts (Abrams, Beers, & Berkow, 1995).

Inefficient reabsorption of intraocular fluid with age results in an increase in the incidence of glaucoma. Untreated, glaucoma leads to blindness. Age-related macular degeneration is a frequent cause of blindness in older adults. The macula is the area of the retina where the most precise visual acuity occurs. Degeneration occurs as a result of any problem that may impair oxygenation or nutrition of the retina and macula. Diabetic retinopathy, in which the retina and the macula are damaged as a result of the pathology of diabetes mellitus, is also a frequent cause of blindness in old age. Although these problems have an increased incidence associated with age, these are pathologic conditions and should be referred and treated as such.

Pain Response

Awareness of and response to pain, especially deep visceral pain, can be markedly diminished with age. Any pain may be underreported for psychological and sociological reasons. As a result, pain in older adults is often undercontrolled, resulting in needless suffering. This diminished report and perception of pain may have life-threatening sequelae. Because care provision depends in large part on the patient's report of complaints and symptoms, emergency treatment is often delayed or may be inappropriate.

Somasthetics or Tactile Sensitivity

Normal aging diminishes and alters the sensation of touch. Changes in dermal cells and their associated neurons interfere with accurate transmission of messages to the nervous system that trigger the sensation of touch. Age is not the only cause of these changes; diseases that occur more frequently with age, such as diabetes mellitus or cerebrovascular accident (CVA) may result in numbness or altered sensation, particularly in the extremities.

Some older adults perceive light touch as burning or painful. As a result, every effort should be made to apply firm gentle pressure when touching the client. Altered perception of the sensations of heat and cold may have serious consequences. Injury to tissues may result from the application of hot pads or cold packs.

Changes in the Skin

Direct inspection of the skin of most older adults confirms typical age-related changes that are often quite pronounced. Elasticity and moisture are diminished both from normal changes and from environmental insults such as excessive sun exposure, smoking, inadequate nutrition, and certain medications (e.g., steroids). These changes cause increased fragility and susceptibility to injury from even modest insults. Therefore care must be taken to minimize any external trauma, no matter how minor.

Increased facial hair in women is associated with depletion of female hormones. Hair distribution is altered, and loss of hair in both sexes may be seen. Self-esteem may be affected negatively by these changes, and the elderly client may be reluctant to socialize or to participate in group activities of any sort.

Subcutaneous fat, especially in the extremities, is decreased, leading to the atrophic or "thinned" appearance of the skin. A common consequence of this normal change is the appearance of purpuric lesions (dark red or purplish macules) representing a small amount of blood under the skin. These lesions arise often after minimal or inapparent trauma and are invariably of no significant clinical consequence. Loss of substantial fat further results in impaired response to temperature change, most notably cold temperatures. A comfortable room temperature for a health care provider may be uncomfortably or even dangerously cold for the elderly client. Reduced size, number, and activity of sweat glands cause poor responses and adjustments to excessive heat. These two normal aging changes result in increased risks of hypo- and hyperthermia. Because the physical and mental alterations associated with these two complications may mimic changes often interpreted as normal in older adults, the consequences of delayed reporting and treatment may be life threatening.

Changes in Kidney and Urinary Function

Kidney function is markedly reduced in normal aging. The most significant physiological change in the aging renal system is its reduced ability to maintain a sufficient glomerular filtration rate (GFR) required for elimination of medications and their metabolites. This well-recognized decline in the GFR as measured by the Creatinine Clearance, though commonly progressive, occurs in as many as two thirds of older persons. In light of this reduction in GFR, the kidneys remain remarkably efficient in their ability to eliminate wastes and to regulate fluid volume and composition. However, when an older adult is impaired by other illness, the renal system may become over-whelmed. In addition, the half-life of many medications prescribed for such illnesses may be extended. This can lead to drug overdose and drug toxicity.

Normal bladder function requires an intact brain and spinal cord, a competent bladder, and active sphincters that can sustain maximum urethral pressure against rising bladder pressure. One also must be able to physically use toileting facilities. With increasing age, bladder volume decreases. The warning time between the desire to urinate and the actual act of urination is shortened and may be lost. Physical impairments commonly associated with aging, such as osteoarthritis, may impair an elder's ability to ambulate to the bathroom, to remove clothing, and to actually use the toilet.

Urinary incontinence, the inability to control the elimination of urine, is common in old age and thus is often accepted quietly by older adults and their health care providers alike. It is estimated that 15% to 30% of the community-dwelling elderly, 30% of all hospitalized elder-ly, and greater than 50% of long-term care residents are incontinent to a significant degree (Abrams et al., 1995). However, incontinence is never normal. Its potential side effects include social isolation, social alienation, and damage to the skin. It is one of the major reasons for admissions to long-term care facilities, as caregivers in the home become unable to deal with the problem.

There is no single explanation for incontinence. Causes and symp-toms vary. *Stress incontinence* occurs when intra-abdominal pressure exceeds urethral resistance. This is usually due to anatomic weak-nesses in the urethral sphincter and bladder neck supports. "Leaking" of urine with coughing, sneezing, laughing, lifting, and so forth, is the most common symptom of stress incontinence. *Urge incontinence* is most often due to central nervous system dysfunction (e.g., stroke or Parkinson's disease) or to local irritating factors (atrophic urethral mucosal changes or infection). The patient senses the urge to void, but cannot inhibit urination in time to reach the toilet. *Overflow inconti-nence* may be due to spinal cord damage, but in the elderly is often due to mechanical blockage of the urethra as in the case of prostatic hyper-trophy. The bladder becomes overdistended, leading to frequent or constant loss of urine. *Functional incontinence* is due to the cognitive inability to recognize the urge to void or to react to the urge. It is also due to the patient's inability to reach the toilet or to remove clothing quickly enough in order to use the toilet. *Iatrogenic incontinence* may be medication induced (diuretic therapy) or the result of physiological alterations such as polyuria associated with elevated blood sugar levels. *Mixed incontinence* occurs when the reasons for the incontinence are multiple.

Just as the types and symptoms of incontinence vary, the mechanisms by which it can be corrected or minimized vary. Noninvasive techniques include ease of toilet accessibility, toilet substitutes (e.g., portable commodes), protective undergarments, scheduled toileting and other behavioral therapies, pelvic muscle conditioning (Kegel exercises), biofeedback, medication, dietary changes (limiting "natural" diuretics such as sugar and caffeine), or combinations of these interventions.

Changes in Gastrointestinal Function and Nutritional Needs

The gastrointestinal system appears to be relatively spared from significant changes in function with normal aging. Oral changes and swallowing are covered in depth in Chapter 6, with additional discussion in Chapter 17. Therefore, the focus here will be on stomach and intestinal function. Decreased peristaltic activity and relaxation of lower esophageal sphincter result in slowed esophageal emptying. Associated indigestion occurs with increased frequency in the aged. Digestive secretions are diminished with age, but this appears to have little effect on digestion. Only an intolerance of large amounts of fat due to decreased pancreatic lipase is clearly recognized. Calorie requirements decline gradually in late life by approximately 12.4 calories per day per year (Kane et al., 1994). However, there is no corresponding decrease in vitamin and mineral requirement. There is no clinical evidence of diminished vitamin absorption due to normal aging changes, and most identifiable deficiencies can be attributable to intake related to dietary alterations or reductions. Specific vitamin deficiency (such vitamin B12) due to diminished absorption occurs with increased prevalence in late life, though this is not considered a normal age-related change. Other deficiencies can be prevented by avoiding inadequate dietary intake of certain minerals such as calcium. Daily multivitamin supplement and frequent small meals can most often correct deficiencies not resulting from pathology. Dietary deficiencies and inadequate nutritional intake may cause both physical and mental changes in the elderly.

Constipation is a frequent complaint in the elderly. It first must be determined that the problem actually exists. Often, there is simply a misconception about what constitutes normal bowel activity. Normal bowel evacuation may be as infrequent as three times per week. However, many persons believe that a daily bowel movement is necessary. Normal elimination should be an easy passage of feces without straining or the feeling that defecation is incomplete. Overuse of laxatives, with an associated reduction of normal colonic action in the absence of these stimulants, is common. Often, and especially in older adults, constipation is related to inadequate dietary intake of fiber and water. Diminished muscle tone and motor function can account for some slowing of wastes through the lower intestine.

In any event, inadequate nutrition and constipation and fecal impaction can cause both physical and mental decline. This symptomatology is often unrecognized or may be erroneously diagnosed and treated. Again, the client should be referred for evaluation of unexplained changes in functional or general health status.

Changes in the Cardiovascular System

Changes in the heart and circulation are among the most noticeable in older persons, but determining their cause is often difficult due to the prevalence of cardiovascular diseases in late life. Venous insufficiency of the lower extremity is a ready example of altered function. This is often thought of as a disease-related change, but it occurs almost universally with advanced age in human beings.

The important measurable changes in physiologic parameters of the cardiovascular system include decreased heart rate, increased cardiac stroke volume, and increased systolic blood pressure with age. Structural and anatomical changes demonstrable with aging include sclerosis of heart valves, increased intimal thickening of the arteries, increased medial fibrosis of arteries, and a resultant decreased compliance of peripheral blood vessels. Tortuosity of larger arteries, such as the aorta, is frequently noted. Many of these changes are associated with atherosclerosis. Gradual decline in the baroreceptor reflexes often results in postural dizziness on rising to the standing position that is typically of only fleeting duration but that can easily be compounded by volume depletion, acute illness, or blood pressure lowering effects of many medications causing syncope or falls.

The increased incidence of coronary heart disease, strokes, hypertension, and congestive heart failure in late life carries very significant implications for morbidity, mortality, and disability in the elderly. Certainly, some of the most common communication disorders in aging result from stroke. These very common chronic diseases also represent areas of true medical progress over the last several decades in terms of prevention, treatment, and health risk modifications.

Changes in the Respiratory System

The normal age-related decline in respiratory capacity is somewhat less variable than most other basic physiological parameters. The most important changes in the respiratory system include decreased elasticity of lung tissue, decline in the activity of the cilia, and a diminished cough reflex. Measurable functional parameters showing a consistent change include decreased vital capacity, decreased maximum oxygen uptake, and increased residual volume.

Although the aging process does result in a reduction in respiratory functioning, "it is difficult to determine how much deterioration in pulmonary function is necessary before speech is affected" (Hollien, 1987, p. 12). These basic age-related changes alone serve to render the older person more susceptible to infections such as pneumonia. In cases of longtime smoking exposure, respiratory functional decline and reduced defenses will typically be much more compromised, even in the absence of clinically demonstrable emphysema or other smoking-related respiratory disease.

Changes in the Musculoskeletal System

Many of the respiratory system changes previously noted result from alterations in musculoskeletal structures. The common symptoms and impaired functions experienced as a result of musculoskeletal changes of normal aging are often considered the most important to the elderly patient. Arthritis, complications of osteoporosis, and nonarticular rheumatism, superimposed on the normal changes of aging in the bones and joints, typically have direct impact on mobility and other important abilities required for self-care.

The hallmarks of age-related changes result from a decrease in flexibility and increase in stiffness of the muscles, joints, and periarticular tissues (such as cartilages). Ambulation and virtually all voluntary body movements are gradually affected, with a progressive slowing of activities. Much of this insidious progression of impaired gross body movements can be ameliorated by regular physical activity. Conversely, physical inactivity does seem to aggravate or accelerate these changes, because loss of muscle tissue may result from disuse.

Osteoarthritis or degenerative joint disease is so prevalent in late life that it is often thought of as an age-related phenomenon. In fact, the noninflammatory, structural deterioration of the joint cartilage that is almost universally present to some extent at very advanced age is often clinically inseparable in its functional presentation from the changes occurring with age.

Common musculoskeletal disorders seen in the elderly include osteoporosis (especially in postmenopausal women), polymyalgia rheumatica, tendonitis, and bursitis. Fibromyalgia is a generalized, somewhat variable disorder of the muscles and the periarticular connective tissues that may account for the most prevalent type of nonarticular rheumatism in late life.

Accurate evaluation and management of the symptomatic musculoskeletal problems of the elderly is imperative in order to prevent functional decline that can threaten even the most basic aspects of self-care and the ability to reside independently.

Changes in the Neurological System

The age-related changes that occur in the central nervous system also present the older individual with gradually progressive impairment of functions, leading to increasing risks of dependency. The number of nerve cells decreases with normal aging; the extent of this loss varies greatly in different areas of the brain. Overall, the brain weight gradually declines with age after the third decade, typically reaching approximately a 10% loss in weight by age 90 (Kane et al., 1994). There also are demonstrable changes in the dopaminergic and cholinergic neurotransmitter systems in the brain, although the significance of these and other identifiable changes have not been satisfactorily determined (Abrams et al., 1995).

A very important age-related change in nerve cell function is the decline in the speed of the action potentials through the nerve fibers. This has been shown to be slowed by approximately 30% between the ages of 20 and 80 years (Kenney, 1988). Peripheral nerves additionally exhibit a gradual loss of the myelin layer, which insulates the axons. This may reduce the precision as well as the speed with which signals are transmitted through the system.

The aging brain also shows a deposition of lipofuscin in nerve cells, deposition of amyloid in cells and blood vessels, and the appearance of senile plaques. Although the latter finding, along with neurofibrillary tangles, is among the hallmark pathological features of Alzheimer's disease, both appear in lesser numbers in the brain with normal aging (Abrams et al., 1995).

As in most other areas of physiologic aging, these changes are a part of the increasing vulnerability of the human organism to a multitude of stresses that can result in premature functional impairment or disability in the older patient. Impaired balance, gait, and peripheral sensory and motor functions represent crucial problems that make a person extremely vulnerable to further disability, especially in key areas such as driving, living alone, and important areas of personal safety.

Dementia is among the most common and serious health problems of late life and becomes increasingly common with advancing age. The dementia syndrome is associated with a significant deterioration of cognition in an alert person that results in impaired function in activities of daily living. Alzheimer's disease accounts for more than 60% of the cases of dementia. The second leading cause is vascular dementia, representing approximately 5% to 20% of cases (Fleming, Adams, & Peterson, 1995).

Common age-related diseases represent serious threats to the declining functions of the normal aging nervous system. Parkinson's disease is a progressive movement disorder involving loss of effective gait, increasing slowness and rigidity of movements, and prominent involuntary tremor. In addition, there is a high incidence of dementia developing in patients with Parkinson's. Cerebrovascular disease and the associated risk of stroke, though theoretically preventable, at least in part, continue to present medical disability to the elderly in epidemic proportions.

Functional Assessment: The Medical Perspective

Functional assessment of communication behaviors is addressed in Chapter 9. However, from a medical perspective, a number of recent publications have emphasized the need to include evaluation of key areas of functional ability in older patients. As Kane et al. (1994, p. 62) indicated in the following equation, "function" is the end result of more than accurate medical diagnosis:

$$\text{Function} = \frac{\text{physical abilities} \times \text{medical management} \times \text{motivation}}{\text{social and physical environment}}$$

Clearly, a thorough patient examination and appropriate laboratory procedures form the cornerstone of any medical evaluation. In the case of the older patient, however, all findings must be interpreted carefully in the light of the kinds of information about normal aging presented in the previous sections. For example, gradual loss of small amounts of weight over an extended time period may not be clinically significant in an 80-year-old woman, although that weight loss must be considered in the context of all other observations and presenting complaints. In contrast, markedly elevated white blood cell counts are abnormal in all age groups and require prompt attention.

Traditional patient examination and laboratory assessment do not provide sufficient information to evaluate health status from a functional perspective. Most recommendations for functional assessment of the geriatric patient include evaluations of (a) activities of daily living, (b) mobility and mobility restrictions, (c) cognitive status (including dementia and/or depression screening), (d) the special senses, (e) urinary continence, (f) nutrition, and (g) a broad range of psychosocial and environmental factors and needs, including caregiver health and burden.

Specific formal or informal assessment protocols for each of these areas have been reviewed by Fleming, Evans, Weber, and Chutka (1995). Additional practical, comprehensive resources for functional geriatric assessment are available (e.g., Gallo, Reichel, & Anderson, 1988; Kane et al., 1994). In view of the content of other chapters in this text, only the activities of daily living and the mobility assessment domains are discussed in any detail here.

It should be first noted that obtaining a comprehensive medical and psychosocial history is essential to the success of a functional assessment of an older adult. As Kane et al. (1994) noted, a number of potential difficulties related to aspects of aging may interfere with the history-taking process. These difficulties are not unique to the assessment process in medicine. Indeed, all health care professionals can expect to encounter some of these history-gathering barriers and must adjust interview techniques appropriately.

Diminished hearing and/or vision may interfere with communication, leading to inaccurate or incomplete data gathering as well as to breakdown in the professional–client relationship. Underreporting of symptoms may result from a variety of factors, including general health beliefs or fears about health problems, depression, cognitive limitations, or actual age-associated changes in physical or physiological responses to disease symptomatology. Many reports of symptoms may appear vague or nonspecific, reflecting the fact that a variety of disease processes may manifest themselves in single, nonspecific complaints such as fatigue or memory loss. Finally, many older adults present with multiple complaints, real or imagined, and the health care provider must probe carefully to distinguish the effects of distinct disorders and/or underlying emotional components.

History gathering does not exist in a vacuum apart from functional assessment activities. Instead, outcomes of certain assessment procedures may point to the need for additional history information. One of the best examples of this interaction can be found in the evaluation of daily living skills, referred to as *activities of daily living* (ADLs) and *instrumental activities of daily living* (IADLs). Both of these terms refer to functional tasks accomplished on a daily basis. ADLs are basic self-care functions; common examples include bathing, dressing, eating, toileting, transfer, and continence. Some scales place communication in this list. ADLs may be assessed informally, through observation and/or report, or may even be evaluated through use of one or more common checklists (e.g., the *Index of Activities of Daily Living*, Katz, Ford, Moskowitz, Jackson, & Jaffee, 1963; the *Barthel Index*, Mahoney & Barthel, 1965). ADLs serve only as indicators of the lower end of the scale of functional abilities. Determination of difficulty in ADLs serves as a starting point for identifying contributing factors and interventions.

IADLs are more complex tasks, involving both cognitive and physical abilities. Many activities fall under the heading of IADLs, including shopping, cleaning, cooking, writing, managing money, and using the telephone, among other activities. Again, both observation and report can be used to assess IADL functioning. One commonly used scale is the Lawton IADL scale (Lawton, Moss, Fulcomer, & Kleban, 1982). Performance of both ADLs and IADLs is heavily influenced by motivational and environmental considerations. Numerous additional ADL and IADL scales have proliferated in the literature in recent years, as functional status has become a critical variable not only in health care but also in research concerning the elderly. Regardless of the assessment approach used, however, all professionals working with older adults should be sensitive to the client's ADL and IADL levels of functioning, as they have a significant impact upon other aspects of performance. Loss of independence is a major determinant of self-esteem and emotional well-being, both factors essential to quality of life.

A related area of major concern in the functional assessment of the geriatric client is mobility. In this context, *mobility* refers to the individual's "capacity to maneuver safely and effectively" (Fleming, Evans, et al., 1995, p. 891). Performance of ADLs and IADLs is dependent in part upon mobility, but the two should be assessed separately. Specific scales are available to detect and quantify mobility limitations (e.g., the *Tinetti Balance and Gait Evaluation,* Tinetti, 1986). However, informal evaluation of gait, balance, shoulder function, and hand function should be performed (Fleming, Evans, et al., 1995). Mobility restrictions can influence the older adult's functioning in virtually all other performance domains. For example, reductions in the frequency and variety of social activities can result in altered communication skills and opportunities. Depression may result from loss of the ability to engage in hobbies or other personally satisfying activities. In addition, the older adult's access to services may be curtailed severely if mobility restrictions become severe.

The bottom line is that, apart from specific disease processes, aspects of aging may alter functioning performance in older adults. Effective health promotion and disability prevention cannot occur without an understanding of these aging changes and their interaction with other health factors.

Health Promotion and Disability Prevention

The foregoing general review of the medical aspects of age-related decline and functional assessment considerations is necessarily brief and should only serve to establish the fundamental nature of the age-related health problems of older patients. All health professionals who work with the elderly should acquire a basic appreciation of the altered presentation of medical problems in this population and the multifactorial nature of their onset and clinical course. That understanding should make clear the importance of a comprehensive, interdisciplinary approach.

The goals of clinical and other interventions on behalf of the health of older adults should evolve from a special set of priorities:

- reducing premature mortality
- reducing mortality from chronic and acute illness
- avoiding iatrogenesis
- extending active life expectancy
- prolonging functional independence
- enhancing quality of life

Each health professional, as a member of the geriatric team, represents a unique part of the diagnostic and therapeutic process for the elderly. Each has the unique opportunity to identify interventions that might lead to important health maintenance, promotion, and prevention strategies. In view of the often critical nature of communication skills in determining an older adult's ability to maintain an independent life-style, this approach and the topics reviewed in companion chapters of this text are of great importance.

References

Abrams, W. B., Beers, M. H., & Berkow, R. (1995). *The Merck manual of geriatrics* (2nd ed.). Whitehouse Station, NJ: Merck Research Laboratories.

Ebersole, P., & Hess, P. (1994). *Toward healthy aging: Human needs and nursing response* (3rd ed.). St Louis, MO: Mosby.

Fleming, K. C., Adams, A. C., & Peterson, R. C. (1995.) Dementia: Diagnosis and evaluation. *Mayo Clinic Proceedings, 70,* 1093–1107.

Fleming, K. C., Evans, J. M., Weber, D. C., & Chutka, D. S. (1995). Practical functional assessment of elderly persons: A primary care approach. *Mayo Clinic Proceedings, 70,* 890–910.

Gallo, J. J., Reichel, W., & Anderson, L. (1988). *Handbook of geriatric assessment.* Rockville, MD: Aspen.

Goldman, R. (1979). Decline in organic function with age. In I. Rossman (Ed.), *Clinical geriatrics* (2nd ed.). Philadelphia: J. B. Lippincott.

Hollien, H. (1987). "Old voices": What do we really know about them? *Journal of Voice, 1*, 2–17.

Kane, R. L., Ouslander, J. G., & Abrass, I. B. (1994). *Essentials of clinical geriatrics* (3rd ed). New York: McGraw-Hill.

Katz, S., Ford, A., Moskowitz, R., Jackson, B., & Jaffee, M. (1963). The index of ADL: A standardized measure of biological and psychosocial function. *Journal of American Medical Association, 185*, 914–919.

Kenney, R. A. (1988). Physiology of aging. In B. B. Shadden (Ed.), *Communication behavior and aging: A sourcebook for clinicians* (pp. 58–78). Baltimore: Williams & Wilkins.

Lawton, M. P., Moss, M., Fulcomer, M., & Kleban, M. H. (1982). A research and service oriented multilevel assessment instrument. *Journal of Gerontology, 37*, 91–99.

Mahoney, F. I., & Barthel, D. W. (1965). Functional evaluation: The Barthel Index. *Maryland State Medical Journal, 14*, 61–65.

Tinetti, M. E. (1986). Performance-oriented assessment of mobility problems in elderly patients. *Journal of the American Geriatric Society, 34*, 119–126.

Williams, M. E. (1994). Clinical management of the elderly patient. In W. R. Hazzard, E. L. Biernan, et al. (Eds.), *Principles of geriatric medicine and gerontology* (3rd ed., pp. 195–201). New York: McGraw-Hill.

Chapter 4

Mental Status and Aging: Cognition and Affect

Daniel J. Johnson

Johnson emphasizes the importance of understanding normal cognitive and affective status in older individuals. He summarizes cognitive changes associated with life span development, then presents a brief discussion of depression and dementia in the elderly. As in the previous chapter, functional assessment of cognition (mental status) and affect (depression inventories) is targeted.

1. *What are some of the issues Johnson identifies as affecting our attempts to define normal cognitive and affective status in older adults? Compare and contrast the "diminished resources" and the "speed of processing" theories of cognitive aging change.*

2. *What can we conclude about age-related changes in IQ, perception, attention, memory, learning, and problem-solving and/or reasoning and executive functions?*

3. *What are the two broad types of dementia identified by Johnson and what characteristics distinguish these types? What are some predictable behaviors at each stage in the progression of Alzheimer's disease?*

4. *How are the behaviors and symptoms of depression differentiated from those of dementia?*

5. *What are the main elements of a mental status examination? Why should speech–language pathologists and audiologists be aware of their client's mental status and the presence and severity of any depression?*

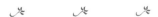

Because of the increasing size of the older population in the United States, practitioners are growing more aware of the need for an understanding of the vast individual variations that exist in the life course of the individual. Although this need for an understanding of normal aging processes applies to all areas of functioning, the cognitive and affective status of aging individuals is particularly important. As Kausler (1988) pointed out: "Cognitive processes direct our attention to specific events present in our environment, enable us to perceive and interpret these events, guide the acquisition of new information about our environment, determine the subsequent memorability of that new information, and [help us] find the means of solving problems created by novel environmental demands" (p. 69). Cognitive processes are directly linked to communication behaviors, and any decline in cognitive functions will typically result in less effective adaptation (Kausler, 1988).

This chapter will provide a summary of cognitive aspects of aging, beginning with a brief introduction to some of the theoretical and applied issues involved in specifying the nature of cognitive aging. Because one critical diagnostic challenge is the differentiation of normal aging from dementia and depression, separate sections will discuss these disorders in depth. Finally, an overview of the components of the mental status examination and commonly used mental status tests will be provided.

Central Issues in Examining Cognitive and Affective Status in Older Persons

Research shows that there are changes in some of the basic cognitive processes involving communication in older adults, including intelligence, attention, memory, learning, problem solving, creativity, and wisdom (Hooker & Shifren, 1995). Unfortunately, specifying the nature of those changes and their impact on the individual adult is not an easy task. A number of factors influence our understanding of normal cognitive aging; a few critical ones will be discussed here.

Studies of changes in brain structure and function in healthy older persons have demonstrated differential effects of aging and selective areas of cognitive vulnerability. Similarly, changes in cognitive ability do not occur uniformly either within or across cognitive domains. In other words, there is substantial variability among older adults, and this variability results in pronounced heterogeneity in performance.

Cohort differences in cognitive strategy and previous learning exacerbate variability.

The heterogeneity of the older population raises interesting questions about what can and should be defined as a normal older adult for the purposes of investigating cognitive functioning. In most instances, normal cognitive and affective function is presumed to exclude the following: history or presence of a *Diagnostic and Statistical Manual of Mental Disorders–Fourth Edition* (DSM–IV; American Psychiatric Association, 1994) disorder; history of any neurologic disease, including head trauma with loss of consciousness; current medical disease that may affect brain function such as diabetes or hypertension; current use or abuse of drugs; use of any medication with central nervous system effects; and any first-degree relative with a psychiatric history (Pucell, Jennifer, Schwartz, Brookshire, & Lewine, 1995). This definition of normalcy can be troublesome, since, as Kausler (1988) pointed out, observed changes in cognitive behaviors across the life span may reflect performance shifts (successful execution of a task) rather than competence shifts (internal capability of the individual). Performance can be highly susceptible to sensory, motor, educational, motivational, stress, mental health, and use/disuse variables.

Physical and psychosocial factors have been shown to influence cognitive performance. Berkman et al. (1993) studied older men and women functioning at overall levels defined as high, medium, and impaired. Significant differences for performance-based examination of both physical and cognitive functions were observed across groups. Low-functioning subjects were almost three times more likely to have an income of less than $5,000 than were the high-functioning group. They were also less likely to have finished high school. The high-functioning group smoked cigarettes less and exercised more than others. They had higher levels of blood glucose concentration and greater peak lung expiratory flow rates. High-functioning older adults were also more likely to engage in volunteer activities, scored higher on scales of self-efficacy and mastery, and reported fewer psychiatric symptoms.

Numerous other studies have explored the interaction between cognitive abilities and other subject variables, with a particular emphasis on functional capacity. Declines in individual function are more likely to occur when general health levels are lower (Emery, Huppert, & Schein, 1995). Obesity is related to loss of functions that require movement or expenditure of energy. Having hearing or vision deficits, a stroke, or arthritis puts one at a greater risk for functional deterioration. Any return to functioning is most likely to occur when premorbid functional status of the individual is high, losses have been recent, and impairments are not severe (Crimmins & Saito, 1993).

Depression is another variable that can affect cognitive function in the elderly. Some older adults report reduced affect, feelings of hopelessness, decreased motivation, difficulty in concentration, and other signs of depression. These persons can be misdiagnosed as having a primary degenerative dementia. However, depressed subjects will often have normal memory test performance, despite an increased incidence of memory complaints. In contrast, subjects with dementia would typically demonstrate poor memory test performance, few memory complaints, and few complaints of depression (Williams, Little, Scates, & Blockman, 1987).

Identification of cognitive change and/or deterioration in older adults may also be influenced by cognitive abilities in early to middle adulthood. Individuals with some cognitive limitations may function successfully in the community throughout most of their life span. However, when they become older, cognitive dysfunction may be exacerbated by aging changes or challenges. Compensatory skills may be overtaxed, and the individual may be at risk for an inappropriate diagnosis of dementia.

Cross-cultural differences also may influence cognitive functioning. Individuals from different cultures show different patterns of participation in social and institutional activities, display different communicative strategies, and may have diverse social and economic experiences of aging. A sociocultural perspective is emerging in cognitive aging research; this research agenda may eventually clarify the differential effects of culture on cognitive style and functioning across the life span (Rogoff & Chavagay, 1995).

The foregoing discussion has acknowledged factors influencing cognitive performance in older adults. Some antecedents of individual differences in age-related change have been described. The following variables have been identified as reducing the risk of cognitive decline in old age (Gribbin, Schaie, & Parham, 1980; Gruber & Schaie, 1986; Grubner-Baldini, 1991; Hertzog, Schaie, & Gribbin, 1978; Schaie, 1984, 1989, 1994):

1. the absence of cardiovascular and other chronic diseases;

2. living in favorable environmental circumstances, as would be the case for those persons characterized by higher socioeconomic status;

3. substantial involvement in activities typically available in complex and intellectually stimulating environments;

4. individual's self-report of a flexible personality style at mid-life as well as flexible performance on objective measures of motor–cognitive perseveration tasks;

5. being married to a spouse with high cognitive status;

6. the maintenance of high levels of perceptual processing speed with old age; and,

7. rating oneself as being satisfied with life accomplishments in mid-life or early old age.

Any discussion of factors associated with reduced risk of cognitive decline in old age raises another issue: To what extent are age differences in cognition observed in the laboratory merely academic concerns? In other words, given the everyday social and environmental demands encountered by most older adults, are complex, time-driven tasks involving considerable amounts of new learning really common? As yet, a clear delineation of the relationship between laboratory cognitive performance and daily functional abilities has not been established for most tasks. Recent studies have attempted to identify factors that predict maintenance of ability with age and/or susceptibility to cognitive pathology, as in dementia (e.g., Malec, Smith, Ivnik, Peterson, & Tanalos, 1996).

Further, if cognitive loss does occur in persons aged 70 years and older, it is possible that a return to independent living functions, both inside and outside of the home, can be achieved through appropriate training. Intervention studies to date demonstrate positive, although short-term, effects (Kausler, 1988; La Rue, 1994). Additional examinations of the outcomes of training designed to maximize ability are needed (Albert, 1994).

Cognition and Normal Aging

Theoretical Models of Cognitive Aging

The search for causes of cognitive change (or lack thereof) in normal older adults has led to a proliferation of theoretical models of cognitive aging. A number of causal factors have been proposed, for example, disuse of selected cognitive skills or age cohort differences in cognitive performance (Hooker & Shifren, 1995). Most models fall into two broad categories (Kausler, 1988). The first group of models postulates "diminished resources" as the underlying cause for cognitive change. Diminished capacity or resource hypotheses suggest that aging deficits are expected only when performance requirements exceed the capacity of older, but not younger, adults. Resource limitations may be related to energy reserves in general, and/or to working memory space available for allocation to specific tasks. A second group of models attributes cognitive change to slowing of the speed of processing of information in the central nervous system (e.g., Salthouse, 1985). Again, these theories assume that negative change or deficit will be evident only with increased rates of processing and/or responding to specific tasks. Generally, one's theoretical orientation does not appear to influence the outcomes of studies of cognitive age differences (Kausler, 1988), although the design of studies may vary according to the experimental hypotheses suggested by each set of theories.

Regardless of theoretical orientation, most researchers agree that cognitive skills fall into two broad categories, originally labeled "fluid" and "crystallized" intelligence (Cattell, 1963; Horn & Donaldson, 1976). *Fluid intelligence* includes those abilities reflecting maturational growth and decline of neural structures; *crystallized intelligence* refers to those abilities that depend on formal and informal life experiences (La Rue, 1992). Selective decrement in some cognitive abilities often is associated with aspects of fluid intelligence (Mitrushina & Satz, 1991; Schaie, 1977).

More recently, Baltes (1993) has reconceptualized these abilities in computer terms in order to look at "the as yet untapped reserves and potentials" (p. 580). In his model, fluid intelligence is now defined as "cognitive mechanics," the neurophysiological architecture or hardware of the brain that is involved in information processing. Elements of cognitive mechanics include the speed and accuracy of sensory processing, short-term memory, discrimination, and categorical skills. Because this hardware is subject to the influences of biologic, genetic, and health factors associated with aging, it is most susceptible to decline. In contrast, "cognitive pragmatics" is more akin to the software of the mind. It reflects intelligence as cultural knowledge acquired through socialization and capable of growth over time. Cognitive pragmatics can include such skills as reading, writing, language comprehension, education, professional skills, and self-knowledge for coping purposes. Thus, it is capable of being used to enhance or compensate for other skill areas.

Intelligence Quotients

It was initially thought that declines in cognition began when persons were in their 20s. A number of major studies of IQ scores of adult volunteers subsequently indicated that alterations in IQ began much later in life (60s or 70s, depending upon the method of measurement). The general pattern is one of improvement in cognitive abilities into the late 30s or 40s, followed by stability throughout the 50s and 60s, and decline only after that point (Hooker & Shifren, 1995; Horn, 1970). Measures of cross-sectional, longitudinal, and cross-sequential research in overall IQ indicate changes of 1 standard deviation or more in the late 60s and early 70s. On the *Wechsler Adult Intelligence Scale–Revised* (Wechsler, 1981), Performance Scale scores drop by more than 1 standard deviation by age 60, and Verbal Scale scores drop by more than 1 standard deviation by age 80 years old (Albert, 1994). In most studies, the relative preservation of verbal skills throughout most of the life span is noted.

Specific Cognitive Domains and Aging

Although various authors conceptualize component cognitive processes differently, most agree that the basic elements of cognition include perception; attention; memory; learning; language; and problem-solving, reasoning, and executive functions. Language changes associated with aging are discussed in Chapter 7. A brief summary of what is known about each of the other domains is provided here. Because the literature in cognitive aging is so extensive, the reader is referred to additional reviews for specific research citations (e.g., Bayles & Kaszniak, 1987; Hooker & Shifren, 1995; Kausler, 1988; La Rue, 1992; Schaie, 1994).

Perception. Perception usually refers to obtaining information through our senses. Perception depends on sensory registration, peripheral feature analysis, and central processes matching patterns to previously stored information (Kausler, 1988). Obviously, visual and auditory perceptual processes can be influenced by altered acuity (sensory registration), as well as a diminished sensitivity to sensory increments. However, both processing at the level of peripheral feature analysis and central pattern matching appear to be slowed in older adults, at least as measured in visual pattern recognition tasks. Visuospatial abilities (e.g., block design, picture completion) also require elements of perception and, like many other cognitive skills, appear well preserved for simple tasks, but increasingly impaired as the other cognitive demands of the task increase (La Rue, 1992).

Attention. Attentional behaviors and changes have received considerable focus in the aging literature; virtually every other cognitive skill, including language and communication, is dependent upon attention for adequate performance. There are a number of terms used to describe component attentional processes. Stankov (1988) identified six such components: concentration, search skills, divided attention, selective attention, attention switching, and vigilance. Most of these can be addressed by considering vigilance, selective attention, and divided attention (Kausler, 1988), which encompass familiar everyday skills and difficulties such as concentration and distractibility.

In normal aging, vigilance, selective attention, and divided attention do not show significant declines before 80 years, as long as tasks remain very simple. However, all three skill areas are negatively affected in older adults by the addition of fatiguing elements (extended vigilance tasks) and by increasing memory demands and/or task complexity, as well as time pressures. Attending skills also appear diminished when stimuli are not personally relevant to the individual. Under these constraints, it takes older adults longer to discriminate meaningful or target stimuli; greater distractibility is evident, as well as difficulty in allocating attentional resources to two events.

Because all testing and treatment situations require adequate attending skills, procedural accommodations must be made for the individual client who is experiencing diminished functioning in these areas. Further, complaints of impaired cognitive functioning in other domains should lead practitioners to probe the attentional demands of daily tasks before drawing any conclusions about cognitive deficit. Subtle attentional changes may be evident in lapses in functioning in everyday activities—lapses that may be misconstrued as signs of generalized diminished functioning or loss of functional abilities for independent living. One example is the divided-attention task of driving while carrying on a conversation with a passenger. Although the older adult's driving skills and conversational skills may be highly functional under usual circumstances, the divided-attention demands of the driving/talking task may result in the older person going through a stop sign or swerving into another lane, behaviors that appear to indicate inadequate functional driving skills.

In addition, specific attentional deficits may be seen in clinical populations, including (a) deficits of alertness or drowsiness, (b) deficits in concentration with wandering attention and distractibility, and (c) unilateral or hemispatial inattention. Practitioners must be able to recognize the difference between normal aging changes in attending skills and specific deficits.

Memory. Some researchers and clinicians link memory and learning, because learning is required if we are to retain knowledge of our interactions with our environment (Kausler, 1988). Both learning and memory refer to perceptual experiences represented and stored in the brain, and thus available to alter future thought and behavior. Nevertheless, it is appropriate to consider learning and memory processes separately.

Memory processes are the most commonly studied aspects of cognitive aging, partly because elderly persons complain frequently of memory impairment and partly because careful manipulation of task memory demands allows researchers to understand better the retained abilities and declining processes of the aging brain. According to La Rue (1992), the memory outcome of information processing requires a series of transformations (processing stages) between sensory registration and long-term memory storage.

The problem in reading the literature and understanding the memory status of the older adult is the variety of terms used to refer to component memory stages and/or processes. It is perhaps simplest to conceptualize memory functions as falling within three broad categories: sensory memory, primary or short-term memory, and secondary or long-term memory (Kausler, 1988; La Rue, 1992; Loring, Lee, & Meador, 1989). *Sensory memory* is the basic stimulus trace, like an echo or image, which lasts only long enough for registration in short-term memory. Short-term memory is temporary, with a 20- to 30-second retention span. It has been viewed as "working memory," in which conscious mental processes are performed, and is analogous to immediate or primary memory. Information is retained here only through effort and rehearsal, prior to being transmitted to one of the long-term stores. Long-term memory is previously learned information and is considered a more permanent storehouse, including both recent and remote memory concepts. Theorists often subdivide secondary or long-term memory elements into semantic, or generic, memory and episodic memory. Semantic memory contains our internal lexicon, a kind of mental dictionary of vocabulary and facts. Episodic memory involves information stored with the context for the occurrence of the event, so that we retain not only the memory of going to a Broadway show but also much additional context information related to the weather, the look of the theater, clothing that was worn, and so on.

Age-associated changes in memory processes are difficult to summarize adequately, because the influences of task differences and modes of response are so pervasive. Deficits are evident earlier in the life span when recall, as compared with recognition, tasks are used. Despite these variations in performance, the following general observations can be provided.

Sensory memory may display age-related deficits due to losses in sensory acuity, with a resulting weakening of the stimulus trace. Short-term or working memory may be more vulnerable to aging processes, because it has a limited capacity for processing and storing information. On simple tasks, working memory skills are retained, at least up to the seventh decade, although some slowing of speed of accessing may be noted. However, when task difficulty increases in any manner—length, complexity of materials, presence of distractors, reduced personal relevance, and/or redundancy—age-related working memory restrictions are identified. This has been found particularly for language processing, as is discussed in Chapter 7.

Secondary memory processes in older adults can be considered from two perspectives: (a) the process of storing new information in long-term memory and (b) access to previously acquired knowledge and event-based memories. Normal older adults appear to be relatively good at retrieving remote events and information from the internal lexicon, as long as the task is nonstressful (Albert, 1994). In fact, passive vocabulary is stable or increases throughout the life span, and older persons are noted for their recollection of past events. However, there is evidence for less extensive and efficient initial processing of new material that must be placed into long-term store (Craik, 1977); shallow processing makes the material more difficult to recover when recall is required. Training in more active use of mnemonic cues produces short-term benefits in recall, but long-term effects are not as strong. Some researchers have suggested that retrieval is at least as great a problem as encoding. It has been speculated that less effective encoding and retrieval may result from limited effort, due to diminished attention and memory. Other researchers have suggested that laboratory tasks may lack relevance, eliciting less subject effort. However, even for everyday memory tasks that are more familiar and naturalistic, age-associated changes are noted (see review in Poon, Rubin, & Wilson, 1989).

Health, sensory acuity, and other variables can affect memory functioning. Older adults' fears and complaints about memory loss typically exceed the deficits they demonstrate in formal testing (Zarit, Cole, & Guider, 1981). Fear of diminished memory functioning may have a major effect on research task performance, because self-consciousness regarding cognitive functioning can alter strategies used in memory tasks.

The patterns of memory performance by elderly individuals demonstrate significant overlap between normal and clinical populations. Formal memory tests poorly differentiate normal aging, dementia, and depression. For this reason, additional information concerning everyday memory performance in normal older adults is needed (Loring et al., 1989). Clinicians must be alert to the presence of memory impairment in older clients, apart from the primary presenting pathology. Sensitivity to client concerns about potentially failing memory and cognitive functions is also needed. Reassurance and reduced task pressure may be required.

Learning, Transfer, and Retention. Learning progresses more slowly for older adults, but does occur (Kausler, 1988). Once new information and/or skills are acquired by the older person, the rate of forgetting appears to be the same as for other age groups. There does appear to be a decline in incidental learning, the acquisition of new information or knowledge when that acquisition is not the focus of the learner's attention. There may also be a decline in transfer and application of previous learning and learning strategies to new situations and tasks. There appear to be few, if any, changes in concept formation as long as tasks are familiar and relatively simple. However, older adults' strategies in concept formation differ, and may be less efficient, than younger adults' strategies. Therapeutic interventions involve elements of new learning coupled with attempts to elicit application of existing skills to new situations. Clinicians must recognize that some older clients may demonstrate a slower learning curve and may require more cuing in transferring learned material and strategies to new situations.

Problem Solving, Reasoning, and Executive Functions. Problem solving and reasoning have been found to demonstrate age-related declines, although some of these declines may be influenced by educational achievement and sociocultural experience. For example, persons with more education show declines later in the life span. A major issue in investigations of problem solving is the degree to which the task represents a real-life challenge or an artificial laboratory construct. For everyday situations, problem solving in healthy, normal older adults may be well preserved. When the same problem-solving skills must be applied to novel information and complex constructs, however, older adults perform more poorly than younger adults. Because some laboratory tasks closely approximate real-life challenges (e.g., a 20-Questions problem-solving task, Denney, 1982), reduced problem-solving efficiency is of some concern.

Executive function is a term that encompasses many of the activities associated with reasoning, problem solving, learning, and concept formation. Executive function involves the individual's skills in planning, initiating, terminating, and shifting purposeful behavior. In addition to the problem-solving and reasoning areas noted here, some older adults evidence difficulty with the planning stages of any activity. There may be age-related changes in the ability to change cognitive set (e.g., increased rigidity, reduced adaptation). Concreteness may be higher. Some older adults may approach any performance task with a conservative response set. In other words, they try to minimize failure, taking few if any risks.

All of these potential age-associated changes in cognitive strategy and problem solving must be considered in the individual client. For individuals coping with a specific communication disorder, many communication situations require problem solving. Tasks should be chosen, as much as possible, to reflect everyday challenges and situations. Active assistance in increasing the efficiency and effectiveness of strategies should be provided (because some benefits to training in problem-solving skills have been reported, Kausler, 1988). It is critical to remember that the social and environmental demands placed upon older adults may be considerably different from the demands imposed in the laboratory. Prior to the onset of a specific disorder, older persons may be able to function with less efficient information processing and problem-solving strategies. It is unreasonable to expect that approaches to learning and functioning that have worked well in the past will suddenly be modified because of a new challenge to the cognitive system.

Dementia

Perhaps the most devastating cognitive problem associated with aging is known as dementia. Although this chapter has focused on cognition in normal aging, one of the major diagnostic concerns of the neuropsychologist and other professionals is determining the difference between nonpathological cognitive change and dementia. Further, researchers continue to explore the degree to which cognitive and language performance in advanced age (i.e., over 80 or 85 years) can be discriminated consistently and reliably from dementia (e.g., Ulatowska & Chapman, 1991).

There are basically two types of dementia: cortical and subcortical (Cummings, 1985; Cummings & Benson, 1983). These types are delineated on the basis of primary site of lesion or neurological degeneration. Cortical dementias are associated with degeneration in neocortical association areas and the hippocampus. In contrast, subcortical dementias are linked to dysfunction in the thalamus, basal ganglia, and rostral brain stem. Because site of lesion differs for these forms of dementia, there are a number of distinguishing characteristics that differentiate the groups of disorders (Bayles & Kaszniak, 1987; Cummings, 1985).

Certainly, motor functions are primary distinguishing characteristics. Patients with cortical dementia show little motor impairment (including speech functions) until the late stages. In contrast, subcortical dementias display dysarthric speech and a wide range of abnormal movement patterns (typically hypokinetic or hyperkinetic). The nature and degree of cognitive impairment also distinguishes cortical and subcortical dementias. Impaired cognitive functions in cortical dementia include aphasia, agnosia, amnesia, acalculia, visuospatial disturbances, and abstraction abilities. In subcortical dementias, common intellectual dysfunctions involve psychomotor retardation, forgetfulness, cognitive dilapidation, impaired insight, and poor strategy formulation. Finally, the two groups differ with respect to awareness or concern about impairments. Persons with cortical dementia typically evidence indifference toward their deficits, whereas individuals with subcortical dementias are more prone to concern about difficulties and resulting depression.

Specific conditions leading to dementia are listed in a variety of sources (e.g., Bayles, 1994; Bayles & Kaszniak, 1987). Of particular interest is the distinction between reversible and irreversible dementias. For example, depression may masquerade as dementia; the term *pseudodementia* is sometimes applied to this condition (see next section). Toxin ingestion, drug interactions, and certain metabolic disorders also can lead to dementia-like symptoms, which are reversible once the underlying medical problem is diagnosed and treated. The three most common forms of dementia seen by communication disorders professionals are Alzheimer's disease, Parkinson's disease, and vascular (or multi-infarct) dementia. Bayles (1994) provided a brief but focused review of the similarities and differences among these three causes of dementia, further differentiating between communication deficits in dementia and those associated with focal cortical lesions (e.g., aphasia). Only Alzheimer's disease will be addressed in any detail in this chapter.

Perhaps the most well known and common type of dementia is known as dementia of the Alzheimer's type (DAT). DAT is a progressive degenerative brain disease associated with characteristic destructive changes within neurons, neuronal loss, and changes in the production and utilization of neurotransmitters and neuropeptides (Ripich, 1991). An estimated 4 million people in the United States are afflicted with this disease. It is the fourth leading cause of death in America. It has been estimated that 14 million persons will have the disease by the year 2050 (Alzheimer's Association, 1993a). Alzheimer's disease usually afflicts persons over the age of 60 years. Ten percent of those over 85 years of age have the disease. Both men and women, all races, and all socioeconomic groups are affected.

Risk factors for DAT are still being investigated. Known factors in order from highest to lowest risk (Katzman, 1993) are family history of dementia, Down syndrome in family, family history of Parkinson's disease, late onset depression, hypothyroidism, head injury, and maternal age greater than 40 years. Genetic factors are of particular interest. It is now known that Apolipoprotein E4 (ApoE4), present in about 25% of the population, is a major genetic marker for DAT susceptibility. What remains unknown is whether or not genetic factors are related to onset of first symptoms after the age of 80 years.

Relatively sophisticated scales for tracking degree of cognitive deficit and associated behaviors and problems in persons with dementia are available (see later discussion of *Global Deterioration Scale for Assessment of Primary Degenerative Dementia,* Reisberg, Ferris, de Leon, & Crook, 1982). There are basically three general stages of symptom progression recognized in Alzheimer's disease (Alzheimer's Association, 1993b). General behaviors associated with the characteristic symptoms of each stage are summarized in Table 4.1. Clearly, performance decrements begin with subtle and inconsistent alterations in memory, orientation, spontaneity, and personality in the first stage, making early diagnosis of probable DAT difficult because of the overlap of these behavioral characteristics with a variety of other disorders and conditions. As DAT progresses, however, the individual becomes increasingly more dysfunctional in daily living activities and more difficult to manage. The final stage is characterized by total dependence and loss of contact with the environment and with caregivers.

Each stage in the progression is also associated with predictable changes in aspects of communication and social functioning. Excellent summaries of the speech–language and communication characteristics associated with these three stages or with the dementia stages of the *Global Deterioration Scale* can be found elsewhere (see Bayles, 1994, and Clark, 1995, respectively). In general, syntactic and phonologic language performance is well preserved through the first and often second stages of DAT. In contrast, semantic and pragmatic aspects of language performance are affected from the very beginning, and may be among the first signs of a change in the individual's behavior. Word retrieval problems are noted early on, along with disorganized conversation and discourse lacking appropriate cohesion and topic initiation and maintenance. As the disease progresses, semantic content becomes massively disrupted, and communication becomes increasingly more vague and difficult to follow. By the third stage, mutism or unintelligible and/or stereotypic utterances predominate.

Differential diagnosis of probable dementia requires team assessment and close examination of all behavioral domains, along with an extensive medical workup designed to eliminate other disorders that may masquerade as dementia. Of particular concern in the differential diagnostic process is the discrimination between dementia and delirium or depression. As noted in the following section, depression often masquerades as dementia.

Table 4.1
Behavioral Characteristics of the Three Primary
Stages in Progression of Alzheimer's Disease

First Stage—2 to 4 years leading up to, and including, diagnosis

Dominant Symptom(s)—recent memory loss

Behavioral Indicators:

- progressive forgetfulness and difficulty with routine chores
- confusion related to directions, decisions, and memory management; may arrive at wrong time or place; constantly checks calendar
- loss of initiative and spontaneity
- disorientation with respect to time and place
- loses objects often, or forgets they are lost
- changes in mood, personality, and judgment
- repetitive actions and statements common

Second Stage—2 to 10 years following diagnosis (longest stage)

Dominant Symptom(s)—increasing memory loss, confusion, and shorter attention span

Behavioral Indicators:

- wandering and restlessness, particularly in late afternoon and evening
- problems recognizing close friends and/or family
- difficulty with thought organization and logical thinking
- increased irritability, fidgeting, and/or teariness
- occasional muscle twitching or jerking
- becomming sloppy, for example, in dressing behaviors and eating skills
- sleeps often but also awakens frequently at night and wanders ("sundowners")
- perceptual–motor problems noted for basic ADLs and IADLs (sitting, setting table)
- increase in paranoia and suspicion
- inability to read signs, write name, perform basic mathematical operations
- impluse control impaired with associated inappropriate behaviors
- changes in appetite
- needs full-time supervision

(Continues)

Table 4.1 *(Continued)*

Third Stage—1 to 3 years

Dominant Symptom(s)—unable to recognize family members or self in mirror

Behavioral Indicators:

- capacity for self-care diminished severely, with total assistance required for bathing, dressing, eating, and toileting
- oral communication disappears, leading to mutism, although groans, screams, and grunts may persist in some patients
- swallowing problems, loss of weight (even with proper diet) (may lead to emaciation)
- bowel and bladder incontinence
- attempts to put everything in mouth; compulsion for touching
- other medical problems may emerge, such as skin infections or seizures
- sleeps more, becomes comatose; eventually dies

Note. From *Stages of Symptom Progression in Alzheimer's Disease,* by Alzheimer's Association, 1993, Chicago: Alzheimer's Association.

Depression and the Elderly

The reported prevalence of depressive symptomatology among the elderly ranges from 5% to 65% in hospital and community populations (Blazer, 1986). Exact figures are difficult to determine because of problems with record keeping, mental health service underutilization by the elderly, and difficulties in accurately diagnosing the difference between true depressive illness and reactions to late life stress or even the normal process of bereavement. Nevertheless, it is believed that depression is the most common emotional disorder seen in older adults. A diagnosis of depression is made only when it can be established that no organic factor initiated and maintained the disturbance. Chronic physical illness, polysubstance dependence (alcohol or over-the-counter drugs), psychosocial stressors (particularly the loss of a loved one), marital separation or divorce, hypothyroidism, and even dementia may contribute as predisposing factors. In major depression episodes, the degree of impairment varies; however, there is always some interference in social and occupational functioning. If impairment is severe, the person may be unable to feed or clothe himself or herself, or maintain minimal personal hygiene.

The behavioral characteristics of major depression are specified in the revised fourth edition of the *Diagnostic and Statistical Manual of Mental Disorders* (DSM-IV, American Psychiatric Association, 1994). To substantiate a diagnosis of depression, five of these symptoms must be present for at least 2 weeks, and either depressed mood or loss of interest must be observed most of the day, nearly every day. Behavioral markers of depression include

1. depressed mood;
2. markedly diminished interest or pleasure in all, or almost all, activities;
3. significant undesired weight loss or gain or a decrease or increase in appetite;
4. insomnia or hypersomnia;
5. psychomotor agitation or retardation;
6. fatigue or loss of energy;
7. feelings of worthlessness or guilt;
8. diminished ability to think or concentrate, or indecisiveness; and,
9. recurrent thoughts of death or suicidal ideation, a suicide plan, or suicide attempt.

The disorder of patients who meet the above criteria without any history of manic episodes is called unipolar depression. If the above criteria are present with a history of a manic episode, the appropriate diagnosis is bipolar disorder, depressed phase.

Depression presents in both young and old adults. In older patients, the cognitive sequelae accompanying depression can be a major source of concern to both patient and family. Generally, depression has only a mild impact on cognition in younger patients. Compared with younger depressives, older patients may show more global cognitive impairment during depressive episodes; at times, these impairments may be severe enough to suggest an organic disorder. Somatic complaints are also more prominent in older depressives (La Rue, 1992).

As noted, it is important to be able to distinguish dementia syndrome of depression, also known as pseudodementia, from true dementia. Usually, pseudodementia can be differentiated from true dementia on the basis of history and mental status examination. The clinical features differentiating pseudodementia from dementia are shown in Table 4.2 (Wells & Duncan, 1981). Patient groups differ in virtually all behavioral domains, including (a) duration of symptoms, (b) complaints of and concerns about dysfunction, (c) degree and type of memory impairment, (d) affective change, (e) mental health history, (f) task performance characteristics, and (g) social and behavioral patterns. A thorough mental status evaluation should be able identify these differential patterns of behavior in order to develop an appropriate diagnosis.

Assessment of Cognitive and Affective Status

The purpose of cognitive and affective assessment is to obtain information needed to characterize a patient's strengths and deficits, identify potential explanations for behavioral patterns, discriminate between normal and disordered and within-disorder types, and provide information for treatment planning. As part of this process, an attempt is made to assess central nervous system disabilities and to distinguish these from emotional and/or environmental influences on behavior. Contemporary approaches for the understanding of mental status assessment of aging populations emphasize the complexity and diversity of aging–cognition relations, potential for learning and behavioral change, and individual differences that exist among older persons (La Rue, 1992).

Clinicians who work with the aged must be aware that their own assumptions about and knowledge of older people and aging processes can influence choice of assessment tasks and diagnostic interpretations. For example, accurate discrimination of normal from abnormal elderly patterns of behavior and cognition depends upon one's understanding of the factors influencing cognitive performance in older adults. There must be recognition of the fact that the relationship of test performance to everyday functioning in later life may be quite limited. Test norms must be interpreted with caution if normative age data for upper age ranges are limited or nonexistent. Examiners must also be able to recognize and accommodate to age-related task performance changes. On a relatively long neuropsychological battery, for example, adjustments may need to be made for a particular older

Table 4.2

Discriminating Features of Dementia and Pseudodementia

Behavioral Domain	Pseudodementia	Dementia
Duration of symptoms	**Short**	**Long**
Complains of and concerns about dysfunction	Usually complains of cognitive loss, with description of concerns, strong sense of distress, and emphasis on disability; tends to highlight failure	Usually complains little about cognitive loss, with complaints being imprecise, appearance of limited concern, and concealment of disability; delights in accomplishments
Memory and attention	Memory loss for recent and remote events usually severe, with memory gaps for specific periods or events common; attention and concentration often well preserved	Memory loss for recent events more severe than for remote events, memory gaps for specific periods unusual; attention and concentration usually faulty
Task performance	"Don't know" answers typical, both in formal testing and orientation tasks; makes little effort to perform even simple tasks and does not try to keep up; marked variability in performance on tasks of similar difficulty	"Near miss" answers frequent in formal testing, with orientation tasks showing mistakes of unusual for usual; struggles to perform tasks, and relies on notes, calendars, and so on, to keep up; performance on tasks of similar difficulty levels consistent
Affective change	Often pervasive	Labile and shallow

Social skills	Loss of social skills often early and prominent	Patients often retain social skills
Behavioral patterns	Behavior often incongruent with severity of cognitive dysfunction; nocturnal accentuation of dysfunction uncommon	Behavior usually compatible with severity of cognitive dysfunction; nocturnal accentuation of dysfunction common
History	History of previous psychiatric dysfunction common	History of previous psychiatric dysfunction unusual

Note. From *Neurology for Psychiatrists*, by C. Wells and G. Duncan, 1981, Philadelphia: F. A. Davis.

client's diminished attending skills. Finally, recommendations for rehabilitation may be biased by one's perception of rehabilitation potential in general in the elderly.

The assessment of mental status is usually preceded by an interview. This interview is used to gain patient history information related to complaints and symptoms. The interview also allows for preliminary determination of a patient's intellectual and psychological functions, assessment of disturbances associated with presenting difficulties, and development of rapport. Usually, the first observations made relate to the patient's appearance and behavior. Mood and affect, like behavior, need to be assessed throughout the examination. Motor function disturbances should be identified. Verbal output can also be a clue to mental status. Abnormalities of thought may be inferred from what the patient is saying. Clues to perceptual abnormalities and sensory deficits may be gathered during this preliminary history-taking process.

Once the interview has been completed and all relevant observations have been made, the mental status examination can proceed. It is the purpose of the mental status examination to refine observations made during the interview. Therefore, the emphasis changes from a concern about the patient's past and observations about spontaneous conversation and behavior to a systematic assessment of neuropsychological functions. Mental status assessment may employ specific evaluation tools, or may consist of selected tasks and procedures designed to explore specific cognitive domains more informally.

If informal tasks are used, it is extremely important to begin with an assessment of attention and concentration. Disturbances in this area will create failures throughout all remaining areas of the mental status examination. Language and speech disorders also must be determined carefully. If specific communication deficits are suspected, a complete speech–language evaluation should be requested to supplement mental status testing. Memory assessment should evaluate both short-term and long-term abilities. An assessment of visual–constructive abilities is also important. Simple problem solving is assessed by asking the patient to solve arithmetic problems. The ability to abstract usually provides a good index of general intellectual abilities. Judgment and insight must be determined. Mood and affect, like behavior, need to be assessed as well.

There are a number of commonly used instruments designed to assess mental status, broader neuropsychological functions, and depression in adults in general and older adults specifically. The reader is referred to La Rue (1992), Strub and Black (1985), and Albert and Moss (1988) for detailed reviews of such instruments. Only selected examples will be provided here.

Assessment of depression in older patients may be accomplished through a variety of testing formats. For example, the *Symptom Checklist-90–Revised* (SCL-90–R, Derogatis, 1992) is a brief, multidimensional self-report inventory designed to screen for a wide range of psychological problems and symptoms of psychopathology. The SCL-90-R can also be used as a progress or outcomes measurement instrument.

Several other instruments are available that offer a range of options. *The Beck Depression Inventory* (BDI; Beck, Ward, Mendelson, Mock, & Erbaugh, 1961) is the most widely used instrument for assessing the intensity of depressive symptoms. It measures cognitive, affective, somatic, and performance-related symptoms of depression in a 21-item self-report format offering multiple choice options. The *Geriatric Depression Scale* (Yesavage et al., 1983) also uses self-report in response to 30 true–false items, with many somatic items eliminated.

The *Revised Hamilton Rating Scale for Depression* (RHAM-D; Warren, 1994) measures specific symptom areas for disruption of family and social life, depressed mood, feelings of guilt, insomnia, nocturnal waking, work and activities, sexual symptoms, loss of weight, agitation, worry, somatic anxiety, gastrointestinal symptoms, general somatic symptoms, hypochondriasis, obsessive–compulsive symptoms, paranoid symptoms, depersonalization, and more. As such, it is a much lengthier and more comprehensive instrument. The *State-Trait Depressive Adjective Checklist* (ST-DACL; Lubin, 1994) is one of the most widely used instruments for measuring feelings of dysphoria, sadness, and psychological distress. The new version of this instrument is composed of seven alternate checklists of 32 or 34 adjectives, and includes a new Trait Mood Scale (e.g., "How do you generally feel?").

A number of assessment tools for evaluation of mental status functioning are also available, including the *Mini-Mental State Examination* (MMSE; Folstein, Folstein, & McHugh, 1975), the *Dementia Rating Scale* (Mattis, 1976), the *Short Portable Mental Status Questionnaire* (SPMSQ; Pfeiffer, 1975), and the *Neurobehavioral Cognitive Status Examination* (NCSE; Kiernan, Mueller, Langston, & Van Dyke, 1987). Only two examples will be discussed in greater detail here.

Perhaps the most commonly used tool is the *Mini-Mental State Examination*. This tool provides brief questions and tasks that sample

orientation, immediate and delayed word recall, attention and calculation, naming, repetition, responses to verbal and written commands,
writing, and visuoconstructional abilities. A total of 30 points can be
achieved. Although a cutoff score of 23 is recommended as an index of
potential cognitive impairment, caution must be exercised in diagnosing individuals whose MMSE scores fall below this point. The
Neurobehavioral Cognitive Status Examination (Kiernan et al., 1987)
assesses six areas of cognition. Following examiner rating of the
patient's alertness and consciousness, questions with varying levels of
difficulty are used to evaluate components of language (fluency, comprehension, repetition, and naming), constructional ability, calculation, memory, and verbal reasoning.

Issues of mental status are critical in tracking the decline in cognitive functions of patients with varying forms of dementia, particularly those with Alzheimer's disease. One of the most commonly used
instruments used to establish level of functioning and of decline is the
Global Deterioration Scale. Patients are assigned a stage from 1 (*no cognitive decline*) to 7 (*very severe cognitive decline*). Each stage is labeled,
and a detailed description of clinical characteristics is provided, both
for assessment purposes and for the development of treatment recommendations. Although Stages 2 and 3 are associated with mild cognitive decline, dementia is not identified until Stage 4 (late confusional),
where cognitive and other deficits begin to interfere consistently in
daily activities.

Conclusions

The older population in the United States is growing, both in numbers
and in the percentage of the total population. For those of us who
serve the needs of aging persons, it is has become imperative to be
able to distinguish normal from pathological changes that are seen in
the elderly. This chapter has reviewed some common theories of cognitive change, identifying known alterations in cognitive functioning
and variables affecting cognition in normal older adults. Dementia,
particularly dementia of the Alzheimer's type, and depression were
also discussed, because they occur with some frequency in older
adults and present significant diagnostic challenges. Finally, the
importance of the mental status examination was highlighted, and elements of mental status testing were reviewed.

Future directions for research related to normal cognitive aging include an increasing emphasis on interdisciplinary investigations, further attempts to understand and identify the relationships between age-related alterations in the brain and in cognitive processes, and enhanced focus on determining factors that predict maintenance of ability with age. Particular emphasis needs to be placed upon determining the effects of variables such as education, overall health, activity level, and feelings of self-efficacy on cognitive functioning in normal older adults. Intervention trials and efficacy studies are needed to determine the outcomes of cognitive interventions designed to modify or enhance memory skills, learning strategies, and problem solving. The interaction between cognition and language for everyday communication needs further exploration.

References

Albert, M. (1994, April). *Neuropsychology of aging and dementia.* San Diego: University of California, San Diego, Department of Psychiatry.

Albert, M. S., & Moss, M. B. (Eds.). (1988). *Geriatric neuropsychology.* New York: Guilford Press.

Alzheimer's Association. (1993a). Is it Alzheimer's? Ten warning signs. Chicago: Author.

Alzheimer's Association. (1993b). Stages of symptom progression in Alzheimer's disease. Chicago: Author.

American Psychiatric Association. (1994). *Diagnostic and statistical manual of mental disorders* (4th ed.). Washington, DC: Author.

Baltes, P. B. (1993). The aging mind: Potential and limits. *The Gerontologist, 33,* 580–594.

Bayles, K. A. (1994). Management of neurogenic communication disorders associated with dementia. In R. Chapey (Ed.), *Language intervention strategies in adult aphasia* (3rd ed., pp. 535–545). Baltimore: Williams & Wilkins.

Bayles, K. A., & Kaszniak, A. W. (1987). *Communication and cognition in normal aging and dementia.* Boston: Little, Brown.

Beck, A. T., Ward, C. H., Mendelson, M., Mock, J., & Erbaugh, J. (1961). An inventory for measuring depression. *Archives of General Psychiatry, 4,* 561–571.

Berkman, L. F., Seeman T. E., Albert, M., Blazer, D., Kahn, R., Mohs, R. C., Finch, C., Schneider, E., Cotman, C., McClearn, G., Nesselroade, J., Featherman, D., Garmezy, N., McKhann, G., Brim, G., Praeger, D., & Rowe, J. (1993). High, usual, and impaired functioning in community dwelling older men and women: Findings from the MacArthur Foundation Research Network on Successful Aging. *Epidemiology, 46,* 1129–1140.

Blazer, D. (1986). The diagnosis of depression in the elderly. *Journal of the American Geriatric Society, 28,* 52–58.

Cattell, R. B. (1963). Theory of fluid and crystallized intelligence: A critical experiment. *Journal of Educational Psychology, 54,* 1–22.

Clark, L. W. (1995). Interventions for persons with Alzheimer's disease: Strategies for maintaining and enhancing communicative success. *Topics in Language Disorders, 15,* 47–65.

Craik, F. I. M. (1977). Age differences in human memory. In J. E. Birren & K. W. Schaie (Eds.), *Handbook of the psychology of aging* (pp. 384–420). New York: Van Nostrand Reinhold.

Crimmins, E., & Saito, Y. (1993). Getting better and getting worse. *Journal of Aging and Health, 5,* 3–36.

Cummings, J. L. (1985). *Clinical neuropsychiatry.* Boston: Allyn & Bacon.

Cummings, J. L., & Benson, D. F. (1983). *Dementia: A clinical approach.* Boston: Butterworth.

Denney, N. (1982). Aging and cognitive changes. In B. B. Wolman (Ed.), *Handbook of developmental psychology* (pp. 102–115). Englewood Cliffs, NJ: Prentice-Hall.

Derogatis, L. (1992). *Symptom Checklist-90–Revised.* Minneapolis: NCS Assessments.

Emery, C. F., Huppert, F. A., & Schein, R. L. (1995). Relationships among age, exercise, health, and cognitive function in a British sample. *The Gerontologist, 35,* 378–385.

Folstein, M. F., Folstein, S. E., & McHugh, P. R. (1975). "Mini Mental State": A practical method of grading the cognitive state of patients for the clinician. *Journal of Psychiatric Research, 12,* 189–198.

Gribbin, K., Schaie, K. W., & Parham, I. A. (1980). Complexity of life style and maintenance of intellectual abilities. *Journal of Social Issues, 36,* 47–61.

Gruber, A. L., & Schaie, K. W. (1986, November). *Longitudinal-sequential studies of marital assortativity.* Paper presented at the annual meeting of the Gerontological Society of America, Chicago.

Grubner-Baldini, A. L. (1991). *The impact of health and disease on cognitive ability in adulthood and old age in the Seattle Longitudinal Study*. Unpublished doctoral dissertation, Pennsylvania State University, University Park.

Hertzog, C., Schaie, K. W., & Gribbin, K. (1978). Cardiovascular disease and changes in intellectual functioning from middle to old age. *Journal of Gerontology, 33*, 872–883.

Hooker, K., & Shifren, K. (1995). Psychological aspects of aging. In R. A. Huntley & K. S. Helfer (Eds.), *Communication in later life* (pp. 99–125). Boston: Butterworth-Heinemann.

Horn, J. L. (1970). Organization of data on life-span development of human abilities. In L. R. Goulet & P. B. Baltes (Eds.), *Life-span developmental psychology: Research and theory* (pp. 423–466). New York: Academic Press.

Horn, J. L., & Donaldson, G. (1976). On the myth of intellectual decline in adulthood. *American Psychologist, 31*, 701–719.

Katzman, R. (1993). Clinical and epidemiological aspects of Alzheimer's disease. *Clinical Neuroscience, 1*, 165–170.

Kausler, D. H. (1988). Cognition and aging. In B. B. Shadden (Ed.), *Communication behavior and aging: A sourcebook for clinicians* (pp. 79–105). Baltimore: Williams & Wilkins.

Kiernan, R. J., Mueller, J., Langston, J. W., & VanDyke, C. (1987). The *Neurobehavioral Cognitive Status Examination:* A brief but quantitative approach to cognitive assessment. *Annals of Internal Medicine, 107*, 481–485.

La Rue, A. (1992). *Aging and neuropsychological assessment*. New York: Plenum.

Loring, D. H., Lee, G. P., & Meador, K. J. (1989). *Issues in memory assessment of the elderly.*

Lubin, B. (1994). *State-Trait Depression Adjective Checklist*. Odessa, FL: Psychological Assessment Resources.

Malec, J. F., Smith, G. E., Ivnik, R. J., Peterson, R. E., & Tanalos, E. G. (1996). Clusters of impaired normal elderly do not decline cognitively in 3 to 5 years. *Neuropsychology, 10*, 66–72.

Mattis, S. (1976). Mental status examination for organic mental syndrome in the elderly patient. In L. Bellak & T. B. Karasu (Eds.), *Geriatric psychiatry* (pp. 79–121). New York: Grune & Stratton.

Mitrushina, M., & Satz, P. (1991). Changes in cognitive functioning associated with normal aging. *Archives of Clinical Neuropsychology, 6*, 49–60.

Pfeiffer, E. (1975). SPMSQ: Short Portable Mental Status Questionnaire. *Journal of the American Geriatric Society, 23,* 433–441.

Poon, L. W., Rubin, D. C., & Wilson, B. C. (Eds.). (1989). *Everyday cognition in adulthood and late life.* New York: Cambridge University Press.

Pucell, D. W., Jennifer, A. J., Schwartz, R. J., Brookshire, J. C., & Lewine, R. J. (1995). Neuropsychological functioning in "normal" subjects. *Neuropsychiatry, Neuropsychology, and Behavioral Neurology, 8,* 6–13.

Reisberg, B., Ferris, S., de Leon, M., & Crook, T. (1982). *The Global Deterioration Scale for Assessment of Primary Degenerative Dementia. American Journal of Psychiatry, 139,* 1136–1139.

Ripich, D. N. (1991). *Handbook of geriatric communication disorders.* Austin, TX: PRO-ED.

Rogoff, B., & Chavagay, P. (1995). What's become of research on the cultural basis of cognitive development? *American Psychologist, 50,* 859–877.

Salthouse, T. A. (1985). Speed of behavior and its implications for cognition. In J. E. Birren & K. W. Schaie (Eds.), *Handbook of the psychology of aging* (2nd ed., pp. 168–194). New York: Van Nostrand Reinhold.

Schaie, K. W. (1977). Toward a stage theory of adult cognitive development. *Aging and Human Development, 8,* 129–138.

Schaie, K. W. (1984). Midlife influences upon intellectual functioning in old age. *International Journal of Behavioral Development, 7,* 463–478.

Schaie, K. W. (1989). Perceptual speed in adulthood: Cross-sectional and longitudinal studies. *Psychology and Aging, 4,* 443–453.

Schaie, K. W. (1994). The course of adult intellectual development. *American Psychologist, 49,* 304–313.

Stankov, L. (1988). Aging, attention, and intelligence. *Psychology and Aging, 3,* 59–74.

Strub, R. L., & Black, F. W. (1985). *The mental status examination in neurology* (2nd ed.). Philadelphia: Davis.

Ulatowska, H. K., & Chapman, S. B. (1991). Neurolinguistics and aging. In D. N. Ripich (Ed.), *Handbook of geriatric communication disorders* (pp. 21–37). Austin, TX: PRO-ED.

Warren, W. L. (1994). *Revised Hamilton Rating Scale for Depression.* Los Angeles: Western Psychological Services.

Wechsler, D. (1981). *Wechsler Adult Intelligence Scale–Revised.* New York: Psychological Corp.

Wells, C., & Duncan, G. (1981). *Neurology for psychiatrists: Dementia.* Philadelphia: F. A. Davis.

Williams, J. M., Little, M. M., Scates, S., & Blockman, N. (1987). Memory complaints and abilities among depressed older adults. *Journal of Consulting and Clinical Psychology, 55,* 595–598.

Yesavage, J., Brink, T., Rose, T., Lum, O., Huang, O., Adey, V., & Leirer, V. (1983). Development and validation of a geriatric depression screening scale: A preliminary report. *Journal of Psychiatric Research, 17,* 37–49.

Zarit, S. H., Cole, K. D., & Guider, R. L. (1981). Memory training strategies and subjective complaints of memory in the aged. *The Gerontologist, 21,* 158–164.

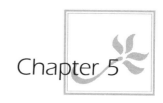

Chapter 5

Hearing in Older Adults

Dean C. Garstecki
Susan F. Erler

Garstecki and Erler point out the significant impact of age-related hearing loss on communication and general well-being, noting that the loss of hearing in the elderly is characterized as being both normal and indicative of a disorder. They review the prevalence of presbycusis, its possible causes, normal changes in the aging auditory system, and the effects of presbycusis on speech perception. The difference between hearing loss and perceived hearing handicap is emphasized, and variables affecting the success of hearing loss management are identified.

1. *Define presbycusis and describe its onset characteristics, common types, and possible causes. In general, what changes in the aging auditory system (from outer ear to auditory cortex) can be expected as a function of the normal aging process?*

2. *What are the effects of presbycusis upon speech perception?*

3. *What is meant by the term* hearing handicap, *how is it measured, and why is it important to understand in older adults with hearing loss?*

4. *In Garstecki and Erler's research, what situations were seen as most difficult by participants with hearing loss? What was the identified relationship between compliance with advice to use amplification and subject variables (e.g., perceived hearing handicap, degree of loss, intelligence, education, financial concerns, and communication management strategies)?*

꙳   ꙳   ꙳

The "normal" hearing condition for older adults is one of sensory deficit. The National Center for Health Statistics (1984) listed hearing loss as the fourth most common chronic condition affecting individuals over age 65, exceeded only by arthritis, high blood pressure, and heart disease. Older adults constitute the largest portion of all individuals who experience hearing loss, and the number of older adults is increasing at a faster pace than any other generation. Because hearing loss potentially has a significant impact on communication and one's general well-being, it is important for clinicians responsible for hearing loss management to be familiar with the prevalence, nature, and consequences of age-related hearing loss.

This chapter begins with a review of hearing loss prevalence data and the characteristics and causes of hearing loss in older adults. This review is followed by a description of age-related changes in auditory system structure and function, including how such changes may be manifested audiometrically and how they may influence speech processing in older adults. Handicap associated with acquired hearing loss is reviewed and approaches and preferences in hearing loss management are discussed.

Age-Related Hearing Loss: Prevalence and Nature of Presbycusis

Prevalence

Epidemiological studies of the Framingham Heart Study cohort indicate a direct relationship between advancing age and hearing loss (Gates, Cooper, Kannel, & Miller, 1990; Moscicki, Elkins, & Baum, 1985). In 1983, a National Center for Health Statistics (NCHS) survey identified 9 million noninstitutionalized United States citizens over age 65 years with self-reported hearing loss. Of these people, 1 in 4 between ages 65 and 74 years and almost 2 of every 5 age 75 years and older admitted having impaired hearing. Across all ages, an estimated 17 million individuals are said to have impaired hearing, indicating that over half of the U.S. population with hearing impairment is age 65 years or older. Goldstein (1984) has contended that a more realistic national estimate would exceed 40 million people.

The U.S. Bureau of the Census (1983) has predicted an increase in the general population from 266 million people in the year 2000 to

300 million in 2030. In the year 2030, as many as 63 million people will reach 65 or more years of age. If prevalence rates remain unchanged, the number of individuals with impaired hearing in the 65- to 74-year-old age group could reach 7 million, with an additional 13 million in the 75 and older age group. Not only will there be a significant number of older individuals in the future, but they will also live longer than past generations. This is particularly true for women (Garstecki & Erler, 1995), who constitute almost 60% of the 65 and older population. By any estimate, the older adult population is large and continuing to expand; in the future, they are likely to represent the majority of clinical populations.

Characteristics and Causes

In the typical life course, hearing loss is evidenced by gradual elevation of pure tone thresholds (Spoor, 1967). Such change may be noted as early as age 30. In another decade, thresholds up to and at 1000 Hz may be within 5 dB of optimal levels and higher frequency thresholds may be elevated. By age 60, pure tone thresholds are elevated across the audiometric test frequency range from 250 Hz to 8000 Hz (see Figure 5.1).

Hearing loss due to the natural aging process is termed *presbycusis*. Presbycusis is characterized by a bilateral decrease in hearing sensitivity, particularly in the higher frequencies. It is a medically irreversible condition that affects auditory signal processing negatively and may influence one's ability to perceive speech. A common complaint among older adults is, "I can hear, but I can't understand," reflecting the unique experience of acquired hearing loss in this age group. Hearing loss may coexist with tinnitus (ringing in the ear) in 15% to 45% of older adults, particularly older men (Gates et al., 1990). Prevalence of presbycusis is slightly greater in males (53%) than in females (47%) (Willott, 1991).

Schuknecht (1974) described four types of presbycusis. *Sensory presbycusis* refers to atrophy of the organ of Corti, which results in an abrupt high-frequency hearing loss. *Neural presbycusis* is characterized by loss of cochlear neurons. The result is a high-frequency hearing loss and decrease in speech recognition ability. *Strial presbycusis* refers to atrophy of the stria vascularis. The result is a flat sensory hearing loss, but with little negative influence on speech recognition ability.

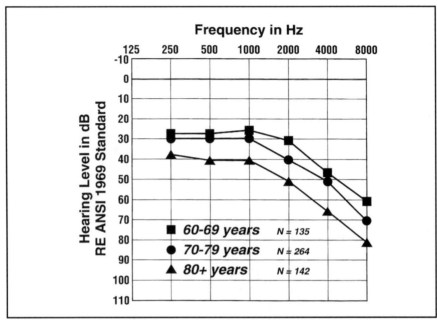

Figure 5.1. Mean hearing threshold levels for men and women combined for three age groups of older people. From "Hearing Status of Ambulatory Senior Citizens," by E. R. Harford and E. Dodds, 1982, *Ear and Hearing, 3*, p. 107. Copyright 1982 by E. R. Harford. Reprinted with permission.

Cochlear conductive presbycusis results in a sloping sensory loss with relatively little degeneration of sensory or neural mechanisms (Dennis & Neely, 1991). These early distinctions have held over time, being confirmed and extended through advanced technology.

The Committee on Hearing, Bioacoustics, and Biomechanics (CHABA, 1988) has suggested that presbycusis results from physiological, pathological, and environmental factors. These may include physiological deterioration, noise exposure, the effects of ototoxic agents, and various medical conditions and treatments. Current theories suggest that presbycusis is caused by biological aging and/or genetic factors (Bentzen, 1983; Gilad & Glorig, 1979; Willott, 1991). Biological aging may result in slow, chronic degeneration of auditory tissue and/or late-emerging factors (e.g., hypoxia due to vascular insufficiency, changes in the immune system, and changes in synaptic function). Genetic factors relate to race and gender as well as to individual differences in metabolism and physiology. Age-related change in the temporal bone and otic capsule, as in the case of otosclerosis, may result in hearing loss. The contribution of everyday environmental noise (sociocusis) to hearing loss may be a factor, but has been difficult to quantify in older adults (CHABA, 1988). In contrast, the effects of various therapeutic drugs, including aminoglycosides (e.g., kanamycin), loop diuretics (e.g., ethacrynic acid), and salicylates (e.g., aspirin) on hearing ability in older adults are well documented (White & Regan, 1987; Willott, 1991).

With an increasing population of older adults, the number of individuals affected by presbycusis will continue to grow. In order to understand more precisely how the process of aging influences hearing, it is helpful to review changes in structure and function of the auditory system.

The Aging Auditory System

System Components

Change in the aging auditory system can occur at various sites along the pathway from the outer ear to the auditory cortex. Nerbonne (1988), Schuknecht (1974), and Willott (1991) have provided comprehensive descriptions of anatomical and physiological change with age in the auditory system.

Outer Ear. Willott (1991) indicated that in the outer ear, cerumen and environmental debris may accumulate over time. Hair growth in and around the external auditory canal opening may accelerate. However, unless the opening to the tympanic membrane is blocked, hearing function will not be affected. The cartilaginous structure of the pinnae and ear canal loses its stiffness over time, increasing susceptibility to ear canal collapse, particularly when pressure is applied to the surface of the pinnae. Earphone placement during routine audiometric assessment of older adults must be monitored carefully. According to Jerger and Jerger (1981), about 33% of all individuals who experience collapsed ear canals are age 65 years and older. Finally, over time the tympanic membrane thickens and loses its elasticity. This condition also has no measurable effect on hearing sensitivity.

Middle Ear. In the middle ear, the tensor tympani and stapedius muscles that control the movement of the ossicular chain may stiffen with age (Nerbonne, 1988; Willott, 1991). This decreases their efficiency in protecting the cochlea from damage due to excessive noise. The stapedial muscle reflex (acoustic reflex) and ossicular chain response to intense sound will appear normal as long as the presbycusic condition is minimal. However, because the acoustic reflex has both sensory and motor components, functioning of the motor components (i.e., middle ear muscles and ossicular chain) may be affected by age. Reflex amplitude and growth may be diminished, particularly on the motor side of the reflex (i.e., uncrossed reflex), because of weakening of the stapedial muscle response and/or dysfunction of the neural circuitry that mediates the reflex. Nevertheless, these changes are not likely to influence hearing sensitivity. The Eustachian tube connecting middle ear air space with the nasal passage will change in elasticity with age, but not enough to result in hearing loss (Chermak & Moore, 1981; Willott, 1991). Alternately, relatively common medical conditions affecting the function of middle ear muscles and joints are likely to alter the acoustic properties of the middle ear system. For example, otosclerosis, a middle ear disease characterized by excessive resorption of bone (J. Jerger & S. Jerger, 1981), may occur in young adults, advancing in severity and handicapping effect in later years. Far advanced otosclerosis in older adults may result in severe to profound sensorineural hearing loss.

Inner Ear. Schuknecht (1974) hypothesized that the cells of the inner ear, like those in other parts of the body, are susceptible to biological aging. However, little is known empirically about such changes in humans. Several theories concerning the aging of the inner ear have been proposed (Jorgensen, 1961; Willott, 1991). One suggests that endogenous ototoxic factors slowly affect auditory system tissues, resulting in hearing loss over time. Another theory suggests that hearing loss may occur because of immune system diseases that present themselves only in later life. Other theories relate inner ear dysfunction to metabolic disorders such as diabetes mellitus, adrenocortical insufficiency, metabolism of selected proteins and lipids, thyroid deficiencies, and alterations in fluid and electrolyte metabolism caused by kidney disorders. Biological aging of the auditory system also may be influenced by genetic factors that affect the body's tissues in general or target the auditory system in particular. Dominant hereditary conditions without associated physical defects may result in high-frequency hearing loss in 1 of every 40,000 individuals. Recessive conditions without associated physical defects may progress from childhood, resulting in severe loss in 1 of every 4,000 adults (Proctor, 1977).

Central Auditory Mechanisms. Finally, central auditory neuron changes may result in central presbycusis (Brody, 1955). Impairment in the central auditory system and/or attenuation of neural input by peripheral pathology could alter auditory signal processing. The result may have unique effects on temporal resolution, frequency resolution, loudness, spatial localization, and speech perception. The auditory brainstem response (ABR) provides electrophysiologic data on brainstem function with insight into the central effects of peripheral presbycusis and biological aging. According to Willott (1991), peripheral presbycusis may be responsible for prolonging wave V latency in older adults; sensorineural hearing loss contributes to this effect, especially in older males. Auditory brainstem response wave amplitudes decrease with age, although it is difficult to separate the influence of sensorineural hearing loss. The middle latency response also is significantly altered in some older adults, which may reflect changes in central auditory processing due to peripheral presbycusis or biological aging. Overall, differences in absolute latencies and amplitudes, interpeak latencies, amplitude intensity functions, and recovery effects between younger and older adults cannot be explained by age alone.

Presbycusis may include higher order signal processing deficits that are correlated with severity of sensorineural hearing loss. For example, discrimination of time intervals for brief stimuli and sound duration in measures of absolute threshold (temporal integration) are negatively affected by sensorineural hearing loss. Problems in temporal perception of binaural time cues may be related to changes in the central auditory system (Gulick, Gescheider, & Frisina, 1989; Willott, 1991). In addition, frequency resolution, or the ability to respond selectively to the frequency components of a complex sound, may decline with age, but this ability is largely dependent on peripheral hearing.

Loudness recruitment is defined as an abnormally steep growth in loudness function that accompanies cochlear impairment (Hallpike & Hood, 1960). It is demonstrated clinically by loudness balancing tasks, Bekesy audiometry, difference limen measures, the Short Increment Sensitivity Index (SISI), measurement of loudness discomfort level, and the middle ear reflex. Although studies of recruitment in older adults have included individuals diagnosed with presbycusis, there is disagreement regarding the prevalence of recruitment in older individuals. Degree of hearing loss and type of cochlear disorder apparently have more to do with the occurrence of loudness recruitment than with the influence of age (Willott, 1991).

Spatial localization, or the process of computing interaural time and intensity information, requires optimal functioning of both peripheral and central auditory mechanisms (Gulick et al., 1989). Peripheral presbycusis interferes with detection of interaural time differences. Conductive hearing loss also negatively influences binaural hearing and, in turn, spatial localization. There are reports of localization difficulties in older adults who do not have significant peripheral presbycusis, suggesting that central mechanisms may have been impaired by age (Willott, 1991).

It appears that many of the problems that older adults encounter in processing frequency, intensity, time, and spatial information may be associated with peripheral presbycusis and vary with the severity of any coexisting sensorineural hearing loss. Peripheral hearing loss distorts or attenuates neural information, decreasing the efficiency of the central auditory system. However, the extent of many performance difficulties suggests an isolated central component that could involve the effects of biological aging or the central effects of peripheral presbycusis (Willott, 1991). Comprehensive assessment of auditory capability in older adults should not stop with pure tone screening or threshold measures. It is also necessary to include measures of speech processing to determine the integrity of the central auditory system. In fact, the central problem may be more handicapping than peripheral hearing loss.

Speech Perception

For many older adults, aging in the absence of significant hearing loss has little effect on speech perception. With hearing loss, speech recognition ability worsens with age, particularly in the presence of background noise (J. Jerger & Hayes, 1977). Helfer and Wilber (1990) reported a strong negative correlation between age and understanding of nonsense syllables in noisy and reverberant environments. For those with cochlear pathology, word recognition ability is consistent with the degree of hearing loss. Individuals with retrocochlear involvement may demonstrate *phonemic regression* (Gaeth, 1948), or unusually poor word recognition ability in comparison with hearing threshold data. Some older individuals may exhibit a rollover of the performance-intensity function; that is, speech recognition ability may decrease with an increase in signal intensity (Olsen, 1991). Rollover occurs more often among individuals over age 80 (Gang, 1976). Marshall (1981) and others have suggested that, although decreases in speech perception ability with age are well documented, causes of such decline are unclear. Because older adult performance on speech recognition tasks declines with advancing age, even when the effects of hearing loss are held constant, it appears that both peripheral and central auditory factors contribute to age-related change.

In contrast, older adult performance on degraded speech perception tasks demonstrates deficits in processing of speech signals that are temporally interrupted, accelerated, filtered, or masked (J. Jerger & S. Jerger, 1981). Although some of these deficits may be explained by peripheral hearing loss, they often cannot be accounted for by perceptual problems alone. Binaural hearing tasks that require integration and synthesis of information can be sensitive to central auditory system deficiencies. Older adult performance on such tasks appears to depend on the nature of the task and hearing loss. Typically, binaural fusion is not greatly diminished if hearing loss is taken into account (Willott, 1991).

There is little evidence that age-related declines in cognitive ability or speed pose serious problems in processing speech and other sounds when older adults are otherwise healthy and listening conditions are favorable. However, under unfavorable conditions, older adults often exhibit perceptual deficits; it is difficult to separate out the influence of diminished cognitive processes under such conditions. Exaggerated deficits in older adults' functioning under difficult conditions (e.g., compressed or masked speech) might be due to overtaxing weakened cognitive or linguistic abilities. Available empirical evidence does not allow this possibility to be ruled out. Further, little is known about speech perception in everyday listening contexts. Clinicians must be aware of variation in performance that is likely to occur within different environments.

In summary, many age-related changes that occur in the structure and function of the human auditory system are predictable and relatively well defined. Some changes have an impact on auditory signal perception; others are observed only under taxing conditions. Cosmetic changes are generally noticeable but essentially inconsequential in their effect on hearing sensitivity. Many changes are internal and invisible, manifested only by alteration of auditory behavior. There is nothing uniform about when changes may occur, where they occur in the system, or their impact on signal processing. However, when changes do occur, they may influence communication and psychosocial functioning in older adults. The next section reviews such hearing handicap in older adults.

Hearing Handicap

Changes in auditory system structure may alter functional performance or behavior and result in restriction of ability to perform normal activities. When this happens, disability occurs. *Handicap* is the disadvantage resulting from an impairment or disability (Hyde & Riko, 1994). Handicap attributable to a hearing condition cannot be predicted by degree, type, or duration of loss alone. Some individuals with mild hearing loss are significantly handicapped, and others with no functional hearing may be minimally handicapped. Weinstein and Ventry (1983) reported that almost one fourth of a group of older adults demonstrating average pure tone thresholds less than 25 dB considered themselves to be handicapped by hearing loss. In contrast, 88% of those older adults with average pure tone thresholds in the 41 to 55 dB range reported hearing handicap. This may be explained in part by Dubno, Dirks, and Morgan's (1984) observation that even adults with "normal" hearing may experience word recognition problems. In addition, it is interesting to note that communication and personal adjustment problems related to hearing loss may not be eliminated by successful hearing aid use (Smedley & Schow, 1990).

Although attempts to define a psychology of deafness have been inconclusive, there is agreement on a range of social and emotional reactions to hearing loss. Erdman, Crowley, and Gillespie (1984) summarized common characteristics of older adults with impaired hearing; these included feelings of stress, low self-esteem, frustration, irritation, embarrassment, and isolation. Older adults may feel stigmatized by hearing loss, isolated from their family, and penalized in their work setting. Some report that hearing loss may affect their communication at work, limiting their ability to advance on the job and interact with their co-workers (Thomas, Lamont, & Harris, 1982). Adults may feel that their self-confidence and personal security have been compromised by hearing loss (Tanner, 1980). In social situations, they may feel at risk for misunderstanding others, inappropriately answering others, or appearing ignorant (Joensen & Saunders, 1984).

A variety of clinical approaches have been proposed for measuring hearing handicap. These include use of arithmetic formulae for converting pure tone threshold data to numeric estimates of hearing handicap, as supported by the American Medical Association/American Academy of Otolaryngology (1979), and use of self-assessment scales and inventories (Erdman, 1993). Of these approaches, self-assessment scale data are of greatest prescriptive value. Self-assessment scales provide an efficient and nonthreatening means of self-disclosure (Erdman, 1993). Scales are composed of items describing personal experiences associated with hearing loss. Contemporary scales address emotional and attitudinal factors that may influence communicative competence. Scales that have been validated for screening purposes include the *Hearing Handicap Inventory for the Elderly–Screening Form* (HHIE–S; Ventry & Weinstein, 1982) and the *Self-Assessment of Communication* (SAC; Schow & Nerbonne, 1982). The HHIE-S is a 10-item questionnaire assessing the emotional and social–situational effects of hearing loss and would be appropriate for use with older adults with acquired, mild-to-moderate hearing loss. The SAC is a 10-item questionnaire assessing personal attitudes about hearing loss and would be appropriate for use with all ages of adults with impaired hearing.

Scales that are useful for diagnostic purposes include the *Communication Profile for the Hearing Impaired* (CPHI; Demorest & Erdman, 1986) and the revised form of the *Hearing Performance Inventory* (HPI; Lamb, Owens, & Schubert, 1983). The CPHI assesses communication performance, the communication environment, use of communication strategies, and personal awareness of problems associated with impaired hearing. The CPHI would be appropriate for determining self-perceived communication problems and the emotional impact of hearing loss in an adult population. Finally, the revised HPI assesses speech understanding with and without visual cues, understanding of low-intensity speech signals, response to communication failure, and social, personal, and occupational aspects of hearing loss. The HPI may be used to measure speech and nonspeech communication skills and the personal effect of hearing loss in an adult population.

Garstecki and Erler (1996) administered the CPHI to over 300 individuals with acquired, mild-to-moderate sensorineural hearing loss to establish a baseline for understanding self-perceived hearing handicap in older adults who are educationally and socioeconomically advantaged. Results suggested that representatives of the sampled group perceived minimal difficulty communicating in social situations, home settings, or under other average conditions, even in the presence of competing background noise. However, they assigned higher importance to effective communication in home and work or work-like settings than in noisier social situations. In the home setting, effective communication is important because it is necessary and unavoidable. Work and business communication (e.g., conversations with bankers, attorneys, physicians, and ministers) is important because it relates to an individual's livelihood and well-being. Communication in social situations tends to be voluntary and, therefore, may be regarded as less important. Older adults may disengage themselves from communicating in selected social situations by rationalizing that they do not care to converse in settings they find challenging due to their hearing loss. Instead, they prefer to assign greater importance to communicating in confined or intimate settings, such as small dinner parties in home settings.

Older adult participants in Garstecki and Erler's (1996) study generally perceived their usual communication environment as unchallenging. They reported little exposure to difficult physical conditions within this communication environment or to challenging communication styles among their usual communication partners. They were not aware of negative reactions by others to any communication problem they might have encountered. Other individuals were perceived as willing to accommodate hearing loss-related needs. These older adults seemed motivated to maintain their communication skills.

In difficult communication situations, older adults preferred to employ positive over negative strategies and to use strategies that were under their volitional control. That is, they preferred to use nonverbal strategies (e.g., positioning themselves for a listening/viewing advantage) rather than verbal strategies (e.g., asking for repetition) or maladaptive strategies (e.g., ignoring others or avoiding communication situations).

In the same study, Garstecki and Erler (1996) examined the older adults' perceived ability to adjust to hearing loss. In general, respondents evidenced positive personal adjustment. Participants demonstrated high self-acceptance and self-esteem and a strong tendency toward accepting negative criticism related to their hearing loss. They revealed little irritation, aggravation, impatience, or annoyance over not always being able to communicate effectively. They reported little depression or stress related to their hearing condition, and were unlikely to withdraw from opportunities for communication or feel isolated in difficult communication settings. However, responses to CPHI scale items dealing with displacement of responsibility for managing hearing loss, exaggeration of responsibility for managing hearing loss, anger, and withdrawal from communication situations demonstrated high variability.

In conclusion, the insidious nature of acquired hearing loss appears to provide time for advantaged older adults with minimal hearing loss to adapt to hearing-loss-related communication and psychosocial problems over time. Although generalization of the results of the Garstecki and Erler (1996) study is limited, data demonstrate that even under favorable conditions, ability to adjust to and accept changes in communication performance with hearing loss may be influenced by communication environment, life-style, and age-related personality factors. These findings underscore the value of utilizing self-report measures in the development of clinical hearing loss management programs.

To optimize one's ability to function with medically irreversible hearing loss, a number of options are available to older adults. Although first consideration is given to hearing aid use, many adults who might benefit from amplification choose not to do so. Instead, they rely on behaviors, such as adjusting volumes, sitting close to a speaker, or avoiding difficult communication situations. The final section of this chapter addresses hearing loss management preferences among older adults.

Hearing Loss Management: Practices and Preferences

Sixty-five percent of all hearing aid owners are age 65 years and older, and almost 60% of this group demonstrate mild-to-moderate hearing loss (Kochkin, 1992). Unfortunately, less than 24% of those individuals who might benefit from use of hearing aids comply with professional advice to acquire them. If the current hearing aid market penetration rate remains unchanged in the year 2030, 16 million adults age 65 and older who could benefit from amplification will not own hearing aids.

A variety of reasons have been offered to explain the traditionally low hearing aid take-up rate. They include severity of hearing loss, advice from hearing professionals, perceived product value (versus cost), and the stigma associated with hearing loss and hearing aid use (Kochkin, 1993).

To better understand how self-perceived hearing handicap may relate to factors influencing decisions to acquire and use hearing aids, a subset of participants in the Garstecki and Erler (1996) study were surveyed regarding their decision to comply with professional advice to use amplification (Garstecki, 1996). Those participants who chose to follow professional advice to obtain hearing aids were described as "compliers," and those who chose not to follow professional advice to obtain hearing aids were "noncompliers." Results indicated that, although differences between compliers and noncompliers were not statistically significant, compliers demonstrated greater hearing loss, higher scores on a measure of general intelligence, higher levels of formal education, and higher annual income than did noncompliers. Interestingly, despite their greater hearing loss, compliers' self-perceived effectiveness in communicating with family members and in quiet settings was significantly greater than that for noncompliers, an observation supporting the benefit of hearing aid use. The "complier advantage" also was demonstrated in work settings and business communication, as well as over a range of average communication conditions. Although some of this success must be attributed to improved signal perception, a resulting psychological boost in self-confidence cannot be ignored.

Compliers preferred to manage their communication problems using verbal rather than nonverbal strategies. That is, they preferred to actively control their communication conditions. This may suggest that hearing aid use bolsters self-confidence or it may reflect innate personality characteristics that led individuals to comply with advice to use hearing aids. Unlike the noncompliers, compliers were more accepting of their hearing loss and were comfortable asking for assistance when experiencing hearing problems.

In addition to compliance issues identified by Garstecki (1996), other factors may influence decisions related to the use of amplification. Although physicians are responsible for surgical and medical treatment of hearing loss, as a group they also have contributed to the low hearing aid take-up rate (Goldstein, 1984). According to Kochkin (1992), physicians influence over 19% of all first-time hearing aid purchasers. Among the older adults surveyed by Garstecki, compliers were less likely to be influenced by their physicians' perception of hearing aid benefit.

According to Kochkin (1992), almost 20% of all nonpurchasers believe that the cost of a new hearing aid exceeds $1,000. In Garstecki's (1996) survey, compliers were less concerned about hearing aid purchase and maintenance costs than were noncompliers. Vanity also was not as much of an issue for compliers as it was for noncompliers. In addition, approximately 20% of all hearing aid users perceived stigma associated with open admission of hearing loss. Compliers tended to ignore any possible stigma associated with hearing aid use. Finally, Kochkin found that, although up to 40% of all new hearing aid users are dissatisfied with either hearing aid performance or their hearing aid dispenser, compliers obviously were not deterred by these factors in purchasing and using hearing aids. Perhaps, as a group, their expectations of dispensers and hearing aid benefit were more realistic than those of noncompliers.

In summary, older adult hearing aid users in the Garstecki (1996) study demonstrated an advantage in communication effectiveness over nonusers despite greater hearing loss. They accepted their hearing loss and took a proactive approach toward dealing with any associated communication problem. They made their decision to use amplification on the basis of self-expected benefit and perceived this benefit as outweighing cost and vanity considerations. They also tended to be tolerant of any shortcomings in the hearing instrument's ability to compensate fully for hearing loss and in the hearing aid delivery system.

Older adults with impaired hearing may also take advantage of clinical programs designed to help them optimize use of sensory aids, deal with personal adjustment to acquired hearing loss, and self-manage problems associated with hearing loss. In these programs, they may learn about assistive listening devices to enhance hearing aid benefit or as a substitute for personal amplification. They also may have an opportunity to acquire strategies for facilitating everyday communication and for repairing communication failure. Such programs may be found in university audiology programs, community hearing organizations, hospitals (most notably within the Veterans Administration Medical Center system), free-standing medical clinics, and as a service provided by private practicing audiologists.

Finally, support groups provide an opportunity for older adults with impaired hearing to learn how to manage consumer issues such as access to public meeting places, telephone communication, and access to closed-captioned films and television programs. Consumer groups provide an opportunity for older adults to socialize with their age peers and to learn how to manage everyday problems related to hearing loss. One of the most successful organized efforts to provide a national support mechanism for adults with acquired hearing loss is the Self-Help for the Hard of Hearing (SHHH) consumer group. This organization has local chapters in most states, a large dues-paying membership, and a journal providing information relating to hearing loss, its effects, and management of hearing loss-related concerns. Although the benefits of a formal affiliation with an adult support group may be readily apparent, relatively few older individuals take advantage of the opportunity to join, regardless of the setting or cost (Marrer & Garstecki, 1985). A more extensive discussion of management issues and approaches can be found in Chapter 18.

Summary

Hearing loss prevalence rates indicate that a substantial portion of the older adult population demonstrates hearing loss due to the natural aging process. Although declines in hearing sensitivity and speech understanding are likely to occur with age, the impact of those changes varies widely among older adults. Auditory deficit may be explained by biological and/or genetic factors influencing structure and function of the auditory system from the pinnae and external canal to the central auditory cortex. The impairment and/or disability created by hearing loss may result in hearing handicap. Such handicap is likely to be associated with change in communication performance that may be influenced by environmental conditions, life-style, and age-related personality factors. Those who choose to use hearing aids appear to derive both a physical benefit (in that sound is easier to hear) and a psychological benefit (in that restored hearing capability appears to bolster self-confidence in everyday communication). If problems remain, older adults should be encouraged to take advantage of rehabilitative services offered in a variety of settings and participation in consumer support group activities.

References

American Medical Association/American Academy of Otolaryngology (AMA/AAO). (1979). Guide for the evaluation of hearing handicap. *Journal of the American Medical Association, 241,* 2055–2059.

Bentzen, O. (1983). Disorders of hearing in the elderly. In R. Hinchcliffe (Ed.), *Hearing and balance in the elderly* (pp. 123–144). New York: Churchill Livingstone.

Brody, H. (1955). Organization of the central cortex. III. Study of aging in human cerebral cortex. *Journal of Comparative Neurology, 102,* 511–556.

Chermak, G. D., & Moore, M. K. (1981). Eustachian tube function in the older adult. *Ear and Hearing, 2,* 143–147.

Committee on Hearing, Bioacoustics, and Biomechanics, CHABA Working Group on Speech Understanding. (1988). Speech understanding and aging. *Journal of the Acoustical Society of America, 83,* 859–895.

Demorest, M. E., & Erdman, S. A. (1986). Scale composition and item analysis of the *Communication Profile for the Hearing Impaired. Journal of Hearing and Speech Research, 29,* 515–535.

Dennis, J. M., & Neely, J. G. (1991). Otoneurologic diseases and associated audiologic profiles. In J. T. Jacobson & J. L. Northern (Eds.), *Diagnostic audiology* (pp. 83–109). Austin, TX: PRO-ED.

Dubno, J., Dirks, D., & Morgan, D. (1984). Effects of age and mild hearing loss on speech recognition in noise. *Journal of the Acoustical Society of America, 76,* 87–96.

Erdman, S. A. (1993). Self-assessment in audiology: The clinical rationale. *Seminars in Hearing, 14,* 303–313.

Erdman, S. A., Crowley, J. M., & Gillespie, G. G. (1984). Considerations in counseling the hearing impaired. *Hearing Instruments, 35,* 50–58.

Gaeth, J. (1948). *A study of phonemic regression in relation to hearing loss.* Unpublished doctoral dissertation, Northwestern University, Evanston, IL.

Gang, R. (1976). The effects of age on the diagnostic utility of the rollover phenomenon. *Journal of Speech and Hearing Disorders, 41,* 63–69.

Garstecki, D. C. (1996). Older adult hearing handicap and hearing aid management. *American Journal of Audiology, 5,* 25–34.

Garstecki, D. C., & Erler, S. F. (1995). Older women and hearing. *American Journal of Audiology, 4,* 41–46.

Garstecki, D. C., & Erler, S. F. (1996). Older adult performance on the *Communication Profile for the Hearing Impaired. Journal of Speech and Hearing Research, 39,* 28–42.

Gates, G. A., Cooper, J. C., Kannel, W. B., & Miller, N. J. (1990). Hearing in the elderly: The Framingham cohort. *Ear and Hearing, 11,* 247–256.

Gilad, O., & Glorig, A. (1979). Presbycusis: The aging ear (Part I). *Journal of the American Audiological Society, 4,* 195–206.

Goldstein, D. P. (1984). Hearing impairment, hearing aids, and audiology. *Journal of the American Speech Language Hearing Association, 9,* 24–35, 38.

Gulick, W. L., Gescheider, G. A., & Frisina, R. D. (1989). *Hearing: Physiological acoustics, neural coding, and psychoacoustics.* New York: Oxford University Press.

Hallpike, C. S., & Hood, J. D. (1960). Observations on the neurological mechanism of the loudness recruitment phenomenon. *Acta Otolaryngology, 50,* 472–486.

Harford, E. R., & Dodds, E. (1982). Hearing status of ambulatory senior citizens. *Ear and Hearing, 3,* 105–109.

Helfer, K. S., & Wilber, L. A. (1990). Hearing loss, aging, and speech perception in reverberation and noise. *Journal of Speech and Hearing Research, 33,* 149–155.

Hyde, M. L., & Riko, K. (1994). A decision-analytic approach to audiological rehabilitation. *Journal of the Academy of Rehabilitative Audiology, Monograph Supplement, 27,* 337–374.

Jerger, J., & Hayes, D. (1977). Diagnostic speech audiometry. *Archives of Otolaryngology, 103,* 216–222.

Jerger, J., & Jerger, S. (1981). *Auditory disorders: A manual for clinical evaluation.* Boston: Allyn & Bacon.

Joensen, J. P., & Saunders, D. J. (1984). Psychological correlates of geriatric hearing loss: Understanding the emotional and behavioral consequences of impaired hearing. *The Hearing Journal, 37,* 39–41.

Jorgensen, B. M. (1961). Changes of aging in the inner ear. *Archives of Otolaryngology, 70,* 154–170.

Kochkin, S. (1992). MarkeTrak III: Higher hearing aid sales don't signal better market penetration. *The Hearing Journal, 45,* 47–54.

Kochkin, S. (1993). MarkeTrak III: Why 20 million in U.S. don't use hearing aids for their hearing loss. *The Hearing Journal, 46,* 26, 28–31.

Lamb, S. H., Owens, E., & Schubert, E. D. (1983). The revised form of the *Hearing Performance Inventory. Ear and Hearing, 4,* 152–159.

Marrer, J. L., & Garstecki, D. C. (1985, February). *Community/clinic management of hearing-impaired aging adults.* Paper presented at the annual meeting of the Illinois Speech-Language-Hearing Association, Chicago.

Marshall, L. (1981). Auditory processing in aging listeners. *Journal of Speech and Hearing Disorders, 46,* 226–240.

Moscicki, E. K., Elkins, E. F., & Baum, H. M. (1985). Hearing loss in the elderly: An epidemiologic study of the Framingham Heart Study cohort. *Ear and Hearing, 6,* 184–190.

National Center for Health Statistics. (1983). *Health interview survey.* Washington, DC: Author.

National Center for Health Statistics. (1984). *Health interview survey.* Washington, DC: Author.

Nerbonne, M. A. (1988). The effects of aging on auditory structures and functions. In B. B. Shadden (Ed.), *Communication behavior and aging: A sourcebook for clinicians* (pp. 137–162). Baltimore: Williams & Wilkins.

Olsen, W. O. (1991). Special auditory tests: A historical perspective. In J. T. Jacobson & J. L. Northern (Eds.), *Diagnostic audiology* (pp. 19–52). Austin, TX: PRO-ED.

Proctor, B. (1977). Diagnosis, prevention, and treatment of hereditary sensorineural hearing loss. *Laryngoscope, 87, Suppl. 7.*

Schow, R. L., & Nerbonne, M. A. (1982). Communication screening profile: Use with elderly clients. *Ear and Hearing, 3,* 135–147.

Schuknecht, H. F. (1974). *Pathology of the ear.* Cambridge, MA: Harvard University Press.

Smedley, T. C., & Schow, R. L. (1990). Frustrations with hearing aid use: Candid observations from the elderly. *The Hearing Journal, 43,* 21–27.

Spoor, A. (1967). Presbycusis values in relation to noise induced hearing loss. *International Audiology, 6,* 48–57.

Tanner, D. C. (1980). Loss and grief: Implications for the speech–language pathologist and audiologist. *Asha, 22,* 916–928.

Thomas, A., Lamont, M., & Harris, M. (1982). Problems encountered at work by people with severe acquired hearing loss. *British Journal of Audiology, 16,* 39–43.

U.S. Bureau of the Census. (1983). *Statistical abstracts of the United States.* Washington, DC: Author.

Ventry, I., & Weinstein, B. (1982). *The Hearing Handicap Inventory for the Elderly:* A new tool. *Ear and Hearing, 3,* 128–134.

Weinstein, B., & Ventry, I. (1983). Audiologic correlates of hearing handicap in the elderly. *Journal of Speech and Hearing Research, 26,* 148–151.

White, J., & Regan, M. (1987). Otologic considerations. In G. Mueller & V. Geoffrey (Eds.), *Communication disorders in aging: Assessment and management* (pp. 36–72). Washington, DC: Gallaudet University Press.

Willott, J. F. (1991). *Aging and the auditory system: Anatomy, physiology, and psychophysics.* San Diego: Singular.

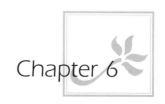

Chapter 6

Age-Related Changes in Speech, Voice, and Swallowing

Anthony J. Caruso
Peter B. Mueller

Caruso and Mueller begin their chapter by stating clearly that clinicians must understand normal age-related changes in speech, voice, and swallowing in order to distinguish such changes from secondary (abnormal) alterations in behavior and to provide effective management. The effects of aging on oral–pharyngeal–laryngeal mechanisms of older adults are described, along with a discussion of the potential impact of such changes on speech, swallowing, and voice behaviors. Although many "normal" changes discussed in this chapter do not impair communication, the authors note that age "differences" in speech and voice may affect daily communicative interactions.

1. *What are some of the age-related structural changes in the oral–pharyngeal mechanism, and what functional effect do these have on swallowing and speech? What are some of the commonly described changes in articulatory timing and positioning associated with an aging system, and do these changes affect intelligibility?*

2. *How do age-related structural changes affect the structure and functioning of the laryngeal mechanism?*

3. *What rationale do the authors offer for clinical consideration of age-associated speech and vocal changes that do not affect intelligibility?*

There is no doubt that significant and measurable changes take place in oral, pharyngeal, and laryngeal mechanisms as sequelae of the aging process. What is less apparent is whether or not these structural changes negatively impact functional performance in speech, voice, and swallowing. Nevertheless, there are sufficient clinical/anecdotal data suggesting that many older speakers are bothered by age-associated alterations in these functions. Therefore, it is necessary for clinicians to be able to discern changes precipitated by normal aging from those that are secondary to the aging process. For the purposes of this chapter, *secondary changes* are those that (a) are caused by physical or emotional abnormalities, (b) can be linked to pharmacological or medical treatment effects, or (c) result from as yet undetected (idiopathic) pathology.

Knowledge of age-related changes in elderly individuals is important to speech–voice clinicians who wish to maximize successful communication for older clients. There is a continually developing database to aid the clinician in making diagnostic or management decisions. These decisions ultimately may have a significant impact on the older client's life adjustment. The major focus of this chapter is to review age-related changes in the oral, pharyngeal, and laryngeal mechanisms associated with two major components of communication (speech and voice), as well as to discuss the impact of such age-related changes on nonspeech functions (swallowing). A word of caution to the clinician: Because of the extreme heterogeneity of the aging process, normative data presented in this chapter must be interpreted cautiously. Moreover, described involutional trends (changes precipitated by normal aging) should not to be generalized to include all or even most older adults.

Changes in Oral–Pharyngeal Mechanism

Structural Changes

Several clinical and postmortem studies have identified important degenerative changes in the oral–pharyngeal mechanism with advancing age (Sonies, 1987). A thorough review of all the senescent alterations in the orofacial mechanisms is beyond the scope of this chapter. We have chosen, however, to discuss selected age-related changes that are (in)directly linked to the orofacial functions of interest (e.g., swallowing and speech). For the most part, the effects of aging on oral–pharyngeal anatomy are predictable and consistent.

One of the most frequently reported age-related changes in the oral cavity is tooth loss and/or compromised dentition. Due to the resorption of the bone in the orofacial mechanism, the amount of bony structures in the oral cavity decreases and teeth are lost. These changes in dental status are compounded by several histologic changes in the oral–pharyngeal mechanism and morphologic changes in neural and muscle tissue and salivary glands. The surface epithelium of the tongue, pharynx, and soft palate, as well as the underlying connective tissue, atrophies (or deteriorates) with age. Moreover, it has been reported that with advancing age, oral mucosa becomes thinner and drier and, consequently, more susceptible to abrasions, traumas, disorders, or disease (Hill, 1984), although some have questioned this speculation (Baum, Caruso, Ship, & Wolff, 1991). Salivary gland mass has been reported to decrease by 25% to 30% with age; however, it is not clear whether salivary flow actually decreases as a direct consequence of aging (Baum et al., 1991). Interestingly, decreased salivary flow is also a common side effect of medications and treatment (e.g., chemotherapy) that are often prescribed to elderly individuals for various medical concerns.

Finally, it appears that certain sensory abilities change with age (see Baum, 1981; Weiffenbach, Cowart, & Baum, 1986). For example, lingual sensation is reduced with age. Additionally, the ability of individuals to perceive pressure on the tongue diminishes as a function of age. Age-related changes in the nervous system may affect neurons in the sensory components of the cranial nerves in addition to subcortical relay nuclei and cortical somatosensory areas (Sabin & Venna, 1984). Unfortunately, little information is currently available to document the effects of aging on the neurobiological aspects of sensory innervation for oral, and particularly, orofacial tissues. In general, however, it appears that somesthetic and kinesthetic sensory abilities are reduced with age. This apparent reduced sensory ability is noteworthy because it is likely to have a negative effect on motor abilities associated with chewing, speaking, and swallowing.

Functional Changes

Swallowing. It is estimated that as many as 6 to 10 million Americans experience disturbances in swallowing to some degree or another (Erlichman, 1989). Moreover, estimates of the prevalence of swallowing dysfunction in elderly individuals range from 16% to 40% (Bloem et al., 1990; Siebens et al., 1986). In light of these estimates, information regarding changes in swallowing with advancing age provides a valuable perspective for the clinician working with elderly clients.

Several recent studies have demonstrated that older (nonpathologic) individuals show altered swallowing performance compared with younger individuals, particularly in temporal parameters of swallowing. Duration of oral and pharyngeal transit time has been reported to be longer (Cook et al., 1994) or more variable (Dejaeger, Peleman, Bibau, & Ponette, 1994) for older versus younger individuals. Bolus velocity during transport is slower for elderly persons than for their younger counterparts. Such alterations in the timing of swallowing reportedly first occur around 45 years of age. With increasing age, overall swallowing duration tends to increase (Robbins, Hamilton, Lof, & Kempster, 1992).

Other qualitative changes in swallowing behavior have been observed in older individuals. The bolus is often held more posteriorly in the oral cavity by older subjects. A significant decrease in pharyngeal clearance (i.e., increased pharyngeal residue counts) has also been reported for elderly individuals (Cook et al., 1994). Postures of the tongue and hyoid bone can be different for elderly versus young subjects (Sonies, Baum, & Shawker, 1984).

A review of the available, albeit limited, literature in aging and swallowing has led many clinicians to conclude that swallowing problems are not a direct result of normal age-related structural changes. For many elderly individuals, age-related changes in swallowing are subtle and not problematic. What is also likely, however, is that secondary aspects of aging (e.g., compromised dental status) may negatively affect a senescent swallowing mechanism. Given this perspective, some elderly individuals may experience occasional swallowing problems in the absence of any significant pathology or underlying disease process. For example, some elderly individuals may be at increased risk for swallowing difficulties if they attempt to transport a bolus that has been inadequately prepared to a swallow-ready consistency (due to tooth loss and/or poorly fitting dentures) through a less elastic pharynx (a known age-related change). Of course, clinically significant swallowing problems may be linked to various pathological conditions. In keeping with the purposes of this chapter, however, we have restricted our discussion to swallowing in nonpathologic elderly individuals.

Speech. Despite the many histologic, morphologic, and neural changes, the ability to produce normal sounding speech appears to be relatively resistant to aging. However, the manner of producing normal sounding speech may be somewhat different for older individuals as compared to their younger counterparts. In many cases, these differences between older and younger speakers are perceptible to listeners, who appear to label these perceived differences as normal variation rather than pathology.

A consistent finding in gerontological communication sciences is that elderly speakers tend to use slower speaking rates than their younger counterparts (e.g., Leeper & Culatta, 1995). Various factors are thought to contribute to this reduction in speaking rate with advancing age. First, relatively long pauses between words are often present during connected or conversational speech of elderly individuals. Second, velocity of articulatory movements during production of sounds and syllables is reduced in elderly speakers. Finally, older speakers tend to produce longer consonant, vowel, syllable and sentence durations when compared to young adults. Although the majority of studies provide evidence for these three factors, there are some contradictory reports (see Caruso, McClowry, & Max, in press); this may be due, at least in part, to the heterogeneity of the aging process.

Studies that examine articulatory placement for sound production are not as extensive as investigations of articulatory timing. Existing findings suggest that elderly speakers have a tendency to produce vowels at places in the oral cavity that are different from young speakers. Moreover, very old (age 80 years or older) speakers shift articulatory placements to approximate the positioning typically associated with the schwa or neutral vowel (Liss, Weismer, & Rosenbek, 1990).

Several explanations for these reported differences between older and young speakers have been offered. For example, the tendency for elderly speakers to neutralize articulatory positioning for vowels is consistent with the documented changes in vocal tract length with advancing age. Others have linked these age-related speech changes with changes in sensorimotor control mechanisms. An alternative explanation has been offered by Amerman and Parnell (1992). Specifically, they suggested that at least some differences in speech production between older and younger speakers may be related to the elderly individuals' "increased caution, concern with accuracy, or more careful monitoring of [speech] motor output" (pp. 72–73).

Another aspect of speech production that has been studied in the elderly is fluency. Most studies have focused on discerning if there is a tendency for normally fluent speakers to become more disfluent with advancing age. In general, these studies are in agreement that the frequency of disfluency does not appreciably change with advancing age (e.g., Caruso et al., in press; Leeper & Culatta, 1995; Yairi & Clifton, 1972).

Changes in the Laryngeal Mechanism

Unlike the previously discussed changes in speech, the effects of senescence on the vocal mechanism and phonation are frequently more apparent. Although vocal signs of senescence are but a small reflection of involution, they are quite obvious to the listener. Subjectively, this is underscored by the prevalent and somewhat stereotypical impression that the voices of old people are characterized by tremulousness, weakness, hoarseness, and altered pitch (Mueller, 1985; Ringel & Chodzko-Zajko, 1987). Most listeners *are* able to differentiate between voices of young and old speakers with at least some degree of success (Hartman, 1979; Horii & Ryan, 1981; Neiman & Applegate, 1990). In two recent studies (Caruso, Mueller, & Xue, 1994; McClowry, Mueller, & Caruso, 1995), both young and elderly listeners were able to judge chronological age of elderly speakers with some accuracy. These studies support anecdotal accounts of the senescent voice.

Although considered to be an inevitable component of the normal aging process, aging of the voice appears to be troublesome to many older people, particularly if they are concerned about potential pathology or if qualitative aspects of their life are affected. To minimize potential errors in diagnosis and management, it is important that the clinician be able to differentiate voice changes precipitated by normal aging from those caused by disease, abuse, or psychopathology. Thus, appropriate counseling for older speakers who express concern about changes in their voice necessitates availability of normative data reflective of how nonpathological aging processes affect the human voice; that is, which aspects of the voice profile fall within normal limits and which do not.

A substantial pool of data concerning the senescent voice has become available, but this pool also reflects the multifaceted nature or heterogeneity of aging. Shadden (in press), in writing about discourse performance in older adults, stated that "one may wonder if the search for normative data in both normal and communicatively-disordered older persons is a futile one." This certainly pertains to phonation, as demonstrated by the variability of voice data collected from elderly subjects. There are, however, some reliable trends that should be of help to the clinician who is attempting to understand the aging voice.

The major acoustic attributes of phonation—pitch, loudness, and quality—are molded by the maturational processes of the laryngo-pulmonary-resonance systems into an adult voice appropriate to the age and gender of the possessor. Barring disease or trauma, the mature vocal instrument will be an effective tool of communication as well as emotional and artistic expression for most of adult life.

The literature pertaining to the effects of aging on the larynx focuses on its various structural and functional components, including the cartilaginous skeleton, intrinsic laryngeal muscles, vocal cords, and nerve and blood supply. In addition to the larynx, the speech- and voice-producing mechanism consists of multiple structurally and functionally integrated components, all of which contribute to phonation but do not age uniformly within and between individuals. Of those components, the respiratory system may be of particular importance. Age-related changes of the respiratory system are discussed in Chapter 3. For the purposes of this chapter, the following discussion is confined to the age-related changes of the structure and function of the larynx. Although available data are not complete and frequently do not relate structural changes to functional events, important patterns are beginning to emerge that promise to facilitate clinical efforts and research direction trends.

Structural Changes

Laryngeal Cartilages. The cartilaginous framework of the larynx undergoes changes from birth into old age, manifested mainly by calcification and ossification (Ardran, 1965; Heatley, Evinson, & Samuel, 1965; Kahane, 1987). These changes occur in both genders, although they are apparent somewhat earlier in the male. Some researchers have also reported age-related changes in the cricoarytenoid joint, which may affect vocal cord approximation and subsequently glottal efficiency (Kahane, 1990).

Nerve and Blood Supply. Although very few data are available regarding the effects of aging on laryngeal blood supply and innervation, changes in both have been observed (Kahane, 1990; Wyke, 1974), and the possibility of decreased neuromuscular control of the larynx as a function of age has been suggested (Linville & Fisher, 1985; Liss, Weismer, & Rosenbek, 1990). However, the functional significance of these findings is as yet undetermined.

Laryngeal Glands. The general consensus seems to be that glands that lubricate the vocal cord mucosa undergo some involutional changes resulting in possible dehydration of the epithelial lining of the cords (Kahane, 1990; Punt, 1974). This could affect the integrity of vocal cord tissue and subsequently its function. Episodes of throat clearing frequently observed in the elderly may be a consequence of this.

Vocal Cords. A number of studies have generated data on the senescent changes of the epithelium of the vocal cords, the lamina propria, and the vocalis muscle (Hirano, Kurita, & Nakashima, 1983; Kahane, 1982, 1983; Kersing, 1986; Mueller, 1985; Mueller, Sweeney, & Baribeau, 1984, 1985; Sato & Tauchi, 1982; Segre, 1971). Although these investigations of the vocal cord components reflect a certain amount of controversy, they nevertheless provide a pool of data on the structural changes that may affect vocal performance in the elderly.

For example, Mueller and his colleagues (Mueller, 1985; Mueller et al., 1984, 1985) compared the morphology of aged male larynges obtained during autopsy with larynges extirpated postmortem from middle-aged men. Results indicated the presence of the normal cadaveric configuration of the glottis in 92% of the controls but in only 19% of the experimental (older) subjects. The older larynges exhibited a preponderance of bowing and sulcus of the vocal cords, as well as what was termed an "arrowhead" configuration of the glottis. These laryngeal changes were considered most likely to be caused by muscle atrophy, resulting in a general decline in the efficiency of the glottal valve. Similar results were obtained by Honjo and Isshiki (1980), who reported marked atrophy of the vocal cords in older males. Changes in the lamina propria are more pronounced in the male than in the female (Kahane, 1990), but because similar data are currently not available for females, these findings should not be generalized to both genders.

In summary, multiple physical changes in the larynx and its components occur with age. Available data do not necessarily pertain to both genders and/or all older adults, are somewhat equivocal, and should be applied with caution when one is interpreting vocal changes characteristic of the senescent voice.

Functional Changes

The numerous age-related changes of the larynx appear to contribute to the phonatory profiles typically associated with many older persons. Data on vocal performance and related measures are summarized in the following paragraphs. Specifically, maximum phonation time, voice quality, vocal jitter/shimmer, and fundamental frequency will be addressed.

Maximum Phonation Duration (MPD). The MPD measure is customarily obtained by requesting a subject to expend the maximum volume of air available for phonation during an effort of sustained phonation. It is reflective of respiratory support and efficiency of glottal valving, although it does not distinguish between these two variables (Kent, Kent, & Rosenbek, 1987). MPD for normal young adults, according to averaged data from a number of studies (Bless & Hirano, 1982; Hirano, Koike, & Von Leden, 1968; Inglis, 1977; Taylor, 1980), is about 30 seconds for males and 24 seconds for females, with considerable variability typical of maximum performance tests. In 40 elderly subjects, MPD values of between 14.6 and 18.1 seconds for males and 14.2 and 14.6 seconds for females have been published (Kreul, 1972; Ptacek, Sander, Mahoney, & Jackson, 1966). Mueller (1982) reported MPDs of 13 seconds for 85- to 92-year-old males and 10 seconds for 85- to 96-year-old females. These data suggest that MPD values produced by the elderly are reduced compared to those of younger persons. Whether or not this reduction significantly affects phonation is subject to speculation.

Voice Quality. Limited data are available on voice quality of the elderly. Perceptual judgments of breathy (Ryan & Burk, 1974) and strained/tense (Ptacek & Sander, 1966) voice qualities have been reported. One study of 227 subjects, ranging in age from 60 to 96 years, found hoarseness in about 30% of the women and 64% of the men

(Mueller, 1978). Hoarseness as well as harshness have also been observed in centenarian females (Mueller, 1990). Changes in vocal cord tissues may introduce vibratory irregularities that could contribute to the voice quality deviations previously noted (Kahane, 1987).

Vocal Jitter/Shimmer. *Jitter* refers to small cycle-to-cycle variations in the vocal cords' vibratory frequency, and *shimmer* refers to amplitude perturbation. Increased pitch perturbations have also been observed in older males (Mysak, 1959). Wilcox and Horii (1980) and Xue (1995) found increased mean perturbation values in both genders. In a study by Linville and Fisher (1985), 70- to 80-year-old females exhibited higher mean jitter values than younger females. The authors speculated as to whether this phenomenon might be attributed to decreasing neuromuscular control or a degree of muscular atrophy. According to Ringel and Chodzko-Zajko (1987), physiologically healthy elderly individuals exhibited less vocal jitter and shimmer than subjects in poor physical condition. Integrity of laryngeal control appears to be associated more with the health status of the individual than with his or her chronological age.

Fundamental Frequency (F_0). Of all the vocal parameters affected by aging, pitch, commonly expressed through measures of fundamental frequency, has been studied most extensively. Results of these investigations, however, are somewhat contradictory. Some investigators have reported a lowering of pitch in older males (Ptacek, Sander, Mahoney, & Jackson, 1966), whereas other data suggest an increased in F_0 in males (Hollien & Shipp, 1972; Mueller, 1985; Mueller et al., 1984; Mysak, 1959; Perello, 1983). The vocal pitch of females has been found to change little with increasing age (Gilbert & Weismer, 1974; McGlone & Hollien, 1963) or to decrease slightly (Benjamin, 1981; Honjo & Isshiki, 1980; Mueller, 1985; Mueller et al., 1984).

Only a few data are available concerning F_0 characteristics of individuals 100 years of age or older. Mueller (1990) found speaking fundamental frequencies (SFF) ranging from 118.7 to 171.5 Hz in a small group of centenarian women. Awan and Mueller (1992) found a mean SFF of 176.92 Hz for 9 women with an average age of 101.7 years. At the time of this writing, no data on centenarian men are available. Figure 6.1 presents a composite illustration of the F_0 data previously discussed in comparison to Aronson's (1980) data for middle-aged men and women.

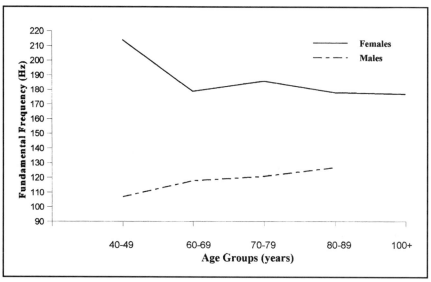

Figure 6.1. Mean fundamental frequency by age groups and sex. (It should be noted that variability of these data is considerable; see Aronson, 1980; Awan & Mueller, 1992; Mueller, 1985; Mueller et al., 1984.)

In conclusion, there appears to be at least a trend for fundamental frequency to increase slightly in males and to decrease somewhat more prominently in females as a function of normal aging. Whether this phenomenon applies to all ethnic populations remains to be seen. Xue and Mueller (1994, 1996) found that elderly Black seemed to present F_o trends similar to those of the White population, but these limited data should not be generalized.

There is strong evidence that laryngeal structure and function are affected by advancing age. However, the precise reasons for the aging of the voice are far from being well understood (Kahane, 1987). Table 6.1 reflects an attempt to present a profile of senescent voice changes.

It should be borne in mind that these changes in laryngeal performance may not necessarily be precipitated merely by the chronological age of the speaker but may more accurately reflect the individual's physiological integrity or biological age. This is underscored by recent investigations suggesting that physically active elderly are judged by listeners to be chronologically younger than their sedate cohorts (Mueller & Xue, 1996; Xue, 1995). Furthermore, because of the heterogeneity of the aging process, these profiles are not universally applicable.

Table 6.1

Age-Related Structural and Functional Changes
in the Vocal Mechanism and Phonation

Structure/Function	Alteration	Comments
Physiological changes		
Laryngeal cartilages	Increased ossification and calcification	Similar for both genders
Nerve and blood supply	Decrease in neuromuscular control and blood supply	Available data are inconclusive
Laryngeal glands	Decrease in output	Thickening of mucous; dehydration
Vocal cords	Atrophy	In males
	Edema	In females
Respiratory support	Decreased	Both genders
Vocal changes		
Vocal quality	Hoarseness	Both genders
Pitch/F_o	Increase	In males
	Decrease	In females
Jitter/shimmer	Increase	Both genders
Maximum phonation duration	Reduced	Both genders

Conclusions

One major recurring theme throughout this chapter is that the variability associated with the aging process is considerable. In essence, what this means for the clinician is that differences among elderly individuals are just as important as differences between older and younger adults. The heterogeneity of aging is reflected in the variability of the data collected from the elderly. It is futile to apply normative data indiscriminately to all older persons. It is also important to keep in mind that an individual's chronological age may not necessarily be congruent with his or her biological age and the integrity of his or her speech-producing mechanism. In order to establish a valid profile of an older person's speech, voice, or swallowing behavior, it is of paramount importance to gather diagnostic data over a period of time. In other words, multiple serial probes more accurately reflect performance than a single, isolated evaluation.

In a recent paper, Caruso et al. (1994) presented data supporting the notion that nonpathological aging processes do not uniformly impinge upon articulatory and laryngeal components of speech production. At least some elderly speakers appear to successfully use articulatory strategies to compensate for an aging voice. The articulatory component may be an important, if not the leading, contributor to the maintenance of a more "youthful" balance among major components of speech production. Compensatory maneuvers may have the potential for promoting youthful-sounding speech. If identifiable, such techniques would have clinical application in cases where preservation of effective and youthful-sounding voice and speech are highly valued (e.g., professional speakers, actors, and salespeople). Articulatory patterns could compensate for and/or offset involutional changes related to vocal aging. Furthermore, these techniques could be taught in an attempt to decelerate age-related changes in speech and voice. What is suggested here is proactive as opposed to the more traditional reactive remediation with the elderly.

We are not suggesting that "old-sounding" voice or speech is necessarily undesirable. However, effective communication is a critical tool for the older adult in the process of life adjustment. For some elderly, this is realized by maintaining their jobs or professions for as long as possible. Effective and appealing (to the listener/consumer) communication patterns are particularly crucial to those who are engaged in competitive professions. Thus, the role of speech–language pathologists who serve the elderly should be broadened to include not only those with identifiable communication problems, but also elderly clients who seek to maintain and even maximize competitive communication skills.

References

Amerman, J. D., & Parnell, M. M. (1992). Speech timing strategies in elderly adults. *Journal of Phonetics, 20,* 65–76.

Ardran, G. (1965). Calcification of the epiglottis. *British Journal of Radiology, 38,* 592–595.

Aronson, A. E. (1980). *Clinical voice disorders.* New York: Decker.

Awan, S. N., & Mueller, P. B. (1992). Speaking fundamental frequency characteristics of centenarian females. *Clinical Linguistics and Phonetics, 6,* 249–254.

Baum, B. (1981). Research on aging and oral health: An assessment of current status and future needs. *Special Care in Dentistry, 1,* 156–165.

Baum, B., Caruso, A. J., Ship, J., & Wolff, A. (1991). Oral physiology. In A. Papas, L. Niessen, & H. Chauncey (Eds.), *Geriatric dentistry: Aging and oral health* (pp. 71–82). St. Louis, MO: Mosby.

Benjamin, B. J. (1981). Frequency variability in the aged voice. *Journal of Gerontology, 36,* 722–726.

Bless, D. M., & Hirano, M. (1982). *Verbal instructions: A critical variable in obtaining optimal performance for maximum phonation time.* Paper presented at the annual convention of the American Speech-Language-Hearing Association, Toronto.

Bloem, B. R., Lagaay, A. M., van Beek, W., Haan, J., Roos, R. A., & Wintzen, A. R. (1990). Prevalence of subjective dysphagia in community residents aged over 87. *British Medical Journal, 300,* 721–722.

Caruso, A. J., McClowry, M. T., & Max, L. (in press). Age-related effects on speech fluency. *Seminars in Speech and Language.*

Caruso, A. J., Mueller, P. B., & Xue, A. (1994). The relative contributions of voice and articulation to listener judgements of age and gender: Preliminary data and implications. *Voice, 3,* 3–11.

Cook, I. J., Weltman, M. D., Wallace, K., Shaw, D. W., McKay, F., Smart, R. C., & Butler, S. P. (1994). Influence of aging on oral–pharyngeal bolus transit and clearance during swallowing: Scintigraphic study. *American Journal of Physiology, 266,* 972–977.

Dejaeger, F., Peleman, W., Bibau, G., & Ponette, F. (1994). Manofluorographic analysis of swallowing in the elderly. *Dysphagia, 9,* 156–161.

Erlichman, M. (1989). Public health service assessment: The role of speech–language pathologists in the management of dysphagia. *National Center for Health Services Research and Health Care Technology Assessment, 1,* 156–161.

Gilbert, H., & Weismer, G. (1974). The effects of smoking on the speaking fundamental frequency of adult women. *Journal of Speech and Hearing Research, 24,* 437–441.

Hartman, D. (1979). The perceptual identity and characteristics of aging in normal adult speakers. *Journal of Communication Disorders, 12,* 53–61.

Heatley, B., Evinson, G., & Samuel, E. (1965). The pattern of ossification in the laryngeal cartilages: A radiological study. *British Journal of Radiology, 38,* 585–591.

Hill, M. W. (1984). The influence of aging on skin and oral mucosa. *Gerontology, 3,* 35–45.

Hirano, M., Koike, Y., & Von Leden, H. (1968). Maximum phonation time and air usage during phonation. *Folia Phoniatrica, 20,* 185–201.

Hirano, M., Kurita, S., & Nakashima, T. (1983). Growth, development, and aging of human vocal folds. In D. Bless & J. Abbs (Eds.), *Vocal fold physiology: Contemporary research and clinical issues* (pp. 22–43). San Diego: College-Hill Press.

Hollien, H., & Shipp, T. (1972). Speaking fundamental frequency and chronologic age in males. *Journal of Speech and Hearing Research, 15,* 155–159.

Honjo, I., & Isshiki, N. (1980). Laryngoscopic and voice characteristics of aged persons. *Archives of Otolaryngology, 106,* 149–150.

Horii, Y., & Ryan, W. (1981). Fundamental frequency characteristics and perceived age of adult male speakers. *Folia Phoniatrica, 33,* 227–233.

Inglis, J. M. (1977). *Obtaining normative data on vocal performance in a group of adult speakers.* Unpublished master's thesis, Utah State University, Logan.

Kahane, J. C. (1982). Age related changes in the elastic fibers of the adult male vocal ligament. In V. Lawrence (Ed.), *Transcripts of the Eleventh Symposium: Care of the Professional Voice* (pp. 116–122). New York: Voice Foundation of America.

Kahane, J. C. (1983). Postnatal development and aging of the human larynx. *Seminars in Speech and Language, 4,* 189–203.

Kahane, J. C. (1987). Connective tissue changes in the larynx and their effects on voice. *Journal of Voice, 1,* 27–30.

Kahane, J. (1990). Age-related changes in the peripheral speech mechanism: Structural and physiological changes. In E. Cherow (Ed.), *Proceedings of the Research Symposium on Communication Sciences and Disorders and Aging* (ASHA Reports No. 19, pp. 75–87). Rockville, MD: American Speech-Language-Hearing Association.

Kent, R. D., Kent, J. F., & Rosenbek, J. C. (1987). Maximum performance tests of speech production. *Journal of Speech and Hearing Disorders, 52,* 367–387.

Kersing, W. (1986). Vocal musculature, aging and developmental aspects. In J. Kirchner (Ed.), *Vocal fold histopathology* (pp. 11–16). San Diego: College-Hill.

Kreul, E. J. (1972). Neuromuscular control examination (NMC) for parkinsonism: Vowel prolongations and diadochokinetic and reading rates. *Journal of Speech and Hearing Research, 15,* 72–83.

Leeper, L. H., & Culatta, R. (1995). Speech fluency: Effect of age, gender and context. *Folia Phoniatrica, 47,* 1–14.

Linville, S., & Fisher, H. (1985). Acoustic characteristics of women's voices with advanced age. *Journal of Gerontology, 3,* 324–330.

Liss, J. M., Weismer, G., & Rosenbek, J. C. (1990). Selected acoustic characteristics of speech production in very old males. *Journal of Gerontology, 45,* 35–45.

McClowry, M. T., Mueller, P. B., & Caruso, A. J. (1995). *Elderly listeners' judgements of age and gender.* Paper presented at the annual meeting of the American Speech-Language-Hearing Association, Orlando, FL.

McGlone, R., & Hollien, H. (1963). Vocal pitch characteristics of aged women. *Journal of Speech and Hearing Research, 6,* 164–170.

Mueller, P. B. (1978). *Communicative disorders in a geriatric population.* Paper presented at the annual meeting of the American Speech-Language-Hearing Association, San Francisco.

Mueller, P. B. (1982). Voice characteristics of octogenarian and nonagenarian persons. *Ear, Nose and Throat Journal, 61,* 33–37.

Mueller, P. B. (1985). What is normal aging? Part XII: The senescent voice. *Geriatric Medicine Today, 41,* 48–57.

Mueller, P. B. (1990). Voice characteristics of centenarian subjects. *Proceedings of the XXIst Congress of the International Association of Logopedics and Phoniatrics, 2,* 414–415.

Mueller, P. B., Sweeney, R. J., & Baribeau, L. J. (1984). Acoustic and morphologic study of the senescent voice. *Ear, Nose and Throat Journal, 63,* 71–75.

Mueller, P. B., Sweeney, R. J., & Baribeau, L. J. (1985). Senescence of the voice: morphology of excised male larynges. *Folia Phoniatrica, 37,* 134–138.

Mueller, P. B., & Xue, A. (1996). Effect of physical activity levels on perceived age and speaking rate of elderly subjects: Preliminary data. *National Student Speech-Language-Hearing Journal, 23,* 63–68.

Mysak, E. D. (1959). Pitch duration characteristics of older males. *Journal of Speech and Hearing Research, 2,* 46–54.

Neiman, G. S., & Applegate, J. A. (1990). Accuracy of listener judgements of perceived age relative to chronological age in adults. *Folia Phoniatrica, 42,* 327–330.

Perello, J. (1983). Characteristics of the elderly voice. *Aging and Communication Bulletin, 16,* 103–114.

Ptacek, P. H., & Sander, E. K. (1966). Age recognition from voice. *Journal of Speech and Hearing Research, 9,* 273–277.

Ptacek, P., Sander, E., Mahoney, W., & Jackson, C. (1966). Phonatory and related changes with advanced age. *Journal of Speech and Hearing Research, 9,* 353–360.

Punt, N. A. (1974). Lubrication of the vocal mechanism. *Folia Phoniatrica, 26,* 287–288.

Ringel, R. L., & Chodzko-Zajko, W. J. (1987). Vocal indices of biological age. *Journal of Voice, 1,* 31–37.

Robbins, J., Hamilton, J. W., Lof, G. L., & Kempster, G. B. (1992). Oropharyngeal swallowing in normal adults of different ages. *Gastroenterology, 103,* 823–829.

Ryan, W., & Burk, K. (1974). Perceptual and acoustic correlates of aging in the speech of males. *Journal of Communication Disorders, 7,* 181–192.

Sabin, T. D., & Venna, N. (1984). Peripheral nerve disorders in the elderly. In M. L. Albert (Ed.), *Clinical neurology of aging* (pp. 425–442). New York: Oxford University Press.

Sato, T., & Tauchi, H. (1982). Age changes in human vocal muscle. *Mechanisms of Aging Development, 18,* 67–74.

Segre, R. (1971). Senescence of the voice. *Eye, Ear, Nose and Throat Journal, 50,* 62–68.

Shadden, B. B. (in press). Discourse behaviors in older adults. *Seminars in Speech and Language.*

Siebens, H., Trupe, E., Siebens, A., Cook, F., Anshen, S., Ilanauer, R., & Oster, G. (1986). Correlates and consequences of eating dependency in the institutionalized elderly. *Journal of the American Geriatric Society, 34*, 192–198.

Sonies, B. (1987). Oral–motor problems. In H. G. Mueller, & V. C. Geoffrey (Eds.), *Communication disorders in aging* (pp. 185–213). Washington, DC: Gallaudet University Press.

Sonies, B., Baum, B., & Shawker, T. (1984). Tongue motion in elderly adults: Initial in situ observations. *Journal of Gerontology, 39*, 279–283.

Taylor, T. J. (1980). *Air flow parameters in college-age individuals.* Unpublished master's thesis, Utah State University, Logan.

Weiffenbach, J., Cowart, B., & Baum, B. (1986). Taste intensity perception in aging. *Journal of Gerontology, 41*, 460–468.

Wilcox, K., & Horii, Y. (1980). Age and changes in vocal jitter. *Journal of Gerontology, 35*, 194–198.

Wyke, B. D. (1974). Laryngeal neuromuscular control systems in singing. *Folia Phoniatrica, 26*, 295–306.

Xue, A. (1995). *A study of selected acoustic parameters of the voice of sedate and physically active elderly speakers.* Unpublished doctoral dissertation, Kent State University, Kent, OH.

Xue, A., & Mueller, P. B. (1994). *Speaking fundamental frequency of elderly African-Americans.* Paper presented at the annual meeting of the American Speech-Language-Hearing Association, New Orleans.

Xue, A., & Mueller, P. B. (1996). Speaking fundamental frequency of elderly African-American nursing home residents: Preliminary data. *Clinical Linguistics and Phonetics, 10*, 65–70.

Yairi, E., & Clifton, N. F. (1972). Disfluent speech behavior of preschool children, high school seniors and geriatric persons. *Journal of Speech and Hearing Research, 15*, 714–719.

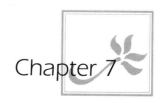

Chapter 7

Language and Communication Changes with Aging

Barbara B. Shadden

Shadden summarizes what is known about language and communication in older adults. The chapter begins with a brief discussion of the potential direct and indirect effects on communication of aspects of aging described in Chapters 2 through 6. The literature on language comprehension and performance in normal older adults is reviewed, and the nature of communicative interactions with the elderly is described. Problems in developing a single definition of normal changes in language and communication in older adults are noted, and the heterogeneity of communication behaviors in the elderly is highlighted.

1. *For the social, physical, and cognitive/emotional aspects of aging considered in earlier chapters, identify the potential impact of such changes on communicative functioning in older adults. In what ways must speech–language pathologists and audiologists accommodate their assessment and intervention approaches to the particular older client?*
2. *What are some of the research dilemmas encountered when attempting to define normal language and communicative performance in older adults?*
3. *What language and communication skills are best preserved across the life span? What variables influence language comprehension in the elderly? For each of the common language domains (syntax, semantics, phonology, morphology, pragmatics/discourse), identify patterns (if any) in the performance of older adults.*
4. *What factors influence the communicative interactions experienced by older adults? What is meant by the "Communication Predicament of Aging?"*

The preceding chapters have provided a series of building blocks in our understanding of the complexities of aging and of the highly individualistic and heterogeneous experiences of older adults in this society. Broad social, physical, and cognitive/emotional aspects of the aging process identified in these chapters may have a profound, although often indirect, influence upon communicative functioning in the elderly. In addition, alterations in auditory status, and in sensory and motor aspects of speech, voice, and related feeding skills, may be concomitants of aging in some individuals. It is fitting that the first section of this text concludes with a chapter specifically addressing language and communication in the elderly.

Central to this chapter are some of the fundamental principles outlined in Chapter 1. First, aging is a developmental phenomenon; second, aging processes and communicative behaviors occur across a continuum. Third, communication is a critical tool for older adults in the process of adaptation and the ongoing struggle to maximize quality of life. Finally, communication behaviors observed in a particular older adult may represent a unique combination of true changes in linguistic functioning as a direct correlate of aging, coupled with compensatory adaptations to other aging realities. Included in these aging realities are the ways in which communication partners interact with older adults. Although it may not be possible at present to tease out clearly which behaviors can be changed and which cannot, practitioners and students must adopt a holistic approach to understanding communicative functioning in the older individual.

Consistent with these premises, the first section of this chapter will examine specifically the manner in which social, physical, and cognitive/emotional changes associated with aging may affect the older adult's ability to use communication effectively on a daily basis (see Chapters 2 through 4). Included in this discussion will be examples of the manner in which speech–language pathologists and audiologists may have to accommodate age-related changes when providing assessment and intervention services. The second section of the chapter examines more closely the growing body of literature concerning language and communication in older individuals (aspects of hearing and voice and speech are considered in Chapters 5 and 6). Individual linguistic components, as well as more broad-based discourse measures, are addressed. The chapter closes with an overview of communicative interactions between older adults and younger partners.

It may be helpful to conceptualize the following discussion as an analysis of variations within a group of persons linked only by chronological age. Because of the arbitrary nature of this grouping, it is critical that clinicians break away from the dichotomy of impaired versus nonimpaired that influences most of our clinical activities. As Garfein and Herzog (1995) have suggested, there is a wide range of levels of functioning in older adults with no known illness or disorder. This variability must provide the context for our interventions with specific communication disorders.

Indirect Influence of Aging on Communication

Aspects of aging may affect an individual's life circumstances and functioning in all arenas. Although this section may appear to focus excessively on diminished functioning, the intent is to clarify those changes that may have secondary effects upon the ability to communicate (Maxim & Bryan, 1994). The information provided is intended to encourage clinicians to move the older client in the direction of "successful aging," at least from the perspective of communication. Successful aging is a rather broad concept that has been characterized by a variety of terms, including robust aging, aging well, productive aging, vitality of functioning, and maintenance of functioning. Recent research supports the concept that successful aging is a multidimensional construct that encompasses social, physical, and mental health (Garfein & Herzog, 1995).

Sociocultural and Socioeconomic Aspects of Aging

The social aspects of aging from the particular perspectives of role changes, transitions, and adaptations are outlined in Chapter 2. Certainly, the majority of older adults experience major alterations in life roles as a result of retirement, shifts in family relationships (loss of active parenting role, shift to grandparent role, loss of spouse), and loss of membership in previous professional or social groups, along with possible shifts in status. The role of caregiver may emerge as a primary focus. In addition, transition dominates the lives of many older adults. For some, transition takes the form of physical relocation, within or outside the home community. Perhaps the most dramatic transition is the residential shift to a long-term care facility. For others, transitions are most apparent in the increased leisure time associated with retirement, the geographical dispersal of friends and family, or even the increasing occurrence of the death of age peers. A social world previously populated by roughly equal proportions of males and females now becomes heavily female dominated. Some persons experience a shift to lower, fixed incomes in times of escalating daily living and health care costs.

Many older adults weather these changes successfully, and there is no impact on social or communicative functioning. For others, transitions and role shifts may have a negative effect on communicative interactions. Social isolation may increase, creating significant loneliness in some elderly persons. Social networks may be reduced, or may have to be rebuilt and modified. Financial restrictions may limit recreational activities, removing a primary source of social contact. Changes in role and status in society may reduce self-esteem; at the same time, the power base for interactions may be skewed negatively away from the older adult (Dowd, 1980). As stereotypes and negative attitudes creep into social exchanges, communication quality may be diminished because the older partner is devalued (Ryan & Capadano, 1978).

Responses to these changes will be highly variable. One older adult may display greater neediness in all social exchanges, placing uncomfortable and excessive demands upon the communication partner, who may, in turn, react by rejecting or avoiding contact. Another older person may withdraw, finding this strategy less emotionally draining than trying to fight what is perceived as an uphill battle against life circumstance. Yet a third may display declining skills and reduced appropriateness of communicative behaviors, due to limited opportunities for maintenance of communicative adequacy. As self-esteem suffers in this process, independent functioning may be reduced and depression may emerge. As Krause (1995) has pointed out, subjective perceptions play a major role in determining how we respond to our environment. If the older individual can find ways to reach out and help others, psychological well-being is enhanced. If the experience of interacting with others is negative, psychological well-being will suffer.

As noted, relocation to a nursing home environment can have a profoundly negative effect on all aspects of individual functioning. These environments are often governed by a series of unwritten rules that regulate patterns of resident-to-resident and resident-to-caregiver communications (Kaakinen, 1995; Lubinski, 1995). Invariably, loss of communicative opportunities and partners results. Mor et al. (1995) noted that becoming a long-term care resident often brings with it adoption of the "sick" role, associated with loss of control, autonomy, and social engagement. The resulting pattern of learned helplessness suggests to the older adult that any assertive action, including communication outreach, is doomed to failure (Decker & Kinzel, 1985; Lubinski, 1991). Negative adaptations do not have to occur (Schroeder, 1986); however, the development of positive adaptive strategies may require some assistance.

The implications of some of these social realities of aging for health care professionals should be obvious. Clearly, the response of the individual client to assessment and treatment will be influenced by access to social partners, the nature of the environment, the adequacy of resources (for both services and social activities), and the attitudes of available communication partners. Clinical management cannot be provided without taking all of these factors into consideration. In addition, the clinician must attempt to determine the degree to which inadequate or inappropriate communicative behaviors are a product of a specific communication disorder, as opposed to learned strategies for coping with other aspects of social aging. Interventions designed to maintain or enhance skills in older persons at risk for communication breakdown must be considered. Greater involvement in caregiver interventions is required; clinicians cannot treat older adults as though they exist in a vacuum. Caregivers are critical ingredients in the success or failure of interventions, and caregivers themselves may have major needs for information and/or support.

Physical Realities of Aging

As stated clearly in Chapter 3, the bottom line in physical aging is that most bodily systems show reduced efficiency over time, with diminished reserve capacity being a major product of these normal changes. Reaction time slows, mobility may be reduced, and fatigue can become ongoing. Sensory limitations—in both vision and hearing—are particularly predictable and significant in their impact upon daily functioning (see Chapters 3 and 5). Changes in speech and voice send clear signals about age to communication partners.

In addition, older adults tend to have chronic and multiple health problems. Because health, cognitive functioning, and emotional well-being are linked, perceived and actual health status have effects far beyond the immediate disorder (C. F. Emery, Huppert, & Schein, 1995; Kaplan, Barell, & Lisky, 1988). In addition, elderly individuals tend to take numerous prescription medications, often supplemented by over-the-counter drugs (Brandell, Brandell, & Hult, 1988). The risks of drug interactions are complicated by changes in the absorption, distribution, metabolism, and excretion of medication-related substances. Thus, overmedication becomes an additional concern.

Although the effects of physical aging upon communication are less obvious that those seen for the social aspects of aging, they are nonetheless real. Difficulties in "getting around" due to general motor slowness, arthritis, health problems, or fatigue may limit access to pleasurable activities that provide opportunities for mental stimulation and communicative interaction. Visual and auditory deficits may reduce or eliminate participation in activities, while also affecting communication directly. Individual strategies for dealing with presbycusic hearing loss vary, as described in Chapters 5 and 18. Some commonly noted responses to changes in auditory status include isolation resulting from decreases in social involvement (Norris, 1981) and limitations in daily functioning (Bess, Lichtenstein, Logan, & Burger, 1989). Chronic and multiple health problems can lead to a preoccupation with oneself and one's health as a topic of communication. Although this consequence can be viewed as an unfortunate negative stereotype, it may have some reality base. If one's activities are curtailed and one is coping with chronic illness and associated fatigue, conversational topics can become limited. The older adult as communication partner may be devalued. Self-image may also change as others react negatively, either to physical appearance or conversational content and focus, further exacerbating the cycle.

Clinicians must be able to recognize the role played by physical aspects of aging in influencing performance during assessments and interventions; appropriate accommodations must be implemented. Accommodations may include adaptation of visual stimuli and room lighting, scheduling of sessions to reduce fatigue, consideration of motor restrictions in designing augmentative communication systems or prescribing specific hearing aids, and close monitoring of mental status and alertness for changes that may indicate excessive medication levels or drug interactions. In addition, treatment programs designed to enhance functional communication must take into consideration the activities in which the older client can engage comfortably; an inventory of such activities and associated physical limitations would be useful.

Cognitive and Affective Changes in Aging

In addition to Chapter 3 of this text, excellent reviews of cognitive and affective aspects of aging can be found in many sources (Bayles & Kaszniak, 1987; Hooker & Shifren, 1995; Hubbard, 1991; Kausler, 1988). Most reviews address such cognitive components as attention, memory, conceptualization, learning, and problem solving, as well as affective disorders such as depression. Any changes in cognition or affect may have an impact on communication directly or indirectly.

There is a consistent pattern to much of the research in cognition and aging. In general, older adults demonstrate little or no decline in attentional or memory skills as long as (a) the task is simple; (b) there are no competing challenges; (c) information to be processed is brief, overlearned, strongly associated, or personally relevant; (d) time constraints are limited; and (e) redundancy is high. In fact, complaints of memory problems are described routinely as more severe than memory difficulties measured in the same individuals in the laboratory. There is some indication that working memory resources become more limited with advanced aging, affecting both language processing and production, as described in subsequent sections. Older adults may learn complex tasks more slowly than younger adults, but retain new learning well. Concept formation and problem-solving skills are minimally affected as long as the tasks represent real-life challenges. The introduction of novel information, complex constructs, and artificial tasks may impair performance. There may also be age-related losses in the ability to change cognitive set, use varied or efficient problem-solving strategies, and exercise appropriate adaptation skills. A conservative approach to task performance, possibly designed to minimize failure, has been noted.

Effects of real or imagined cognitive changes associated with normal aging may influence communicative and social participation in a variety of ways. Anxiety about mental decline may lead some older individuals to withdraw from activities and social situations because of concerns that cognitive deficits may be revealed. Other older adults may change communication strategies to compensate for cognitive alterations. Situation-specific effects of cognitive change on communication may emerge. For example, a highly educated older adult who previously took advantage of every opportunity to attend lectures and similar stimulating events may now find such activities more difficult to process, and thus more tiring; the obvious response is to reduce or eliminate such participation. Communication itself is a highly adaptive process; changes are made constantly to accommodate to listener reactions and environmental context. This aspect of communication in aging has not been studied extensively, but it is reasonable to assume that some older adults with reduced adaptive skills may become less adequate communication partners.

Depression in older adults is discussed in Chapters 2 and 4. Although data suggest that depression may be no more prevalent in the elderly than in other age groups, these figures may be suspect due to the limited utilization of mental health services by older persons. The impact of depression on communication is evident across the life span. Depressed individuals use shorter, less elaborated language, show reduced nonverbal affect, and initiate communication and social activity less often. Cognitive effects are also seen (Lichtenburg, Ross, Millis, & Manning, 1995).

Clinicians must be aware of possible age-related changes in selected cognitive skills or the presence of affective disturbances so that specific communication disorders can be differentiated from other changes in functioning. Alterations in processing and/or learning styles and strategies may need to be accommodated. For example, repetition and simplification of instructions may be required with one client; another may need increased task demonstration and opportunities to practice or become familiar with treatment or testing materials. Motivation may be affected by emotional state and/or attitudes toward self-worth. In particular, an older adult's performance anxiety related to the actual testing or treatment context may require greater reassurance on the part of the examiner and different approaches to feedback. Otherwise, fear of performance failure may inhibit some older clients from responding, rather than risk error or a display of deficit. In addition, clinicians must be vigilant for evidence of underlying affective disturbances, such as depression, or diminishing cognitive skills that reflect a shift toward the pathological end of the cognitive aging continuum. Mental status should be monitored. The need for team interventions and appropriate referral is evident.

Linguistic Comprehension and Production in Older Adults

What do we actually know about language and communication in older adults, or about the nature of communicative interactions involving the elderly? Although there has been a proliferation of research addressing language and aging in recent years, there are few definitive answers concerning the nature of language change associated with the normal aging process. Given the marked variations in the social, biological, and cognitive processes of aging found across individuals, this lack of definitive answers is not surprising. An understanding of methodological and theoretical challenges in measuring communicative behavior in older adults is essential for any practitioner wishing to interpret the research literature.

Research Dilemmas

A variety of dilemmas confront researchers attempting to define changes in language and communication associated with normal aging processes. These dilemmas have been outlined by a number of authors (e.g., de Santi & Obler, 1991; Holland, 1990). Perhaps the single greatest difficulty stems from the pronounced heterogeneity in this population. Older adults have lived longer than the rest of the population and thus have accumulated a diverse set of life experiences that may influence all aspects of performance. In addition, each is particularly susceptible, in a highly individual way, to the many aging influences identified throughout this text. Defining a homogeneous population of older adults for participation in a given study is close to impossible.

Worse yet, if one has defined a homogeneous population, it is probable that one has ruled out as many presumably "negative" subject variables as possible. If we take only healthy, highly educated, normally hearing, visually intact, economically comfortable elderly persons as our subjects, we may be measuring the performance of what Ringel and Chodzko-Zajko (1990) referred to as "geriatric supermen." In fact, there is undoubtedly a natural selection process, based on which older adults actually volunteer for participation in research studies. The question must then be asked: Are these the "normal" older adults whom we wish to establish as a reference point for all other clinical populations? Clearly, the answer is "no." Because there are no simple solutions, the clinician must read the literature carefully with respect to subject selection attributes.

There are also significant questions about the actual criteria for defining aging, along with strong evidence that subsets within the older population exist and produce distinct behavioral patterns. Most studies use some measure of chronological age as their yardstick for defining or segmenting older subjects from younger subjects, despite any support for the idea that ages 65 or 70 years are valid break points in the life span. In fact, the only chronological age distinction that may have validity in linguistic research is a separation of older-old (over 80 or 85 years) from younger-old age ranges (Ulatowska & Chapman, 1991). Instead of chronological age, Ringel and Chodzko-Zajko (1988, 1990) have argued for the development of a biological yardstick of aging, in which biological health and disease exist on a continuum that, in part, defines the extent of the effects of aging upon any given individual. Other subgroups within the older population might relate to institutionalization, education, income, ethnic group, and gender.

Another frequently cited research dilemma is the problem of research design selection. A true life span approach to exploring language and communication requires use of a longitudinal design. Only in this fashion can we explore intraindividual changes that emerge over the course of many years. There are few longitudinal studies of language and communication. As a result, there is poor definition of behavior within the middle years of the life span. Longitudinal explorations of linguistic functioning can also be contaminated by the state of theoretical understanding of language and communication constructs at the beginning of the study. A longitudinal study of life span language changes begun in the 1960s, for example, would probably focus extensively on syntactic aspects of performance, with little or no attention to discourse and pragmatic measures.

In contrast, the cross-sectional research design (comparing younger and older samples) is relatively easy to complete but difficult to interpret. Individuals within a given age group form an age cohort, with a number of shared life experiences that cannot readily be compared with those of persons in a different age cohort. For example, college degrees in individuals who are currently over 65 are comparatively uncommon. In contrast, the college degree is rapidly becoming the norm for many persons in their 20s. On a more subtle level, age cohorts have different traditions of social interaction and are at different points in the life cycle with respect to their expectations of others.

These and many other age cohort factors can influence discourse performance in particular.

One final research concern warrants discussion—the virtual absence of data concerning differential age-related patterns of language performance and communicative interactions in diverse cultures. The gerontological literature has only recently begun to focus on the fact that the experience of aging and attitudes toward older persons are very different across ethnic groups (Jackson & Ensley, 1995). Although extensive data suggest that communicative behaviors and clinical interactions vary markedly across ethnic and cultural groups (e.g., Battle, 1993), there is virtually no information about the nature of clinical interactions with communicatively disordered older adults from non-White backgrounds. Research is needed to clarify further a number of aspects of multicultural aging, including (a) prevalence of communication disorders, (b) access to and utilization of speech–language pathology and audiology services in non-White populations, (c) alterations in assessment and intervention strategies needed to accommodate to cultural variations in older clients, and (d) language and communication changes in culturally and linguistically diverse groups. For now, clinicians must make every effort to accommodate ethnic variations that may influence the older person's functional and communicative status, inside and outside of the treatment room.

Theoretical Considerations

Implicit in the above discussion is a recognition of the complexity of both aging and communicative processes. The neural substrates for language and the intricate interactions between linguistic and cognitive systems to produce adequate communication are still not well understood. When this is coupled with a continuing search to pinpoint the underlying neurophysiological mechanisms of aging, it is not surprising that many questions remain unanswered. It is not unreasonable, for example, to expect that age concomitants, such as loss of neural plasticity and reductions in working memory, will influence higher level linguistic and communicative performance (Ulatowska & Chapman, 1991). In fact, many current theories of language performance in aging incorporate the idea of challenges to the central nervous system—working memory restrictions, generalized cognitive resource reductions, and/or problems in resource allocation—to explain communicative behaviors.

Some researchers have proposed that there are nonlinear modifications in cognitive functions associated with selected changes in the brain and associated differential slowing of activity (Albert, Duffy, & Naeser, 1987). Certainly, we know that specific language functions (e.g., phonology, syntax) are more lateralized, localized, and automatic than are broader language abilities involving semantics and pragmatics. Because advanced biological aging of the brain is typically diffuse and bilateral, phonology and syntax should show relative preservation, whereas semantic and pragmatic organization should be more disrupted (Kempler, Curtiss, & Jackson, 1987). Further, it is not unreasonable to suspect the presence of individual differences in the aging of biological structures and systems responsible for language and communication. Such individual differences might account for the presence of subgroups of communicators within the elderly population, such as verbose versus taciturn individuals (Arbuckle, Gold, Frank, & Motard, 1989; Critchley, 1984). Chapman and Ulatowska (1991) have proposed that mechanisms such as general cortical disinhibition and subcortical deterioration, respectively, may explain these subgroups.

Finally, researchers and clinicians must always be alert to the need to distinguish between change resulting from deficit and change resulting from compensatory strategy. For example, modifications in narrative style in story telling may represent a positive change resulting from life experience, a deficit in underlying cognitive organizational processes, or a compensatory strategy on the part of a lonely older adult hoping to hold the attention of a communication partner.

Despite all of these concerns, defining the spectrum of linguistic and communicative behaviors in the elderly remains an important task. The following sections summarize available research literature, examining first those skills that appear to be preserved, followed by an overview of language comprehension. Language production will be addressed from the perspective of the traditional linguistic domains of semantics, syntax, and pragmatics, with the discussion of pragmatics focusing on discourse production. Because of the extensive literature, the reader is referred frequently to representative or summary references.

Most of the earliest investigations of language change in aging were by-products of an interest in changes in intelligence across the life span (Maxim & Bryan, 1994); as a result, research tended to focus on lexical comprehension or production at the word and sentence levels, particularly as related to memory deficits. Further, models of language behavior 20 years ago were more structurally oriented than those currently in vogue. Early reports emphasized a relative preservation of language performance as individuals aged, except for aspects of lexical performance (Myerson, 1976). Speech and voice production received greater attention, as their acoustic and physiological attributes could be measured more readily (Benjamin, 1988).

As theories of both aging and language behavior became more sophisticated, researchers and clinicians began to recognize and analyze the fact that a primary characteristic of communication in the elderly was its variability and heterogeneity (Albert, 1980). More sophisticated attempts to explore the interaction between language, cognition, and other individual variables have emerged and continue into the present.

What Is Preserved?

In general, some linguistic and communicative functions appear to be preserved in several domains. Automatic, highly overlearned language functions, such as those used in greetings and social discourse, appear relatively unaffected by aging. In addition, passive vocabulary (e.g., word recognition) and other basic lexical and semantic skills (e.g., retention of underlying semantic meanings) remain relatively unimpaired, or improve through adulthood, at least until very advanced stages of aging (Cooper, 1990; O. B. Emery, 1985, 1986). Kynette and Kemper (1986) reported no differences in type-token ratios across the age span, and Walker, Roberts, and Hedrick (1988) actually noted increases in type-token ratios in older women. An increase in lexical diversity was also suggested by Obler's (1980) identification of elaborated output in oral Cookie Theft picture descriptions. Glosser and Deser (1992) indicated that use of lexical cohesive ties and lexical production errors did not distinguish age groups. Phonological and morphological elements and rule systems, although receiving limited research attention, do not appear to be disrupted in aging. As a result, these traditional linguistic elements will not be discussed further. Finally, some basic pragmatic skills appear to be retained well into old age.

Language and Discourse Comprehension

Recent longitudinal research suggests a slight but consistent decline in language comprehension as individuals move from their 30s through their 50s into their 70s (Obler, Au, & Albert, 1995). Decline is evident primarily when tasks place stress upon the cognitive/linguistic systems by increasing cognitive demands or removing cues normally used to facilitate comprehension. Sentence-level deficits in comprehension of complex syntactic constructions are also reported for comparisons of pre-middle-aged and older adults (O. B. Emery, 1985, 1986) and in comprehension and imitation of syntactic constructions by older subjects (Kemper, 1986, 1987).

More recent investigations of language comprehension have focused on processing of longer text-based material in a variety of formats. This focus was stimulated by Cohen's (Cohen, 1979; Cohen & Faulkner, 1981) early work, which revealed that text comprehension reflected a complex interaction of cognitive, experiential, and linguistic factors that could be manipulated to determine the contributions of selected elements. Recently, von Eye, Dixon, and Krampen (1989) summarized four sets of variables influencing discourse comprehension in older individuals. *Subject characteristics* include specific memory impairments, other cognitive skills, prior knowledge of topic or context, and verbal abilities and deficits. *Task demands*, particularly influential in determining performance, include type of recall task (free, cued, immediate, delayed); recognition; demands for summarization, inference, or thematic identification; and other interpretive challenges. *Text material design* also controls performance, depending upon such variables as organization of material, redundancy and plausibility, type of text (narrative vs. expository), propositional density, propositional ties, lexical and syntactic complexity, modality of presentation (written vs. verbal), rate and prosodic alterations, presence of competing noise, and associated imagery. Finally, *orienting components,* such as attentional demands, subject instructions, and recommendations for use of cuing or acquisition strategies, influence performance.

Recent studies and literature reviews regarding discourse comprehension can be found in a number of sources (e.g., Adams, Labouvie-Vief, Hobart, & Dorosz, 1990; Dixon, Hertzog, Friesen, & Hultsch, 1993; Drevenstedt & Belleza, 1993, 1990; Kahn & Cordon, 1993; Wingfield, Wayland, & Stine, 1992). Across studies and variables, two conclusions can be drawn about discourse comprehension in older adults. First, discourse comprehension is highly variable across tasks and across subjects. Second, age-related decrements in discourse comprehension emerge reliably only when task challenges are increased and/or when normal linguistic and prosodic cues are reduced, distorted, or eliminated. The consistency of the latter finding has led some researchers to conclude that the one factor common to all the conditions producing decrements in text comprehension in older subjects is the presence of increased demands upon working memory resources and, more generally, resource allocation for challenging tasks (Hartley, 1988; Kahn & Cordon, 1993; Light & Anderson, 1985). In a recent study of metaphor and idiom comprehension and interpretation based on paragraph length material for presentation (Vogel, Sugar, & Cardillo, 1995), older adults performed less well than younger adults, with the older subjects producing more unrelated and literal errors and more restatements. Results are described as supporting the idea of limitations in the processes of active retrieval and analysis of new information in the context of previously acquired and stored information.

Individual differences continue to play a major role in understanding discourse comprehension in older adults. Education and continued mental activity have been shown to influence performance. Discourse comprehension, as evidenced in essay and story recall tasks, also may be subject to differences in strategy. Adams (1991; Adams et al., 1991) found that older subjects were more integrative, interpretive, and reconstructive in dealing with narrative material. Clinicians must recognize that all of the discourse task variables described earlier can influence the comprehension performance of a specific older client; further, task selection can be manipulated to maximize treatment outcomes.

Semantics

Some basic elements of lexical comprehension and production appear to remain relatively unchanged across the life span. However, there is evidence that other semantic skills are more vulnerable to aging influences than the more focal performance skills involving syntax and phonology. Summaries of semantic changes associated with aging, particularly in the context of memory impairment, can be found in Benjamin (1988), Au and Bowles (1991), Goulet, Ska, and Kahn, (1994), and Bayles and Kaszniak (1987).

Most changes in basic word- and sentence-level semantic performance are associated with some form of decline in word-finding skills

(Albert, 1980; Obler & Albert, 1981, 1984). One of the most commonly used tasks is confrontation naming. In general, most studies report a slowing in naming skills, along with an increase in naming errors (Au & Bowles, 1991). Goulet et al. (1994) reviewed 25 studies exploring picture naming in older subjects. Although close to half of the studies reported that older persons were less accurate than younger adults in naming skills, results within and across studies showed considerable variability. Some variability might be attributed to research design differences and/or problems, but additional discrepancies resulted from subject characteristics. Health and education were particularly influential, along with actual chronological age. Neils et al. (1995) also examined the performance of 323 older persons on the *Boston Naming Test* (Goodglass & Kaplan, 1983) in an attempt to tease out the influence of specific variables. Three variables, education, age, and living environment, contributed 32% of the variance in performance and interacted predictably. Given the high prevalence of word retrieval deficits in adult neurologically impaired clients, particularly in individuals with mild language deficits, declines in word-finding skills in normal older adults present major diagnostic challenges.

Other aspects of semantic performance have also been studied. Word fluency skills are reduced in older subjects, although the relationship between word fluency and word retrieval in discourse is not clear (Heller & Dobbs, 1993). Some studies have suggested that fewer proper nouns and more high-frequency nouns are used in discourse. Older subjects access categorical information more slowly and generate fewer categories in free categorization tasks. Word association behaviors change, with more syntactically linked ("sit" . . . "down") and idiosyncratic ("sit" . . . "chicken soup") associations replacing the young adult use of dominant semantically linked ("sit" . . . "stand") associations. This is an intriguing finding, in that some aphasic individuals, as well as persons with dementia, also produce idiosyncratic language. How can clinicians distinguish an idiosyncratic, but acceptable, word production from a disordered one? Is the ultimate test the individual's ability to provide a logical explanation for the response?

There are also questions about the effectiveness of coding of new lexical information; at least some findings indicate that older adults' encoding strategies demonstrate less imagery, organization, and elaboration (Benjamin, 1988). At best, one can conclude that active word retrieval, generation, and divergent semantic processes may be affected in some older adults, particularly when speed and memory demands are introduced. Semantic behaviors also play a major role in the amount, quality, and efficiency of communicating information in extended discourse. This role will be discussed in a later section.

Syntax

Syntactic functioning in older adults has been studied fairly extensively, partly because of the relative ease of measurement of syntactic skills and partly because breakdown in syntactic performance under selected conditions provides clues about underlying system capacities and challenges. Issues of length, complexity, and accuracy have been addressed. Maxim and Bryan (1994) recently completed an extensive study of aspects of syntactic performance in the conversational discourse of older adults. No younger adults were tested; the authors' intent was to begin to provide normative data about syntactic characteristics of the older population.

In one study, Maxim and Bryan (1994) found that older men produced fewer sentences than older women, but the number of sentences per conversational turn and pronoun usage was similar. Complex sentences were used with minor difficulty; error rates increased with higher complexity. Although all subjects evidenced the ability to monitor errors, the old-old subgroup made fewer repairs in relationship to errors and produced fewer errors (a finding attributed to use of more frequently occurring clausal structures). Core grammar elements included extended use of ellipsis and reliance on more coordinating, rather than subordinating, conjunctive units.

Research findings related to syntactic functioning in the elderly are somewhat variable. Most studies of syntactic functioning compare young with old groups, although some longitudinal work has been reported. Utterance length, although highly variable, appears to be reduced in older adults, possibly because of an increase in use of sentence fragments (Chafe, 1982; Cohen & Faulkner, 1986; Critchley, 1984; Shewan & Henderson, 1988; Walker et al., 1988). No change in syntactic complexity has been identified as a function of age in some studies (e.g., Cooper, 1990; Glosser & Deser, 1992; Labov & Augur, 1993; Shewan & Henderson, 1988; Ulatowska & Chapman, 1991; Walker et al., 1988). In a few instances, increased complexity and elaboration of syntactic form in both written and spoken picture description tasks has been noted (Obler, 1980; Obler & Albert, 1981). Elaboration was characterized by more complex, embedded sentences, more noun modification, more words in general, and higher noun/verb ratios, with increased use of prepositional phrases reported in a study by Cooper (1990).

In most studies of syntactic complexity, however, researchers have reported reduced complexity with advancing age across a wide variety of experimental tasks, including sentence imitation, written and oral discourse production, text comprehension and imitation, and life span diary studies. Much of the work in this area has been carried out by Kemper and colleagues (e.g., Kemper, 1988, 1990; Kemper, Kynette, Rash, O'Brien, & Sprott, 1989; Kynette & Kemper, 1986). Because reduced complexity is particularly apparent for left subordinate clauses, it is speculated that working memory restrictions play a major role in this aspect of linguistic performance. Some of Kemper's work has explored this hypothesis; greater syntactic complexity and length are correlated with higher education and better memory skills on the *Wechsler Adult Intelligence Scale–Revised* (Wechsler, 1981) digit span task. In addition, the fact that narratives of older adults are judged to be clearer and more interesting than those of younger adults suggests that conscious choice of story-telling strategies may result in reduced complexity.

Pragmatics and Discourse

The *pragmatic domain* is typically defined as involving the use of language in social contexts (Roth & Spekman, 1984). Within pragmatics, discourse tasks are particularly appealing as research and clinical tools because they reflect language used for a variety of purposes or functions. In addition, each discourse type (narrative, procedural, expository, conversational) requires a complex interaction of cognitive and linguistic skills to produce an informative and clear communication. Thus, task challenges can be manipulated to probe the functional integrity of the older adult's language and cognition. Further, discourse performance may be linked directly to both verbal and nonverbal cognitive performance as well as to rated competence, when competence is defined in terms of learning, planning, and problem-solving skills in coping with environmental challenges (North & Ulatowska, 1981; North, Ulatowska, Macaluso-Haynes, & Bell, 1986).

Many of the syntactic and semantic findings reported earlier come from discourse-based studies. Additional domains of interest in this section will be verbal fragmentations, cohesion, information, discourse organization, and conversation. Only selected highlights of research findings will be presented, given the extent and often contradictory nature of outcomes.

Verbal Fragmentation. The terms *verbal fragmentation* and *verbal disruption* refer to interruptions in the smooth flow of speech and information content in discourse, often believed to reflect word retrieval deficits or more general language and cognitive formulation problems (Yairi & Clifton, 1972). Although verbal fragmentations and associated semantic and phonologic errors have been studied in adult neurologically impaired populations, less is known about normal older adults. This is unfortunate in view of the fact that optimal clinical management of specific neurological disorders requires some knowledge of the verbal disruptions produced by normal older speakers.

Fluency characteristics have been described as cues to speaker age (Ptacek & Sander, 1966). In general, a number of studies have noted increased uncertainty behaviors or verbal fragmentations in the discourse of older persons (Chafe, 1982; Schow, Christensen, Hutchinson, & Nerbonne, 1978; Yairi & Clifton, 1972). In at least two studies (Pindzola, McCloskey, & Moran, 1989; Walker et al., (1988), frequency of occurrence of types of disfluent behavior, from most to least common, were interjections, followed by revisions and repetitions. In the latter study, frequency of interjections and revisions significantly differentiated young and old adults. In contrast, Cooper (1990) examined disfluencies produced during a picture description task performed by adults aged 20 to 78 years. The only fluency difference noted was the older speakers' use of longer pauses. Clearly, both task and classification scheme for analyzing verbal fragmentations can influence outcomes, as can individual differences.

Cohesion and Coherence. *Cohesion* is typically defined as structural or linguistic linkages across text elements and is measured by analyzing the presence, nature, and adequacy of cohesive ties. Although at least five major cohesive categories have been described by Halliday and Hasan (1976), analyses of older adults' discourse productions have tended to focus on referential cohesion. A few investigations have also considered text coherence, usually measured through impressions of the speaker's maintenance of the thematic unity of the text.

In a recent study by Chapman, Ulatowska, King, Johnson, and McIntire (1995), no significant differences in referential cohesion skills were noted when older (over 80 years) and younger adult control subjects (aged 47 to 78 years) were compared. Glosser and Deser's (1992) older subjects also experienced no problems with lexical cohesion or reference, although they did appear to have difficulty with the global thematic coherence of their discourse productions, as defined by the relationship of verbal output to the general topic of conversation. Glosser and Deser suggested that these difficulties may indicate a breakdown in memory processes and/or executive control, reflecting the interaction of linguistic and nonlinguistic cognitive factors.

Despite these findings, most studies of referential cohesion have noted a decrease in adequate referential skills in older adults, particularly evident in the increased use of indefinite terms (Cannito, Hayashi, & Ulatowska, 1988; Cooper, 1990; North et al., 1986; Obler, 1980; Ulatowska & Chapman, 1991). Disrupted reference (indefinite, nonspecific, ambiguous) was particularly seen in older-old subjects. Inflated pronoun use and escalating pronoun reference problems with increased task complexity have also been noted (North et al., 1986). Clinical differentiation of normal and pathological use of reference can be difficult. The following utterance was produced by a normal older subject in describing a sequence of cartoon pictures: "The girl was crying so he went up it to help resolve that situation but he got in trouble when it caught his shirt." It would be tempting to classify this speaker as communicatively disordered.

Informational Content. Communication of information is at the core of discourse production. Information analyses in normal elderly and clinical populations have considered the amount, quality, and efficiency with which information is communicated. Results of studies using normal older adults have tended to yield conflicting outcomes at times, due both to individual variability and to differences in the measures used to analyze information. However, the issue of informativeness is critical to understanding the behaviors seen in clinical populations, particularly in individuals with dementia.

Earlier research (e.g., Obler, 1980) indicated a possible increase in the number of themes in a written picture description task when subject age progressed from the 50s to the 70s. Cooper (1990) manipulated the presence or absence of time constraints and found no differences in the information produced by older, as compared with younger, subjects. Despite these findings, the general pattern appears to be a slight decline in the amount, type, and efficiency of information communicated across the life span, with the old-old demonstrating the greatest age effects.

The work of Ulatowska and colleagues has provided us with most of our data concerning information elements in the discourse of older adults (e.g., Cannito, Hayashi, & Ulatowska, 1988; North & Ulatowska, 1981; North et al., 1986; Ulatowska, Cannito, Hayashi, & Fleming, 1985; Ulatowska & Chapman, 1991; Ulatowska, Hayashi, Cannito, & Fleming, 1986). Their work supports some of the following conclusions. First, older-old subjects produce less information (propositions, procedural steps) than younger-old or young adults. Second, the oldest groups of subjects appear to demonstrate reduced informational relevance, particularly with increased discourse task challenges. Third, in most instances, older-old subjects produce different types of information (e.g., less setting information) with reduced accuracy in narrative structure elements and propositions. However, in a recent study comparing older-old adults with Alzheimer's patients and matched younger control subjects (Chapman et al., 1995), Alzheimer's subjects produced more disruptive and fewer frame-supporting propositions than the other two groups; the normal groups did not differ.

The concept of communication efficiency is viewed by some researchers as a critical analysis domain. Measures of efficiency tend to focus on the rate of communicating information, and are highly variable (Shewan & Henderson, 1988). There is some evidence for a slight decline in communication rate with advancing age (Benjamin, 1988; Schow, Christensen, Hutchinson, & Nerbonne, 1978). Communication efficiency is also related to the concept of verbosity. *Verbosity,* or loquacity, is of particular interest in the elderly because of common stereotypes of the garrulous, conversation-dominating older individual. When asked to describe how to use an American supermarket, one 71-year-old adult spoke for 23 minutes on the subject; in contrast, a second 74-year-old woman produced three sentences: "Get a cart, find what you need, and check out and pay for the items." Both subjects were classified as "normal"; clearly, individual differences in quantity of verbal output exist.

Verbosity has been defined and measured in a variety of ways in the clinical and research literature. Gold and colleagues (Gold, Andres, Arbuckle, & Schwartzmann, 1988; Arbuckle et al., 1989) have used the construct of verbosity to characterize off-target communicative behavior in older persons, defining off-target verbosity as any failure to remain focused on the preceding conversational topic, and further quantifying behaviors in terms of the degree of digression (extent of verbosity) present. Gold and colleagues identified three subgroups of older speakers—extended talkers, controlled talkers, and nontalkers—and reported that verbose characteristics were correlated with cognitive, situational, and personality attributes. There is also evidence that verbose older adults do not constitute a single population, but instead may be subdivided into those who present critical information first versus those who extend information throughout the discourse.

Organizational Elements. *Organizational elements* of discourse refer to the individual's cognitive/linguistic strategies in following accepted "rules" for a particular task (e.g., preserving the episode or story grammar structure of narratives, producing essential steps in the appropriate order in procedures). Ulatowska and research colleagues (see previous references) have concluded that, with some exceptions, these organizational or macrostructural elements of discourse are retained well throughout the life span, particularly for relatively simple tasks. Some older-old subjects display qualitative differences in the type of information selected for inclusion, or the style of communication (descriptive versus narrative). However, while narrative framing abilities distinguish older-old adults from persons with Alzheimer's disease, these abilities do not differentiate older-old and younger "normal" adults (Chapman et al., 1995).

Adequate discourse organizational skills do not ensure a person's ability to deal with what are referred to as *superstructural discourse activities,* such as outlining, defining a theme, producing summaries, and providing a statement of gist or moral of a story. Older adults do evidence performance decrements in complex tasks involving superstructural awareness, and these deficits are more pronounced in the older-old (Ulatowska & Chapman, 1991). Problems with producing summaries, morals, or themes are consistent with Glosser and Deser's (1992) finding that older adults experienced breakdown in their ability to maintain coherent reference to the general topic of the communication.

Conversation. *Conversation* is the basic medium of communicative exchange. Early reports of conversational skills in older adults relied heavily on anecdotal data to describe subgroups (e.g., verbose vs.

taciturn) or increased egocentrism (Helfrich, 1979; Looft & Charles, 1971). Differences in topic-switching strategies and pauses during turn shifts were also noted. Although the literature concerning conversational skills of normal older adults is relatively sparse, it appears that basic conversational skills remain intact (in the absence of other aging variables affecting performance and/or pathology).

For example, Hutchinson and Jensen (1980) identified appropriate topic maintenance/switching skills and turn-taking behaviors in cognitively intact older nursing home residents. Their observation has been supported by Boden and Bielby's (1983, 1986) findings that conversational regulation and orderly turn taking were maintained with facility in older communicators. Older partners were more effective than young adults at latching one turn to the next, using reference to their past and to common events to integrate conversational elements of the conversation, and manipulating topics from the other speaker's turn to expedite a topic shift. This partner sensitivity has been demonstrated in barrier communication tasks as well. In two studies (Molfese, Hoffman, & Yuen, 1981–1982; Siegel & Gregoria, 1985), no differences in time and/or accuracy of task completion were noted for older, as compared with younger, dyadic partners; appropriate speech style accommodations were made by older speakers. Only Hupet, Chantraine, and Nef (1993) reported a difference between old and young partners in dyadic communications. Although both groups benefitted from task repetition, older partners were slower to benefit, requested partner elaboration less often, required more collaborative communication, and interpreted partner references more idiosyncratically.

One issue raised by these studies is the possibility that older adults use different conversational and communicative strategies with different content, when compared with younger adults. Conversations between young and old married couples were analyzed by Gould and Dixon (1993). Strategy and content differences were apparent. Younger couples used shorter clauses and were more likely to situate events in a particular time frame and provide factual detail. Older couples discussed more subjective topics and employed a monologue conversational format more frequently than younger couples. This study is intriguing in light of two other aspects of conversational behavior—topic content and communicative strategy—that have been investigated in older adults.

There are some very common stereotypes about the content or common topics addressed by older adults in conversation, as well as about typical conversational partners. Topics frequently described by older adults (about other older adults), health professionals, and children of older parents include health, family, the past, and the weather (Shadden, 1988). In the same study, respondents reported perceptions that older people talk mostly with family. Recently, Stuart, Vanderhoof-Bilyeu, and Beukelman (1994) studied older adult conversations. Topics included frequent references to friends, more than family (although there were gender differences), and to food, household routines, games, and sports. Surprisingly, women were more likely than men to discuss games and sports. In essence, it is necessary to challenge assumptions about restricted topical content, as well as about specific topics, addressed in elderly conversations.

The second point raised by the Gould and Dixon (1993) study relates to differences in communicative strategy. Obler (1980) described older adults as master story tellers. Boden and Bielby (1983, 1986) supported this conclusion, noting the highly effective manner in which older adults use historical events and social experiences as a topic-organizing framework, in order to establish intimacy and express accumulated experience and wisdom functionally and effectively (see Chapter 14). In essence, the function of communication may change with aging, bringing modifications in communicative strategy. It is not surprising that Kemper (1990) found that older adult narratives were described as clearer and more interesting than those of younger adults.

Communicative Interactions: Negotiating a Shared Reality

The preceding section addressed conversation primarily from the perspective of the behaviors of the older adult. However, Schroeder (1986) has pointed out the need for closer examination of the reality constructed between older and younger communicators, suggesting that communication problems encountered by many older adults may be more directly attributable to younger partners' attitudes and behaviors. To close out this chapter, the impact of attitudes, stereotypes, and expectations upon communicative interactions will be reviewed briefly from the perspective of breakdown in speech style accommodations and setting-specific rules and regulatory beliefs affecting communication.

Younger adults tend to devalue communicative exchanges with older adults (Dowd, 1980). To a large degree, this devaluation reflects general attitudes and stereotypes about the elderly as cognitively challenged and thus less competent, as hearing impaired, as restricted in topics and partners, and as verbose or inappropriate, among other negative attributes (Shadden, 1988). Respondents in Shadden's study expressed a wide range of opinions about the actual communication skills of older adults. Some comments reflected an awareness of heterogeneity in communication behaviors and strategies. Other responses were highly negative, for example, "Older persons are self-centered. They don't listen. They also can't hear but that's different from not listening" (Shadden, 1988, p. 20). Interestingly, generalized devaluation does not extend to actual ratings of older versus younger communicators when communication samples are provided. In such contexts, ineffective older communicators may be less likely to be viewed negatively on personal traits than comparably ineffective younger communicators (Ryan & Johnston, 1994). Perhaps a kind of reverse ageism is operating, along with lower expectations for older communicators.

Attitudes toward aging and the elderly can lead to the use of different styles of communication with older adults. Most of these styles or strategies reflect under- or overaccommodation to the older partner's real or perceived aging attributes (Ryan, Giles, Bartolucci, & Henwood, 1986). *Accommodation* refers to changes in speech style made in order to acknowledge the partner and enhance communicative success. *Underaccommodation* occurs when perspective-taking skills that are required for successful communication are reduced or eliminated, and suggests the younger partner's disinterest in the communicative interaction. The result is a predictable breakdown in the interaction. For example, a family member may consistently ignore a grandparent's hearing loss, making no attempt to accommodate appropriately to ensure effective communication.

Overaccommodation occurs when one modifies one's speech style to a stereotypical perception of the older partner (e.g., shouting, using oversimplified language). Overaccommodation may be triggered by numerous cues, as summarized in the research of Ryan and others (e.g., Ryan, Bourhis, & Knops, 1991; Ryan & Capadano, 1978; Ryan & Cole, 1990; Ryan, KwongSee, Meneer, & Trovato, 1992; Ryan & Laurie, 1990). Such trigger cues include institutional setting, role as care recipient, visible signs of aging and/or frailty, use of assistive devices, memory lapse (even if normal), old-sounding speech and voice, and reduced hearing. When partners accommodate to a stereotype or external cues, one result may be inappropriate use of speech registers variously termed "elderspeak" (Cohen & Faulkner, 1986), "patronizing speech" (Ryan et al., 1991), and/or "secondary baby talk" (Caporael, 1981). In general, these speech registers involve oversimplification of language form and vocabulary, exaggerated suprasegmentals, increased volume, higher pitch, more imperatives, and frequent repetition.

Use of variations of elderspeak is judged differently, by both recipients and impartial observers, depending upon the actual cognitive deficits of the older partner. For example, follow-up studies by Caporael (Caporael & Culbertson, 1986; Caporael, Lucaszewski, & Culbertson, 1983) provided data suggesting that cognitively more impaired residents were more likely to appreciate "baby talk," and that these speech styles were perceived as conveying nurturance, but not respect. When scripts of interactions with older adults were presented to subjects, patronizing speech was viewed as showing less respect and lower professional competence, while yielding less resident satisfaction (Ryan et al., 1991; Ryan, Orange, & MacLean, 1993). Respondents judged patronizing speech to be associated with high pitch and exaggerated intonation, along with communication-detracting nonverbal behaviors.

The literature cited above, along with many additional studies, has established that these negative interactional patterns are realities in older communication. Devaluation of older partners and inappropriate speech style accommodations can lead to what has been termed the "Communication Predicament of Aging" (Orange, Ryan, Meredith, & MacLean, 1995). The communication predicament occurs when the older adult not only loses opportunities for communication but also is reinforced for reacting in age-stereotyped ways, resulting in loss of self-esteem and further limitations of social interaction, and an increased likelihood of learned helplessness. A vicious cycle is established.

Inappropriate and detrimental communicative patterns are particularly evident in nursing home settings (Lubinski, 1995). What is interesting is that recent research has established that a variety of unwritten rules and self-regulating beliefs also influence resident-to-resident communications in such settings (Kaakinen, 1995). In general, the influences are negative, limiting frequency and nature of social and communicative interactions. Additional research is needed to clarify the realities constructed between older persons and communication partners of all ages in all settings.

Conclusions and Future Directions

Clearly, heterogeneity is the single common denominator in any description of changes in language and communication in older adults. Aspects of social, physical, and cognitive/affective aging may indirectly influence the frequency and adequacy of involvements in communicative interactions. Attitudes and stereotypes may alter choices of speech style used by conversational partners, often in the direction of negative or demeaning communications. Although neurological substrates of aging may bring subtle reductions in discourse comprehension under difficult task conditions, expressive language skills appear highly variable. Active naming performance appears to decline across the life span, and syntactic complexity may be reduced. Communication of information content, referential skills, verbal fluency, and organization of discourse may show decrements; however, these effects are shown consistently only with considerably advanced age. In contrast, story telling skills may increase.

The dilemma in specifying the nature of language and communication was described at the beginning of this chapter. It is difficult to determine the extent to which observed communicative behaviors are the result of normal aging changes in language systems, indirect responses to life alterations, and/or strategies adopted to deal with aspects of the individual's life situation. Hopefully, ongoing research will continue to clarify those factors contributing to language and communication performance in older adults. In the meantime, practitioners must begin to tease out the influences of normal aging from true pathology, and must be more assertive in accommodating assessments and interventions to the individual older client. The remainder of this text provides models for and innovative examples of management of communication problems in the elderly.

Webb, Schreiner, and Asmuth (1995) have argued convincingly that "no skill serves the older adult better than the ability to communicate effectively with others in face to face interactions [in which they can] literally alter the reality in which they find themselves" (p. 159). As communication disorders professionals, we are committed philosophically to the importance of communication. Yet it is all too easy to get caught up in the intricacies of a speech–language or hearing disorder, losing sight of the larger issues of the aging individual as a communicator in a particular environment, with specific partners and unique assets and liabilities. Interventions designed to maintain or enhance communicative adequacy in "normal" older adults are being reported with increasing frequency in the literature (e.g., Hyde, 1988; Praderas & MacDonald, 1986). Perhaps it is time for speech–language pathologists and audiologists to assume a broader perspective concerning their roles and responsibilities with respect to older adults.

References

Adams, C. (1991). Qualitative age differences in memory for text: A life-span developmental perspective. *Psychology and Aging, 6,* 323–336.

Adams, C., Labouvie-Vief, G., Hobart, C. J., & Dorosz, M. (1990). Adult age differences in story recall style. *Journal of Gerontology, 45,* P17–27.

Albert, M. (1980). Language in normal and dementing elderly. In L. Obler & M. Albert (Eds.), *Language and communication in the elderly* (pp. 145–150). Lexington, MA: D.C. Heath.

Albert, M., Duffy, F. H., & Naeser, J. (1987). Nonlinear changes in cognition with age and their neuropsychologic correlates. *Canadian Journal of Psychology, 41,* 141–157.

Arbuckle, T. Y., Gold, D., Frank, I., & Motard, D. (1989, November). *Speech of verbose older adults: How is it different?* Paper presented at the annual meeting of the Gerontological Society of America, Minneapolis.

Au, R., & Bowles, N. (1991). Memory influences on language in normal aging. In D. N. Ripich (Ed.), *Handbook of geriatric communication disorders* (pp. 293–306). Austin, TX: PRO-ED.

Battle, D. E. (1993). *Communication disorders in multicultural populations.* Boston: Andover Medical Publishers.

Bayles, K. A., & Kaszniak, A. W. (1987). *Communication and cognition in normal aging and dementia.* Boston: Little, Brown.

Benjamin, B. J. (1988). Changes in speech production and linguistic behavior with aging. In B. B. Shadden (Ed.), *Communication behavior and aging: A sourcebook for clinicians* (pp. 164–181). Baltimore: Williams & Wilkins.

Bess, F. H., Lichtenstein, M. J., Logan, S. A., & Burger, M. C. (1989). Comparing criteria of hearing impairment in the elderly: A functional approach. *Journal of Speech and Hearing Research, 32,* 795–802.

Boden, D., & Bielby, D. D. (1983). The past as resource: A conversational analysis of elderly talk. *Human Development, 26,* 308–319.

Boden, D., & Bielby, D. D. (1986). The way it was: Topical organization in elderly conversation. *Language and Communication, 6,* 73–89.

Brandell, M. K., Brandell, R. K., & Hult, R. (1988). Pharmacology and aging. In B. B. Shadden (Ed.), *Communication behavior and aging: A sourcebook for clinicians* (pp. 121–134). Baltimore: Williams & Wilkins.

Cannito, M. P., Hayashi, M. M., & Ulatowska, H. K. (1988). Discourse in normal and pathological aging: Background and assessment issues. *Seminars in Speech and Language, 9,* 117–134.

Caporael, L. R. (1981). The paralanguage of caregiving: Baby talk to the institutionalized aged. *Journal of Personality and Social Psychology, 40,* 876–884.

Caporael, L. R., & Culbertson, G. H. (1986). Verbal response modes of baby talk and other speech at institutions for the aged. *Language and Communication, 6,* 99–112.

Caporael, L. R., Lucaszewski, M. P., & Culbertson, G. H. (1983). Secondary baby talk: Judgments of institutionalized elderly and their caregivers. *Journal of Personality and Social Psychology, 44,* 746–754.

Chafe, W. L. (1982). Integration and involvement in speaking, writing, and oral literature. In D. Tannen (Ed.), *Spoken and written language: Exploring orality and literacy* (pp. 35–54). Norwood, NJ: Ablex.

Chapman, S. B., & Ulatowska, H. K. (1991). Aphasia and aging. In D. N. Ripich (Ed.), *Handbook of geriatric communication disorders* (pp. 241–254). Austin, TX: PRO-ED.

Chapman, S. B., Ulatowska, H. K., King, K., Johnson, J. K., & McIntire, D. D. (1995). Discourse in early Alzheimer's disease versus normal advanced aging. *American Journal of Speech-Language Pathology, CAC Supplement, 4,* 124–129.

Cohen, G. (1979). Language comprehension in old age. *Cognitive Psychology, 11,* 412–429.

Cohen, G., & Faulkner, D. (1981). Memory for discourse in old age. *Discourse Processes, 4,* 253–265.

Cohen, G., & Faulkner, D. (1986). Does 'Elderspeak' work? The effect of intonation and stress on comprehension and recall of spoken discourse in old age. *Language and Communication, 6,* 91–98.

Cooper, P. Y. (1990). Discourse production and normal aging: Performance on oral picture description tasks. *Journal of Gerontology, 45,* P210–214.

Critchley, M. (1984). And all the daughters of musick shall be brought low: Language function in the elderly. *Archives of Neurology, 41,* 1135–1139.

Decker, S. D., & Kinzel, S. (1985). Learned helplessness and decreased social interaction in elderly disabled persons. *Rehabilitation Nursing, 10,* 31–32.

de Santi, S., & Obler, L. K. (1991). Methodological issues in research on aging and language. In D. N. Ripich (Ed.), *Handbook of geriatric communication disorders* (pp. 333–347). Austin, TX: PRO-ED.

Dixon, R. A., Hertzog, C., Friesen, I. C., & Hultsch, D. F. (1993). Assessment of intraindividual changes in text recall of elderly adults. In H. H. Brownell & Y. Joanettte (Eds.), *Narrative discourse in neurologically impaired and normally aging adults* (pp. 77–101). San Diego: Singular.

Dowd, J. J. (1980). *Stratification among the aged.* Monterey, CA: Brooks-Cole.

Drevenstedt, J., & Bellezza, F.S. (1993). Memory for self-generated narration in the elderly. *Psychology and Aging, 8,* 187–196.

Emery, C. F., Huppert, F. A., & Schein, R. L. (1995). Relationships among age, exercise, health, and cognitive function in a British sample. *The Gerontologist, 35,* 378–385.

Emery, O. B. (1985). Language and aging. *Experimental Aging Research, 11,* 3–60.

Emery, O. B. (1986). Linguistic decrement in normal aging. *Language and Communication, 6,* 47–64.

Garfein, A. J., & Herzog, A. R. (1995). Robust aging among the young-old, old-old, and oldest-old. *Journal of Gerontology, 50B,* 277–287.

Glosser, G., & Deser, T. (1992). A comparison of changes in macrolinguistic and microlinguistic aspects of discourse production in normal aging. *Journal of Gerontology, 47,* P266–272.

Gold, D., Andres, D., Arbuckle, T., & Schwartzman, A. (1988). Measurement and correlates of verbosity in elderly people. *Journal of Gerontology, 43,* P27–34.

Goodglass, H., & Kaplan, E. (1983). *The Boston Naming Test.* Philadelphia: Lea & Febiger.

Gould, O. N., & Dixon, R. A. (1993). How we spent our vacation: Collaborative storytelling by young and old adults. *Psychology and Aging, 8,* 10–17.

Goulet, P., Ska, B., & Kahn, H. J. (1994). Is there a decline in picture naming with advancing age? *Journal of Speech and Hearing Research, 37,* 629–642.

Halliday, M. A., & Hasan, R. (1976). *Cohesion in English.* London, England: Longman.

Hartley, J. T. (1988). Aging and individual differences in memory for written discourse. *Language, Memory, and Aging, 3,* 36–57.

Helfrich, H. (1979). Age markers in speech. In R. Klaus, H. Scherer, & H. Giles (Eds.), *Social markers in speech* (pp. 63–107). Cambridge, England: Cambridge University Press.

Heller, R. B., & Dobbs, A. R. (1993). Age differences in word-finding in discourse and nondiscourse situations. *Psychology and Aging, 8,* 443–450.

Holland, A. L. (1990). Research methodology: Part I. Implications for speech–language pathology. In E. Cherow (Ed.), *Proceedings of the Research Symposium on Communication Sciences and Disorders and Aging* (ASHA Report No. 19, pp. 35–39). Rockville, MD: American Speech-Language-Hearing Association.

Hooker, K., & Shifren, K. (1995). Psychological aspects of aging. In R. A. Huntley & K. S. Helfer (Eds.), *Communication in later life* (pp. 99–125). Boston: Butterworth-Heinemann.

Hubbard, R. W. (1991). Mental health and aging. In D. N. Ripich (Ed.), *Handbook of geriatric communication disorders* (pp. 97–111). Austin, TX: PRO-ED.

Hupet, M., Chantraine, Y., & Nef, F. (1993). References in conversation between young and old normal adults. *Psychology and Aging, 8,* 339–346.

Hutchinson, J. M., & Jensen, M. (1980). A pragmatic evaluation of discourse in normal and senile elderly in a nursing home. In L. K. Obler & M. L. Albert (Eds.), *Language and communication in the elderly* (pp. 59–73). Lexington, MA: D. C. Heath.

Hyde, R. B. (1988). Facilitative communication skills training: Social support for elderly people. *The Gerontologist, 28,* 418–420.

Jackson, J. J., & Ensley, D. E. (1995). Minority elders really ain't all alike. In R. A. Huntley & K. S. Helfer (Eds.), *Communication in later life* (pp. 127–156). Boston: Butterworth-Heinemann.

Kaakinen, J. (1995). Talking among elderly nursing home residents. *Topics in Language Disorders, 15,* 36–46.

Kahn, H. J., & Cordon, D. (1993). Qualitative differences in working memory and discourse comprehension in normal aging. In H. H. Brownell & Y. Joanettte (Eds.), *Narrative discourse in neurologically impaired and normally aging adults* (pp. 103–114). San Diego: Singular.

Kaplan , G., Barell, V., Lisky, A. (1988). Subjective state of health and survival in elderly adults. *Journal of Gerontology, 43,* S1114–1120.

Kausler, D. H. (1988). Cognition and aging. In B. B. Shadden (Ed.), *Communication behavior and aging: A sourcebook for clinicians* (pp. 79–106). Baltimore: Williams & Wilkins.

Kemper, S. (1986). Imitation of complex syntactic constructions by elderly adults. *Applied Psycholinguistics, 7,* 277–288.

Kemper, S. (1987). Life-span changes in syntactic complexity. *Journal of Gerontology, 42,* 323–328.

Kemper, S. (1988). Geriatric psycholinguistics: Syntactic limitations of oral and written language. In L. L. Light & D. M. Burke (Eds.), *Language, memory, and aging* (pp. 58–76). New York: Cambridge University Press.

Kemper, S. (1990). Adults' diaries: Changes made to written narratives across the life span. *Discourse Processes, 13,* 207–133.

Kemper, S., Kynette, D., Rash, S., O'Brien, K., & Sprott, R. (1989). Life-span changes to adults' language: Effects of memory and genre. *Applied Psycholinguistics, 10,* 49–66.

Kempler, D., Curtiss, S., & Jackson, C. (1987). Syntactic preservation in Alzheimer's disease. *Journal of Speech and Hearing Research, 30,* 343–350.

Krause, N. (1995). Negative interaction and satisfaction with social support among older adults. *Journal of Gerontology, 50B,* P59–P73.

Kynette, D., & Kemper, S. (1986). Aging and the loss of grammatical forms: A cross-sectional study of language performance. *Language and Communication, 6,* 65–72.

Labov, W., & Auger, J. (1993). The effect of normal aging on discourse: A sociolinguistic approach. In H. H. Brownell, & Y. Joanette (Eds.), *Narrative discourse in neurologically impaired and normal aging adults* (pp. 115–133). San Diego: Singular.

Lichtenburg, P. A., Ross, T., Millis, S. C., & Manning, C. A. (1995). The relationship between depression and cognition in older adults: A cross-validation study. *Journal of Gerontology, 50B,* P25–P32.

Light, L. L., & Anderson, P. A. (1985). Working-memory capacity, age and memory for discourse. *Journal of Gerontology, 40,* 737–747.

Looft, W. R., & Charles, D. C. (1971). Egocentrism and social interaction in young and old adults. *Aging and Human Development, 2,* 21–28.

Lubinski, R. (1991). Learned helplessness: Application to communication of the elderly. In R. Lubinski (Ed.), *Dementia and communication* (pp. 142–151). New York: Decker.

Lubinski, R. (1995). State-of-the-art perspectives on communication in nursing homes. *Topics in Language Disorders, 15,* 1–19.

Maxim, J., & Bryan, K. (1994). *Language of the elderly: A clinical perspective.* London: Whurr.

Molfese, V. J., Hoffman, S., & Yuen, R. (1981–1982). The influence of setting and task partner on the performance of adults over age 65 on a communications task. *International Journal of Aging and Human Development, 14,* 45–53.

Mor, V., Branco, K., Fleishman, J., Hawes, C., Phillips, C., Morris, J., & Fries, B. (1995). The structure of social engagement among nursing home residents. *Journal of Gerontology, 50B,* P1–P8.

Myerson, M. D. (1976). The effects of aging on communication. *Journal of Gerontology, 31,* 29–38.

Neils, J., Baris, J. M., Carter, C., Dell'aira, A. L., Nordloh, S. J., Weiler, E., & Weisiger, B. (1995). Effects of age, education, and living environment on Boston Naming Test Performance. *Journal of Speech and Hearing Research, 38,* 1143–1149.

Norris, M. L. (1981). Social impact of hearing loss in the aged. *Journal of Gerontology, 36,* 727–729.

North, A. J., & Ulatowska, H. K. (1981). Competence in independently living older adults: Assessment and correlates. *Journal of Gerontology, 36,* 576–582.

North, A. J., Ulatowska, H. K., Macaluso-Haynes, S., & Bell, H. (1986). Discourse performance in older adults. *International Journal of Aging and Human Development, 23,* 267–283.

Obler, L. K. (1980). Narrative discourse style in the elderly. In L. K. Obler & M. L. Albert (Eds.), *Language and communication in the elderly* (pp. 75–90). Lexington, MA: D. C. Heath.

Obler, L. K., & Albert, M. L. (1981). Language and aging: A neurobehavioral analysis. In D. S. Beasley & G. A. Davis (Eds.), *Aging: Communication process and disorders* (pp. 107–121). New York: Grune & Stratton.

Obler, L. K., & Albert, M. L. (1984). Language in aging. In M. L. Albert (Ed.), *Neurology of aging* (pp. 245–253). New York: Oxford University Press.

Obler, L. K., Au, R., & Albert, M. L. (1995). Language and aging. In R. A. Huntley & K. S. Helfer (Eds.), *Communication in later life* (pp. 85–97). Boston: Butterworth-Heinemann.

Orange, J. B., Ryan, E. B., Meredith, S. D., & MacLean, M. J. (1995). Application of the Communication Enhancement Model for long-term care residents with Alzheimer's disease. *Topics in Language Disorders, 15,* 20–35.

Pindzola, R. H., McCloskey, L., & Moran, M. J. (1989, November). *Communicative fluency in aged persons.* Paper presented at the annual convention of the American Speech-Language-Hearing Association, St. Louis, MO.

Praderas, K., & MacDonald, M. L. (1986). Telephone conversational skills training with socially isolated, impaired nursing home residents. *Journal of Applied Behavior, 19,* 337–348.

Ptacek, P. H., & Sander, E. K. (1966). Age recognition from voice. *Journal of Speech and Hearing Research, 9,* 273–277.

Ringel, R. L, & Chodzko-Zajko, W. J. (1988). Age, health, and the speech process. *Seminars in Speech and Language, 9,* 95–107.

Ringel, R. L, & Chodzko-Zajko, W. J. (1990). Some implications of current gerontological theory for the study of voice. In E. Cherow (Ed.), *Proceedings of the Research Symposium on Communication Sciences and Disorders and Aging* (ASHA Report No. 19, pp. 66–74). Rockville, MD: American Speech-Language-Hearing Association.

Roth, F. P., & Spekman, N. J. (1984). Assessing the pragmatic abilities of children: Part I. *Journal of Speech and Hearing Disorder, 49,* 2–11.

Ryan, E. B., Bourhis, R. Y., & Knops, U. (1991). Evaluative perceptions of patronizing speech addressed to elders. *Psychology and Aging, 6,* 442–450.

Ryan, E. B., & Capadano, H. L. (1978). Age perceptions and evaluative reactions toward adult speakers. *Journal of Gerontology, 33,* 98–102.

Ryan, E. G., & Cole, R. (1990). Evaluative perceptions of interpersonal communication with elders. In H. Giles, N. Coupland, & J. Weimann (Eds.), *Communication, health, and the elderly* (pp. 172–190). Manchester, England: University of Manchester Press.

Ryan, E. B., Giles, H., Bartolucci, G., & Henwood, K. (1986). Psycholinguistic and social psychological components of communication by and with the elderly. *Language and Communication, 6,* 1–24.

Ryan, E. B., & Johnston, D. G. (1984, November). *The influence of communicative effectiveness on evaluations of younger and older adults speakers.* Paper presented at the annual meeting of the Gerontological Society, San Antonio, TX.

Ryan, E. B., KwongSee, S., Meneer, W. B., & Trovato, D. (1992). Age-based perceptions of language performance among younger and older adults. *Communication Research, 19,* 423–443.

Ryan, E. B., & Laurie, S. (1990). Evaluations of older and younger adult speakers: The influence of communication effectiveness and noise. *Psychology and Aging, 5,* 514–519.

Ryan, E. B., Orange, J. B., & MacLean, M. (1993, August). *Evaluations of communication accommodation in individuals with dementia.* Paper presented at the annual meeting of the American Psychological Association, Toronto.

Schow, R. L, Christensen, J. M., Hutchinson, J. M., & Nerbonne, M. A. (1978). *Communication disorders of the aged: A guide for health professionals.* Baltimore: University Park Press.

Schroeder, A. B. (1986, November). *An analysis of the interaction patterns of the elderly: The deterioration of relationships.* Paper presented at the annual meeting of the Speech Communication Association, Chicago.

Shadden, B. B. (1988). Perceptions of daily communicative interactions with older persons. In B. B. Shadden (Ed.), *Communication behavior and aging: A sourcebook for clinicians* (pp. 12–30). Baltimore: Williams & Wilkins.

Shewan, C. M., & Henderson, V. L. (1988). Analysis of spontaneous language in the older normal population. *Journal of Communication Disorders, 21,* 139–154.

Siegel, G. M., & Gregoria, A. W. (1985). Communication skills of elderly adults. *Journal of Communication Disorders, 18,* 485–494.

Stuart, S., Vanderhoof-Bilyeu, D., & Beukelman, D. (1994). Differences in topic reference in elderly men and women. *Journal of Medical Speech-Language Pathology, 2,* 89–104.

Ulatowska, H. K., Cannito, M. P., Hayashi, M. M., & Fleming, S. G. (1985). Language abilities in the elderly. In H. K. Ulatowska (Ed.), *The aging brain: Communication in the elderly* (pp. 125–140). San Diego: College-Hill Press.

Ulatowska, H. K., & Chapman, S. B. (1991). Neurolinguistics and aging. In D. N. Ripich (Ed.), *Handbook of geriatric communication disorders* (pp. 21–37). Austin, TX: PRO-ED.

Ulatowska, H. K., Hayashi, M. M., Cannito, M. P., & Fleming, S. G. (1986). Disruption of reference in aging. *Brain and Language, 28,* 24–41.

Vogel, D., Sugar, J., & Cardillo, J. (1995, November). *Idiom explanation by older persons.* Paper presented at the annual convention of the American Speech-Language-Hearing Association, Orlando, FL.

von Eye, A., Dixon, R. A., & Krampen, G. (1989). Text recall in adulthood: The roles of text imagery and orienting tasks. *Psychological Research, 51,* 136–146.

Walker, V. G., Roberts, P. M., & Hedrick, D. L. (1988). Linguistic analyses of the discourse narratives of young and aged women. *Folia Phoniatrica, 40,* 58–64.

Webb, L. W., Schreiner, J. M., & Asmuth, M. V. (1995). Maintaining effective interaction skills. In R. A. Huntley & K. S. Helfer (Eds.), *Communication in later life* (pp. 159–179). Boston: Butterworth-Heinemann.

Wechsler, D. (1981). *Wechsler Adult Intelligence Scale–Revised.* New York: Psychological Corp.

Wingfield, A., Wayland, S. C., & Stine, E. A. (1992). Adult age differences in the use of prosody for syntactic parsing and recall of spoken sentences. *Journal of Gerontology, 47,* P350–356.

Yairi, E., & Clifton, N. F. (1972). Disfluent speech behavior of preschool children, high school seniors, and geriatric persons. *Journal of Speech and Hearing Research, 15,* 714–719.

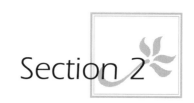

Section 2

Intervention Approaches: A Continuum of Care Settings and Service Delivery Models

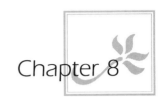

Chapter 8

The Continuum of Care Settings and Service Delivery Models

Joan K. Glickstein

Glickstein's chapter introduces the management section of this text by iden-tifying the continuum of care settings for health care provision to older adults. Evolving models of service delivery designed to accommodate to expanding service delivery sites and rapidly changing reimbursement policies are described. Glickstein urges that, because additional changes in govern-ment regulations and funding systems can be expected over the next 5 to 10 years, speech–language pathologists and audiologists need to stay current and to recognize that, like it or not, health care provision has become a true business.

1. The traditional continuum of care settings and services reflects a rather linear model with little overlap across settings and service providers. How have changes in reimbursement policy and health care delivery models influenced this continuum? What new roles have been assumed by hospitals? By long-term care facilities? By home-based programs? How has competition for the subacute care market influenced service delivery?

2. Define managed care and identify the role of case management in man-aged care systems and the different models for case management service delivery. How is managed care affecting speech–language pathology and audiology service delivery? What changes might be projected for the future?

❧　　　❧　　　❧

It is impossible to understand why certain health care services are delivered at some sites and not at others without some basic understanding of our health care system. The United States has traditionally viewed the delivery of health care services as both medically and crisis oriented. Our current health care delivery system is based on one principle: the cure and eradication of disease. At the time of its inception, this was quite reasonable considering that, in 1900, individuals over age 60 constituted 6.4% of the population and individuals over 65 constituted 2.9% (Gelfand, 1988). The U.S. census did not begin recording persons 100 years or older until 1980. In that year, the census reported 25,000 persons 100 years of age or older. The average age of the U.S. population jumped from 27.9 years in 1979 to 31.5 in 1985. It is this shift in the aging cohort, along with changes in family structure and life-styles, that created the need for continuums of care. It is the cost of providing the services within the continuum that has forced the change in our health care delivery systems. In turn, there has also been a shifting of care settings.

The development of service settings capable of accommodating a crisis-oriented care system created a somewhat arbitrary and artificial division between those services delivered in the hospital and those delivered at other sites. Koff (1988) described two representations of care systems, one linear and one circular. The linear approach is inflexible and does not clearly illustrate appropriate goals for those in need of chronic care. On the other hand, a circular, client-centered configuration has the potential for utilizing a variety of services throughout the trajectory of acute and chronic illness.

Figure 8.1 illustrates the traditional continuum of care settings and the overlapping of services that has occurred within the last 8 years. Table 8.1 lists the traditional services provided in each of the care settings and their expected outcomes. In this traditional service delivery configuration, persons with acute conditions are serviced in acute care facilities (hospitals) and those with long-term conditions are serviced in long-term facilities (nursing homes). There is little or no interaction between service providers. With the exception of those natural linkages that occur through religious affiliation, linkages between settings on either a formal or informal basis are rarely considered. Note that the expected outcome of service delivery at all sites is progression of the client/patient to a higher level of function, creating the impression that rehabilitation services are to be limited to those persons who can demonstrate significant (measurable) gains within a specified time

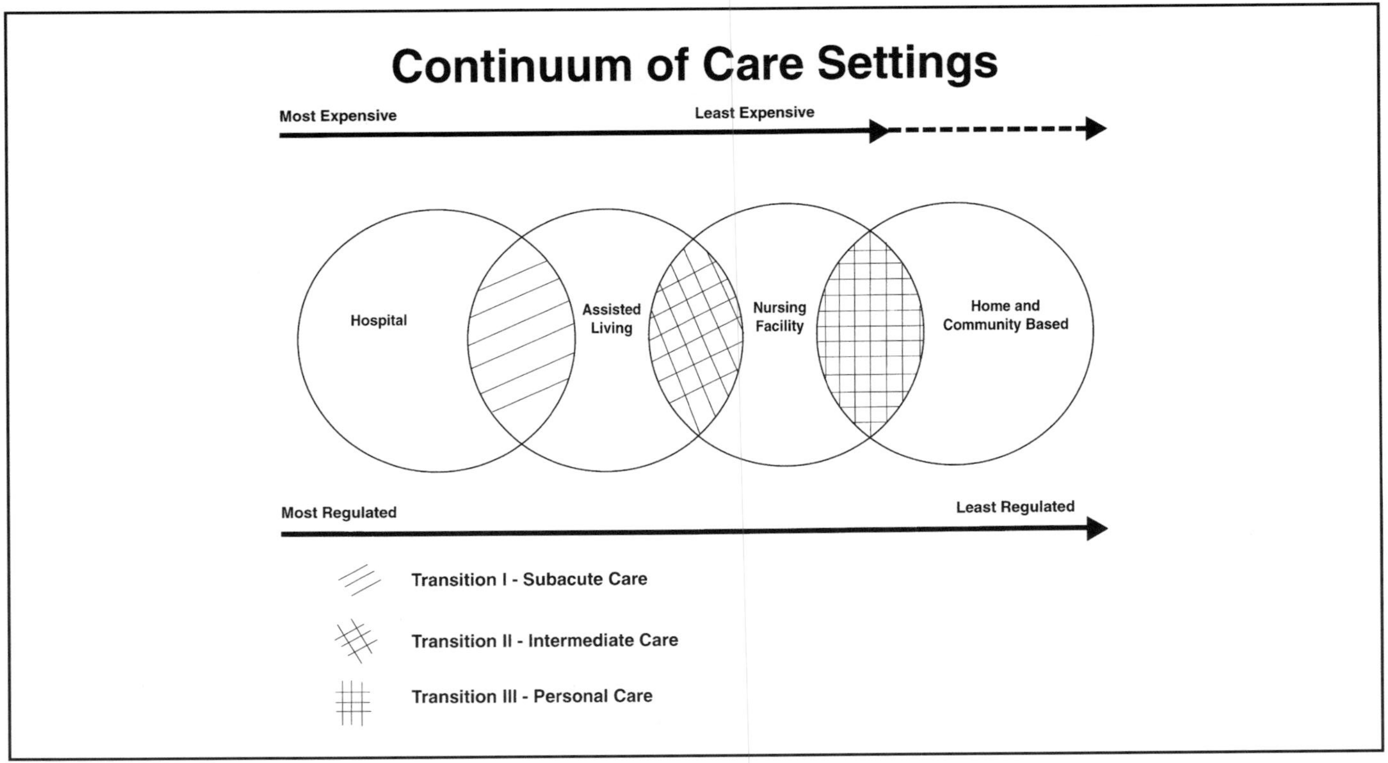

Figure 8.1. Continuum of care settings. *Note.* From *Reimbursable Geriatric Service Delivery: A Functional Maintenance Therapy System*, by J. Glickstein and G. Neustadt, 1992, Gaithersburg, MD: Aspen. Copyright 1994 by GNI. Reprinted with permission.

Table 8.1
Traditional Service Sites and Patient Needs

Site	Patient Type	Needs	Outcomes Expected
Hospital (acute care)	Head trauma, CVA, myocardial infarction	*Medical:* risk for medical instability high *Nursing:* multiple and/or complex rehabilitation needs, potential for high medical acuity skilled nursing *Rehabilitation services (OT, PT, SLP):* high potential based on diagnosis	Progress to higher level of function
Nursing facility (long-term care)	CVA, myocardial infarct, persons who are unable to sustain themselves in community and require general nursing supervision	*Medical:* risk for medical instability low *Nursing:* multiple needs are routine, potential for high medical acuity or skilled nursing on a limited basis *Rehabilitation services (OT, PT, SLP):* potential based on diagnosis	Progress to higher level of function
Assisted living (reduced function)	Dementia, frail elder, persons who are unable to live independently and do not require general nursing services	*Medical:* outpatient medical services for medically stable conditions *Nursing:* may require home health visits *Rehabilitation services (OT, PT, SLP):* need varies based on diagnosis	Progress to higher level of function
Home and community-based (independent living)	Dementia, frail elder, persons who are unable to live independently and do not require general nursing services	*Medical:* outpatient medical services for medically stable conditions *Nursing:* general nursing *Rehabilitation services (OT, PT, SLP):* need varies with diagnosis	Progress to higher level of function

Note. CVA = cerebrovascular accident; PT = physical therapy; OT = occupational therapy; SLP = speech–language pathology.

frame. In practice, this system rations services by denying service to those with chronic or long-standing conditions and those who need minimal service to maintain their current level of function.

Current trends in aging and the demands of the 1987 Omnibus Budget Reconciliation Act (OBRA) to maintain the individual's quality of life in long-term care facilities has forced a shift in the focus of care from acute to chronic and from episodic to long term. This shift in focus, along with changes in public policy and funding, has led to a blending of services and an overlapping of service delivery sites. The major impetus for this change has been the funding stream.

Speech–language pathology, with its roots in medicine and the medical model, has been slow to adapt. Among communication specialists, traditional thinking holds that persons with speech–language disabilities are to be treated only in the acute stages of their disability and persons with long-standing speech–language disabilities are not appropriate candidates for therapy. The result of such thinking has been denial of speech–language services to a segment of the adult population most in need of communication. Perhaps of even greater consequence is the veil of invisibility that has developed around the field itself.

Changes in Reimbursement Policy that Have Affected Changes in Care Settings

Of all the major public programs available in this country, Medicare is by far the largest and most controversial. Although the Medicare system is, in fact, an insurance program, it is viewed by many as a public health program designed as a give-a-way to the elderly. Few people realize that approximately 10% of the Medicare dollar goes to service disabled individuals under the age of 65, or that all persons who pay into the social security system also pay into the Medicare Part A system. Further, Part B of Medicare is both optional and requires a monthly premium that is community rated.

Talk about "changes" or "reform" to the act started on the day the Medicare bill was passed by Congress and has continued ever since. The first forced steps in change in the payment system occurred in 1983 with the advent of diagnosis-related groups (DRGs), a prospective payment system based on the classification of patient illnesses in terms of expected lengths of hospital stay. DRGs were the government's answer to runaway hospital costs. The DRG is a complicated listing of primary and secondary diagnoses that places hospital inpatients into 470 groups. The groups are clinically coherent and homogeneous with respect to resource use. The Health Care Finance Administration (HCFA) bases its Medicare Part A hospital reimbursement levels on DRGs. Under the DRG system, a hospital is compensated for a pre-determined number of days per patient; the hospital is required to absorb the costs of extended-stay patients. In response to the DRG system, hospitals reevaluated their patient care and reduced the number of patient days accordingly.

HCFA then began expanding the Medicare prospective payment system to post-hospital care. The objective was to determine the feasibility of making payments to the hospital or third-party comprehensive Part A payer for inpatient and post-hospital care that would not be contingent on actual use of post-hospital services. Such payments would continue to be based on some type of DRG. The extended prospective payment system would bundle hospital, skilled nursing facility, home health care, and rehabilitation hospital services into a single prospective payment for the entire episode of care.

The next step was to develop a payment system for long-term care similar to the one used in acute care. The designation of RUGs, or Resource Utilization Groups, was the government's response. The RUG system is a classification of individuals by medical condition and Activities of Daily Living (ADL) dependencies. The RUG II payment system is based on the relationship between the care needs of defined groups of individuals and the cost of resources used for their care. Although RUGs are being used in a number of states, the RUG system is not yet the law of the land.

While Congress looks for ways to cut back and/or contain the costs of health care services, service providers continue to look for new market niches in an effort to assure their future survival and profitability. The first big break for hospitals came in 1988. At that time, the Department of Public Welfare recognized distinct-part medical rehabilitation units of general hospitals as separate inpatient providers under the Medical Assistance Program and paid these units under Medicare principles of cost reimbursement, freeing the distinct part from the DRG. Prior to this change, these units were considered part of the acute care hospital and were paid under the DRG prospective payment system. Because the medical rehabilitation units are recognized as separate providers and paid under a retrospective cost reimbursement system, the hospitals receive compensation for the high costs associated with comprehensive rehabilitation.

The certified distinct part (CDP) provides "subacute care," defined as "a comprehensive inpatient program for the individual who has had an acute event as a result of an illness, injury, or exacerbation of a disease process; has a determined course of treatment; and does not require intensive diagnostic and/or invasive procedures. The severity of the individual's condition requires an outcome-focused interdisciplinary approach utilizing a professional team to deliver complex clinical interventions (medical and/or rehabilitation). These highly specialized programs promote quality care through efficient and effective utilization of health care resources" (McDowell, 1995, p. 4). In essence, the CDP creates a mechanism for the acute-care hospital to maximize reimbursement of Medicare patients by creating a facility within a facility. For hospitals with acute rehabilitation programs that are experiencing declining census, adding subacute rehabilitation programs can be a survival strategy.

Changes in Service Delivery Sites

Hospitals

Although the DRG was designed to be used with the Medicare population to determine equitable Medicare Part A reimbursement, the effect of the DRG was to shorten the stay of all hospital patients. The resulting reduction in bed use forced hospitals to take a new look at their customer and service base. Patients left "quicker and sicker." With fewer dollars from inpatients, the hospital had to find new market niches to cover their costs. In the search for new markets, hospitals began to take ownership of outreach programs that were home and community based and to add new specialty units to the existing plant. A comparison of Configuration 1 and Configuration 2 (Figure 8.2 and Figure 8.3) illustrates the hospitals' move into new markets and the shifting of provider settings.

Note that in Configuration 1, the hospital provides both inpatient and outpatient care and may have a tangential relationship to a nursing facility. The customer base is the acute care patient. The relationship with the nursing facility is typically limited to mutual patient referral via the social services department, and the two institutions do

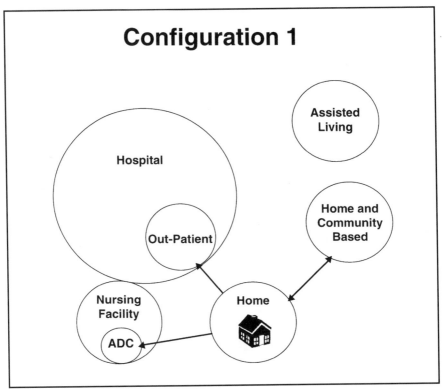

Figure 8.2. Configuration 1: Traditional service provider settings and markets. *Note.* From *Reimbursable Geriatric Service Delivery: A Functional Maintenance Therapy System,* by J. Glickstein and G. Neustadt, 1992, Gaithersburg, MD: Aspen. Copyright 1994 by GNI. Reprinted with permission.

not compete for customers. Adult day-care (ADC) is housed within the nursing facility. Assisted living and home- and community-based services are independent and have no linkage with the hospital.

Whereas hospitals have seen their future in outpatient departments, nursing homes have moved in a different direction. Many nursing homes saw an opportunity in the early 1980s to provide a public service and possibly increase their revenue and client base by providing space for adult day-care. With the Alzheimer's disease movement and growing recognition of the need for adult day-care services for confused adults, space for such services was eagerly sought. Adult day-care was seen by many family members as an opportunity for respite and as an inexpensive alternative to nursing home or

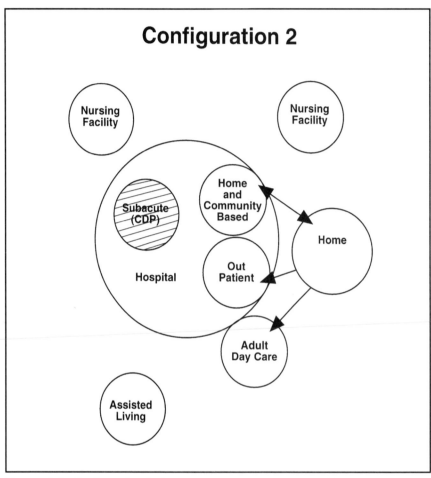

Figure 8.3. Configuration 2. Opening new hospital markets. *Note.* From *Reimbursable Geriatric Service Delivery: A Functional Maintenance Therapy System,* by J. Glickstein and G. Neustadt, 1992, Gaithersburg, MD: Aspen. Copyright 1994 by GNI. Reprinted with permission.

assisted living placement. While offering the caregiver temporary respite at an affordable cost, adult day-care offered nursing facilities an opportunity to provide a needed community service and to build a new customer base.

Configuration 2 (Figure 8.3) illustrates some of the changes brought about by the DRG and the CDP. In this configuration, the hospital retains the traditional customer base and develops a certified distinct part (CDP). Patients are discharged from the traditional part of the hospital and moved to a unit called subacute. The hospital subacute patient is typically one who may or may not be at risk for medical instability, who requires the services of the rehabilitation physician, nursing, and therapy, and whose expected outcome is discharge to the community. All of the services in the subacute unit are geared toward the medical (physical) rehabilitation of the patient. Patients in this unit all qualify for a skilled level of care, which is billed accordingly. This means that patients who would have been discharged to some type of extended care facility for service are now retained by the hospital. In essence, the hospital has gone into direct competition with the nursing facility by retaining patients longer and providing services that would otherwise be provided in a long-term care setting.

The hospital has also begun to compete with traditional home- and community-based programs by adding outreach programs. Services may be offered either directly from the hospital or off-site. For example, the hospital's physical plant would be modified to include offices and other space needed for the provision of services. Alternatively, the hospital might choose to develop satellite facilities within the community, staffed by members of the hospital corporation. Free-standing satellite facilities offer many of the services of the parent hospital but on a limited basis. Some hospitals have set up shop in shopping malls, offering walk-in services and free health screens. In its search for expanding markets, the hospital corporation may establish a tangential link with an adult day-care facility by offering space and/or programs.

Nursing Facilities

Note that in Configuration 2 (Figure 8.3), both the nursing facility and assisted living facility are left on their own. Without linkages and/or support from other health care systems, it becomes more difficult and more costly to establish a firm customer base. To counter a perceived threat to their own market, nursing facilities opted to establish CDPs of their own. Nursing facilities are going head-to-head in competition with hospitals for patients who require intensive rehabilitation services, changing the service delivery provider sites to those shown in Configuration 3 (Figure 8.4). In this configuration, it is the nursing facility that provides the continuum with the exception of acute hospital care.

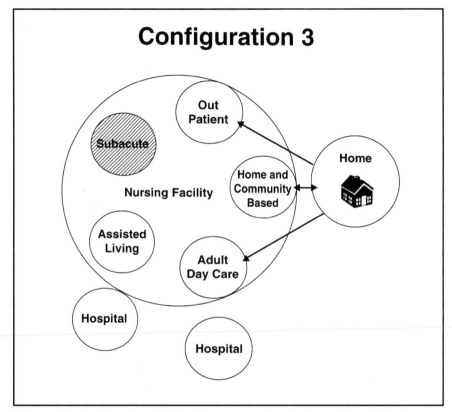

Figure 8.4. Configuration 3: Opening new nursing facility markets. *Note.* From *Reimbursable Geriatric Service Delivery: A Functional Maintenance Therapy System*, by J. Glickstein and G. Neustadt, 1992, Gaithersburg, MD: Aspen. Copyright 1994 by GNI. Reprinted with permission.

The nursing home industry saw entry into the subacute market as a way of attracting new customers and capturing revenues above the usual Part A dollars for residents who required a higher level of skilled services than those seen in the traditional nursing home population. Large nursing home chains started to diversify aggressively into subacute care in the form of distinct, low-cost subspecialty programming. Programs such as medical rehabilitation, ventilator care, traumatic brain injury, and other traditionally high-cost hospital programs are marketed directly to insurance companies and case managers as part of managed care plans. These programs have been effective in moving patients out of hospitals and into nursing facilities.

Medicare currently reimburses nursing facilities at the lower of their costs or charges subject to certain routine cost limits. Because the calculation of these limits is based on the costs of average staffing provided in the late 1980s, skilled nursing facilities that provide true subacute care almost certainly exceed these limits. Therefore, for a nursing facility to successfully provide a Medicare reimbursed subacute unit, the facility must ask for and receive an exception to their routine cost limits. Between 1989 and 1993, the number of nursing facilities that have filed for exceptions to the routine cost limits and developed subacute distinct parts has increased significantly due to the aggressiveness of many of the larger chains and the opportunities perceived in the new managed care markets.

One barrier to nursing home subacute care is the 3-day hospital rule that prevents Medicare from covering care in skilled nursing facilities unless the individual has been hospitalized for 3 days. HCFA is currently looking into the feasibility of waiving the 3-day rule for subacute care. Project supporters say many types of patients, including at-home ventilator patients who develop a temperature and need observation, can be managed just as well in a subacute nursing facility setting as in a hospital. It is not unusual for some patients to go a hospital for the 3-day stay so that they can qualify for subacute care in a nursing facility. Currently, the cost of care in a nursing facility is significantly less than in a hospital. If outcome studies indicate positive or equal results in both hospital and nursing home settings, it will be the cost of care that determines the location of the subacute unit.

While the nursing and hospital industries continue their battle over who will provide subacute care, nursing facilities continue to extend their claim on the continuum by adding outpatient, home- and community-based, and assisted living services. In Configurations 1 and 2 (Figures 8.2 and 8.3), assisted living is identified as a separate service delivery site. In Configuration 3 (Figure 8.4), we see assisted living provided in the nursing facility. Assisted living was added to the list of services as a separate entity when regulations establishing admissions criteria and preadmission screenings for admission to nursing homes were established. Residents of assisted living or personal care facilities require assistance in activities of daily living, cannot function independently in their own home, but do not require 24-hour nursing services. The funding stream has been through private pay and Medicaid. Delivery of rehabilitation services has been on an "as needed" basis. Some nursing facilities have identified separate wings as "assisted living" areas and provide rehabilitation on an out-patient basis through their own rehabilitation departments.

Home Health Care

There are two methods of delivering health care services in the home. The first is through a home health agency and the second is as an out-patient benefit in the home. Although both methods are reimbursed through Medicare, the laws regarding each benefit are quite different.

The Medicare home health agency (HHA) benefit was established by the Social Security Amendments of 1965 (Public Law 89-97) and became effective July 1, 1966. It was originally conceived as a stage in the continuum of care following hospitalization, where the patient's recovery and rehabilitation could be continued effectively at home at a lower cost than at the hospital or in a nursing facility. The evolution of home health from an acute benefit to a long-term care benefit began during the 1970s. Demand for home health care has increased due to the growing number of elderly in the population, especially in the number of Medicare enrollees 85 years or older; the shift from acute to chronic illness needs; increased life expectancy; and an increasingly complex array of expensive and sophisticated medical technologies that can be administered in the home. These factors, combined with the liberalization of the HHA benefit through legislative changes, have helped to make home health the fastest growing component of Medicare spending. Between 1974 and 1990, total HHA payments grew from $141.5 million in 1974 to $3.7 billion in 1990 (Helbing, Sangl, & Silverman, 1992). Among the more significant changes in the law were (a) the Social Security Amendments of 1972 (Public Law 92-603), which eliminated the 20% coinsurance for HHA services furnished under Part B; and (b) OBRA 1980 (Public Law 96-499). Highlights of these acts include the following:

- elimination of the 3-day prior hospitalization requirement as a condition for the receipt of HHA services;
- elimination of the requirement to meet the Part B deductible before Medicare payments for HHA services under Part B can be initiated;
- elimination of the 100 visits per year limit on HHA visits; and

- permission for proprietary HHAs to furnish Medicare-covered services in states not having licensure laws (as a result of this provision, the number of proprietary agencies certified to participate in the Medicare program increased from 165 in 1980 to 1,841 in 1985).

Very simply put, both Medicare hospital insurance (Part A) and supplementary medical insurance (Part B) programs cover HHA services without a deductible or coinsurance charge. Currently there is no limitation on the number of HHA visits covered under Medicare, no prior hospitalization requirement, and no limit to the benefit as long as the beneficiary meets the eligibility criteria for care.

Health services in the home may also be delivered by agencies other than HHAs. However, under Medicare regulations, these services are billed under Part B outpatient services and are subject to all of the Part B regulations, including the deductible and coinsurance. This particular benefit has far-reaching implications for nursing facilities and for hospitals, because it makes it possible for these entities to provide services in the home without having to incur the additional cost involved in a new layer of regulations, staffing, and bookkeeping.

Comprehensive Outpatient Rehabilitation Facilities (CORFs)

Comprehensive Outpatient Rehabilitation Facilities (CORFs) are freestanding nonresidential facilities established and operated exclusively for the purpose of providing diagnostic, therapeutic, and restorative services to outpatients only. CORFs provide rehabilitation services under Part B of Medicare. They are medical in nature, in that they must be operated by or under the supervision of a physician. Although the overwhelming majority of CORF clients require rehabilitation services that are acute or compensatory in nature, there is nothing in the Medicare guidelines that precludes a CORF from establishing maintenance programs. In fact, the Medicare guidelines clearly articulate the CORF's right to establish such programs. A 1989 HCFA transmittal provided guidelines for speech–language pathology and occupational therapy services for submission of claims for outpatient therapy to intermediaries. Section 502.1 B (Maintenance) discussed the documentation necessary to justify a claim for maintenance therapy.

The final paragraph stated: "Your maintenance program will be considered established when it has been designed to fit the patient's level of function and when instructions to the patient and supportive personnel have been completed sufficient for them to safely and effectively carry it out. Give reasonable assurances that this has occurred. After that point, the services will not be considered reasonable and necessary."

Providing the Continuum: Managed Care and Other Integrating Mechanisms

Integrated health care service systems is the term used for those systems having a single point of entry and providing multiple services. An HMO is an integrated service system. Configuration 4 (Figure 8.5) illustrates one type of integrated health care service system with a single point of entry. Ideally, the objective of such a configuration is the efficient delivery of high-quality services that are cost-effective, that do not overlap, and whose goal is to assure users their highest level of independent function. These are more or less the espoused goals of many of today's managed care plans. The objective of managed care is to form integrated delivery systems with other local providers to establish referral chains for patients with changing care needs at a cost savings. Keeping these goals and objectives in mind, one can begin to understand the importance of the linkages shown in Configurations 2 and 3 (Figures 8.3 and 8.4). In a prospective or gate-keeping payment system, the company that can provide "the biggest bang for the buck" is the one that will get the contract.

It is important to recognize that *managed care* is not a term used to identify a single entity or service delivery system. Rather, it is a term used to cover a broad array of payment, provider, and service systems that can be combined in a multitude of ways. Managed care may be viewed on a continuum, with a number of plan types offering an array of features that vary in their abilities to balance access to care, cost, quality control, benefit design, and flexibility. The common thread that seems to run through most, but not all, managed care contracts is a prospective payment system based on a per capita basis. That is, a service provider will receive a predetermined amount of money for agreeing to care for a given number of persons in a specified time frame. The service provider receives that money whether or not the patient is actually treated.

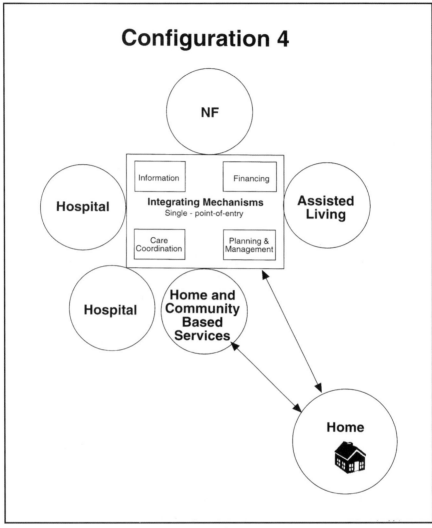

Figure 8.5. Configuration 4: An integrated health care service system with a single point of entry. *Note.* From *Reimbursable Geriatric Service Delivery: A Functional Maintenance Therapy System*, by J. Glickstein and G. Neustadt, 1992, Gaithersburg, MD: Aspen. Copyright 1994 by GNI. Reprinted with permission.

As managed care attempts to define itself, service providers look for ways to fit into the system, and the line between cost and profit continues to shrink as more rehabilitation companies take the plunge into establishing contracts with managed care companies. Establishing a relationship with a managed care entity is relatively straightforward. The rehabilitation company must determine what the payer is looking for, what the needs are in the community, and if anyone else is supplying the service. Before entering into negotiations with a managed care company, the rehabilitation company must have all of the facts regarding the type of patients the payer serves, their rehabilitation needs, the cost of servicing this population, and the risks involved in accepting a per capita contract. It is important that pricing and payment schedules are spelled out contractually. The rehabilitation provider must also know all of the service authorization requirements, as unauthorized services will result in no payment. Contracts should also include a "no cause cancellation" clause. This gives the rehabilitation provider a way out if the negotiated price is too low to care for patients properly.

Case Management

Case management has been called many names, such as case coordination, care coordination, care management, and resource coordination. Case management differs from care planning in that care planning may be one task of the case or care manager. As defined by Kane (1988), case management is "the coordination of a specified group of resources and services for a specified group of people" (p. 5). Kane went on to identify the sequential tasks of case management as follows:

1. case finding or screening to identify people in the target population who may require services;

2. comprehensive, multidimensional assessment to determine any individualized unmet needs;

3. care planning, which requires decisions about how the needs identified in the assessment can be met;

4. implementation of the plan;

5. monitoring both the progress of the client and the adequacy of the services given under the plan; and

6. formal reassessment at intervals to gauge continuing need.

In short, the case manager is the gate keeper at the point of entry to any integrated system of care. Depending upon the system, the case manager may be a social worker, a physician, a nurse, or any other designated professional.

Case management services have been provided to Medicaid recipients living at home since 1981. Section 2176 of the 1981 Omnibus Budget Reconciliation Act (P.L. 97-35) gave the Department of Health and Human Services the authority to grant waivers to states on Medicaid plans. It was reasoned that home- and community-based services could be provided to persons who are Medicaid eligible and determined to be nursing home certifiable at a lower cost than the services provided in an institution.

In the regulations governing the waiver authority, *case management* is defined as "a system under which responsibility for locating, coordinating, and monitoring a group of services rests with a designated person or organization" (Greenberg et al., 1983). Throughout its history, case management has had dual sets of goals. One set relates to service quality, effectiveness, and service coordination. The other set relates to goals of accountability and cost-effective use of resources. Case management has been looked at by both consumer-oriented groups and cost controllers as a way of bridging the information gap, ensuring the equitable delivery of high-quality needed services and eliminating unnecessary services. Kane (1988) stated: "Depending on the design of the system, case management can increase the quality and the efficiency of care . . . [by] generating better information about the outcomes for individual clients; generating better information about the performance of service providers; identifying gaps and duplications; and gaining greater control over quality" (p. 5).

From the beginning, case management was a popular and readily acceptable concept to a variety of health care providers. Austin (1993) felt that case management was accepted because "it has not been viewed as a systemic reform, but as a function that can be incorporated into ongoing delivery systems without changing structural relationships among providers" (p. 17).

A key to case management effectiveness in the areas of system development and cost containment is the case manager's authority to allocate resources in the development of care plans for clients. Austin (1983) described three basic types of case management models, each having its origins in the way care planning is implemented.

1. Broker model—Brokers do not have dollars to allocate on behalf of their clients. They make referrals and follow up with their

clients and the providers. In this model, there is no guarantee that the services or providers recommended will be the ones received.

2. Service management model—The case manager has fiscal responsibility for allocation of service dollars, usually a specified percentage of nursing home costs. It is the case manager's responsibility to develop care plans within predetermined cost caps. This is the model found in Medicaid home- and community-based waiver (2176) programs.

3. Managed care model—The financial responsibility and liability for expenditures are shifted to the provider through capitated provider contracts. If the provider can deliver services at a cost lower than the dollar amount in the contract, the provider keeps the surplus. However, if the cost exceeds the amount agreed upon, the provider must assume the excess costs.

The major responsibilities of the case manager in each case are care planning and resource allocation. Case managers function as resource allocators and distributors in their local delivery systems. They potentially operate with considerable power and authority.

Managed Medical Care

Managed medical care is an outgrowth of the private sector, dating back some 60 years. In the 1970s, prepaid group and solo practice plans were recast into a popular marketable entity called a Health Maintenance Organization (HMO), with the development of Preferred Provider Organizations (PPO) later in the same decade. Both prepaid group and individual practice associations ushered in a new kind of corporate health care delivery in the United States. For the first time, physicians shared the risk of financing health care for an enrolled population. In return, physicians were offered the choice between billing and collecting a fee-for-service from the patient or having the HMO pay the physician directly out of prepaid per capita payment (capitation) for health care services. These models led to widespread dissemination of managed care plans. HMOs assumed responsibility for providing a comprehensive range of health services to voluntarily enrolled populations at a fixed annual premium.

A major factor in the overall success of HMOs was the willingness of physicians to accept financial risk in providing health and medical care services to groups of subscribers. If HMO physicians incurred expenses exceeding budgeted costs, then part or all of the shortfall would have to be absorbed by the physicians. On the other hand, any excess in revenues over expenditures could be shared by physicians. Enrollees were to achieve savings in health insurance premiums mainly by reduction in the number of unnecessary hospital admissions and length of hospital stays. By combining coverage for outpatient and inpatient care in a single premium, HMOs reduce hospitalization utilization by shifting some services to a less expensive ambulatory setting.

HMO physicians always share the risk for overutilization of medical care. They are also subject to corporate influences, such as those arising from mergers, buy outs, and diversification, as well as to having their services marketed to the public.

Structure of Health Maintenance Organizations (HMOs)

An HMO is a corporate entity that (a) has an organized system for providing health care in a geographic area, (b) accepts responsibility to provide or otherwise assure the delivery of an agreed-upon set of basic and supplemental health maintenance and treatment services, (c) has a voluntarily enrolled group of persons, and (d) is reimbursed through a predetermined, fixed, periodic prepayment made by or on behalf of each person or family unit enrolled in the HMO without regard to the amounts of actual services provided (from the report of the Committee on Interstate Commerce on the Health Maintenance Organization Act of 1973, Public Law 93-22, in which the term is legally defined).

HMOs are considered alternative health delivery systems that provide comprehensive health care services. They emphasize preventive and primary health care as a means of reducing health costs. HMOs can have a variety of forms, names, and sponsors and may be either for profit or nonprofit. They may be based in a hospital, medical school, or private clinic, and may be publicly or privately owned, consumer owned, union owned, or physician owned. There are five basic HMO formats. These models differ on the basis of how the HMO relates to its participating physicians.

Staff Model. In the staff model, physicians are employed directly by the HMO. Staff model HMOs have a greater degree of control over the practice patterns of their practitioners, and as a result, can better manage and control the utilization of health services.

Group Model. In the group model, the HMO contracts with a separate medical group entity, and the medical group is compensated on a capitation basis for each individual enrolled by the HMO.

Individual Practice Association (IPA). In the IPA, the HMO purchases from physicians who are independent contractors rather than employees of or partners in the group. Also, the physicians continue to practice in their own offices, so the number of HMO delivery sites is greatly expanded.

Network. In the network format, the HMO contracts with more than one group practice to provide physician services to its members. These group practices may be broad based, multispecialty groups. An example of this type of HMO is Health Insurance Plan of Greater New York, which contracts with many multispecialty physician group practices in the New York area.

Direct Contract. In the direct contract format, the HMO contracts directly with individual physicians to provide physician services, attempting to recruit broad panels of community physicians to provide physician services as participating providers. These HMOs usually recruit both primary care and specialist physicians and typically use a primary care case management approach (also known as a gatekeeper system).

Social Health Maintenance Organizations (SHMOs)

The SHMO is a newer version of the traditional HMO. SHMOs provide a wider range of services than traditional HMOs. Although they structure service delivery along a modified but traditional medical model, they include social and rehabilitative services. Allied health professionals provide most of the rehabilitation in SHMOs. Rehabilitation services are offered solely to disabled individuals who are considered likely to experience functional improvement. However, SHMOs offer more flexibility for allocating resources among interventions that are not ordinarily considered medically necessary, but that may be critical in maintaining independence, such as grab bars and ramps.

Summary

As care settings and service providers begin to overlap, the lines between acute and chronic care begin to converge. The newest market, transitional care (subacute, intermediate, personal), represents the next battleground for Medicare dollars. While hospitals and nursing facilities compete for the subacute dollars, a variety of aggressive for-profit companies are looking to move into nontraditional settings where regulation is either weak or nonexistent. However, the movement from most regulated to least regulated settings has prompted the government to begin development of an entirely new set of regulations. Questions relating to the least expensive versus the most cost-effective service delivery system are yet to be addressed. One thing is certain; the health care stakes are enormous for everyone from the consumer to the provider. The challenge for the consumer is access to quality care. The challenge to the service provider is to stay in the game.

Communication disorders specialists must stay abreast of the times. They must be aware of changes in government regulations and funding systems in order to maximize service delivery. Prospective payment systems under managed care leave no room for "frills." If speech–language pathologists and audiologists cannot prove their worth through documented outcomes, their services will either be eliminated or be provided through "more cost-effective methods." In the 1990s, the business of health care is neither health nor care. It is business! As specialists in communication disorders, clinicians and universities must join forces to develop a database on functional outcomes, clinical pathways, and the use of auxiliary personnel. All of this must be put into the context of a funding and health care delivery system that is in flux.

References

Austin, C. D. (1983). Case management in long term care: Options and opportunities. *Health and Social Work, 8,* 16–30.

Gelfand, D. E. (1988). *Adulthood and aging: The aging network: Programs and services* (Vol. 8, 3rd ed.). New York: Springer.

Glickstein, J., & Neustadt, G. (1992). *Reimbursable Geriatric Service Delivery: A Functional Maintenance Therapy System.* Gaithersburg, MD: Aspen.

Greenberg, J., et al. (1983). *An analysis of responses to the Medicaid home and community based long term care waiver program (Section 2176 of PL 97-35).* Washington, DC: National Governors Association, State Medicaid Information Center.

Health Maintenance Organization Act of 1973, Public Law No. 93-22.

Helbing, C., Sangl, J., & Silverman, H. A. (1992). Home health agency benefits. *Health Care Financing Review, Annual Supplement,* 125–148.

Kane, R. (1988). Introduction. *Generations, 12,* 5.

Koff, T. H. (1988). *New approaches to health care for an aging population. Developing a continuum of chronic care services.* San Francisco: Jossey-Bass.

McDowell, T. (1995, February). Study finds Medicare savings in subacute care. *Subacute Care Report, 1,* 1–7.

Omnibus Budget Reconciliation Act of 1980, Public Law No. 96-499.

Omnibus Budget Reconciliation Act of 1981, Public Law No. 97-35.

Omnibus Budget Reconciliation Act of 1987, Public Law No. 100-203.

Social Security Amendments of 1965, Public Law No. 89-97.

Social Security Amendments of 1972, Public Law No. 92-603.

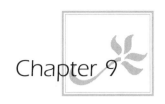

Chapter 9

Functional Communication Assessment and Outcomes

Paul R. Rao

In earlier chapters, several authors have addressed issues of functional assessment specific to their disciplines. In Chapter 9, Rao explores broad issues of functional assessment of the elderly as these issues apply specifically to speech–language pathology. The effects of age-related changes in behavior and skills are acknowledged, and principles of functional assessment are outlined. A description of some commonly used functional communication assessment tools is provided.

1. *How do aspects of aging affect the manner in which we approach functional communication assessment in older adults? In addition to the examples provided by Rao, what other normal aging changes may have an impact on assessment procedures?*

2. *How does the World Health Organization's classification of impairment, disability, and handicap influence the way in which we view communication disorders in older adults, and the assessment approaches we adopt for each level of this classification?*

3. *What is the focus or purpose of functional communication assessment, as defined by an American Speech-Language-Hearing Association (1990) panel? How does functional communication assessment differ from more traditional skills assessments?*

4. *Describe the basic elements of a functional communication assessment, as defined by Rao. Select three commonly used functional communication measures described in this chapter and compare them in terms of purpose, scope, measurement domains, and scoring properties.*

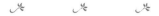

F unctional assessment and functional outcomes have become the buzzwords of the health care industry in recent years. Related concept and practice patterns have been debated at the level of public policy, federal legislation and regulations, and accreditation standards: Third-party guidelines are being modified to include mandates for measurable functional outcome (Frattali, 1992). DeJong (1987) summarized the concerns of functional assessments and outcomes in three dimensions: (a) independence, (b) productivity, and (c) wellness. Each of these dimensions can be framed in terms of a question related to the consumer of services: "First, can a person live *independently,* i.e., can a person live in a relatively unstructured environment with a minimum of hands on care or supervision? Second, can the person live actively and *productively* not only in terms of gainful employment, but also in terms of contributions to family and community life? Finally, can a person remain *free of preventable complications* that result in downstream health care utilization, especially hospital care?" (DeJong, 1987, p. 261). These questions take on particular significance when the target behavior is communication and the target recipient group is the elderly. Communication disorders professionals are working to apply the terms and concepts of functionality to communication assessments and interventions for all age groups. In the case of older adults, concepts of functional communication and outcomes must be framed within the context of the heterogeneity of this population and the varied aspects of aging influencing behavior in a given individual.

This chapter addresses functional communication and assessment in the elderly through an integration of the consumer and the clinical perspectives. As background, the first sections review gerontological considerations and age-related changes that may have an impact on the conduct and interpretation of a functional communication assessment. The World Health Organization's (WHO; 1980) classification of impairment, disability, and handicap is provided as a framework for looking at levels of functioning and the different assessment required at each level. In the second portion of the chapter, functional communication and functional communication assessment are defined further. Distinctions between traditional comprehensive communication assessment and functional communication assessments are discussed. Both informal and formal functional communication assessment approaches—involving client, significant other, and additional members of the rehabilitation care team—are presented. Case examples illustrate how appropriate functional assessment can lead to reduction in disability and handicap, despite a chronic impairment of specific skills.

Context for the Functional Communication Assessment of Older Adults

Consumer Perspectives

In "Harassing the Elderly," Karen DeCrow (1993) asked, "Why do young psychiatrists demean patients with tests that dismiss a life full of experience?" (p. 11A). DeCrow was referring to her observations of mental status exams being administered periodically throughout the day to her 83-year-old mother, who had been admitted to the hospital for observation following an unexplained fall. What was striking about DeCrow's indictment was how "on the mark" her criticism was of the content, style, and administration of many geriatric assessment tools. They seem more designed to entrap than to assess the elderly. Here was a young neurology resident of 25 interrogating a cultured, educated, but clearly anxious, elderly woman. "What time is it?" with no clock visible from the bed. "What day is it?" with no calendar in the room. "Spell the word 'world' backwards." Not a functional query. "How many children do you have?" (The skeptical resident verified the answer with the embarrassed daughter who was observing this "testing.") Mental status exams may be necessary, but this demeaning exercise is heaped upon at-risk elderly clients with as much regularity as meals and often with as much caring as tray delivery. These tests may resemble the give-and-take one might encounter in a functional communication assessment, but they do not exemplify quality functional assessment.

Batavia (1991), a consumer, attested to the fact that consumers *are* interested in both the process and outcomes of the services that they receive: "They want the process to be conducted in a dignified manner, and not to be in any way degrading. In this regard, it is important that the consumer be informed about the process of functional assessment and how it affects the overall plan of care" (p. 9). By serving as an active partner/team member, the consumer can contribute to assessing his or her progress and to setting functional goals. Health care workers and older patients must work together to ensure that these functional goals maximize productivity, creativity, well-being, and happiness (Friedan, 1993).

Gerontological Considerations and Age-Related Changes

U.S. health care has added years to life. According to the most recent census report (U.S. Bureau of the Census, 1990), there are 30 million Americans 65 or older and our overall life span is creeping upward and now stands at 75 years and 5 months. Today, more than ever before, the focus on aging and rehabilitation is on "adding life to years" or, as Friedan has suggested, living well, more than simply living. She described this change as truly evolutionary, since the new emphasis will be on productivity, not just survival.

Williams (1990), the guru of the National Institute on Aging, has suggested that this goal of aging is fundamentally a rehabilitative one: to restore and/or maintain the maximum degree of independence possible for each older person. His personal optimistic note to facing the millennium is as follows: "We now know, from much recent research as well as everyday observations, that the majority of older persons, even those with some partially disabling conditions, can maintain good overall vigor in very late years—the nineties at least and possibly longer" (p. 5). The results of the Baltimore longitudinal study (cited in Williams, 1990) show that most of the organs of the human body do not wear out. It also shows that through use, such as physical exercise and mental activity, much of previously lost function due to inactivity can be regained, with measurable benefits to muscle, bone, heart, and mind.

Thus a rehabilitation focus is clearly the preferred approach for the gerontologist seeking to extend the life span and for the communication disorders professional seeking to maximize personal independence and dignity and to contribute to a satisfactory quality of life (Granger, 1984). As holistic health care givers, speech–language pathologists (SLPs) and audiologists must treat the whole person. In doing so, they must factor in a number of important aging realities.

The first aging reality is the heterogeneity of the older population. Ruth Weg (1986), a noted professor of gerontology, offered some particularly sage reflections on this topic: "Aging is multidimensional. It is everything that relates to being a human being. What is most fascinating about looking at aging processes is that they are not the same, even in groups of persons the same ages. The older we get the more different we become from one another. We are living out a unique inheritance that each of us has, with a unique set of life experiences. We need to begin to assess people in terms of their functional ages. Chronology is the least reliable indicator of all" (p. 3).

A second set of aging realities pertains to stereotypes about attitudes toward older individuals. In a "My Turn" piece in *Newsweek* (Rubinstein, 1991), the 72-year-old author warned us about the hype of the golden years. "They are not the best of times. It's just that the alternative is even worse" (p. 13). Pessimism permeates his column, which presents his perspective as popular '90s realism. Such pessimism contrasts sharply with other positive stereotypes of aging, those depicting a time of unlimited freedom from responsibilities and cares, of self-growth and actualization. The truth probably lies somewhere in the middle—aging is no bane or boon, but is often a decremental biologic and psychosocial process. However, the presence of decrement or change does not lead inevitably to disability, nor is it predictable in any individual older adult. Care must be taken that "ageism," in any form, does not influence service provision.

As Rubenfield (1986) pointed out at the 1984 Conference on Aging and Rehabilitation, older persons are actually under the double jeopardy of the prejudices of "ageism" and "disabilityism." Williams (1990) documented many examples of these prejudices on the part of consumers and professionals alike. For example, physical therapists assessing hypothetical patient descriptions indicated that they would be much less aggressive in their treatment goals for an older, compared to a younger, patient with the same condition. Studies of medical advice on preventive measures also indicate less vigorous efforts by physicians with older, compared to younger, patients. Do we believe that "you can't teach old dogs new tricks?" Concerns about age biases and their impact on patient outcomes and quality of care prompted the Joint Commission on the Accreditation of Health Care Organizations (1995) to build into its new accreditation standards a mandate that rehabilitation staff working in facilities caring for an elderly population must demonstrate specific competencies (knowledge, skills, and abilities) unique to that population.

Chapters 2 through 7 of this text identify many aspects of aging that may positively or negatively influence the older individual's function and life adaptation. Table 9.1 outlines some of the known

Table 9.1
Age-Related Changes

Biological[a]	Psychological	Social
Muscle strength	Slow learning pace	Negative view of aging
Cardiac function	More repetitions	Less frequent referrals
Pulmonary function	Rehabilitation skepticism	Self-ageism
Orthostatic changes	Self-doubt	Financial barriers
Peripheral vascular resistance	Outcome doubt	Smaller circle of friends

Note. From "Introduction," by K. Brummel-Smith, 1990. In B. Kemp, K. Brummel-Smith, and J. Ramsdall (Eds.), *Geriatric Rehabilitation.* Boston: College Hill.
[a]The biological functions all reflect a decrement/reduction of normal function.

age-related changes in the elderly that may affect audiologist's and speech–language pathologist's rehabilitation efforts. The physiologic changes may result in an older person being fatigued more and, as a result, having reduced endurance. The psychologic changes may result in an elderly person requiring more repetitions and time to learn a given new task. In addition, the professional may encounter the psychological barrier of the older adult being suspicious of the clinician's own abilities, the value of rehabilitation, and/or whether one has enough time left to adjust to a change in condition.

The functional assessment of older adults requires the SLP and audiologist to be cognizant of the above gerontological considerations, as well as age-related changes. This requires a unique clinical perspective, because the elderly population in general has such unique needs. Do we adapt the test situation for the obvious visual and auditory challenges our elderly clients face? Do we conduct shorter sessions to obviate fatigue? Lezak (1983) cautioned that clinicians should be sensitive to the psychological orientation that elderly persons may bring to a test or other structured task. The biological, psychological, and social factors noted in Table 9.1 should help to sensitize the clinician. Lezak noted that the most important factor in the assessment may be enlisting the cooperation of the elderly client: "With no school requirements to be met, no jobs to prepare for, and usually little previous experience with psychological tests, a retired person may reasonably not want to go through a lot of fatiguing mental gymnastics that may well make him look stupid to the youngster in the white coat sitting across the table. Particularly if they are not feeling well or are concerned about diminishing mental acuity, elderly persons may view a test as a nuisance or an unwanted intrusion into their privacy" (p. 118). It is important to anticipate these feelings and let the patient know before, during, and after the test that such misgivings are perfectly natural and understandable. Lezak suggested testing older clients with meaningful and nonthreatening materials, such as playing cards. Elderly persons sometimes have little patience for activities that have no apparent relevance to their daily lives, and many structured tasks and tests are filled with such unfamiliar activities. To this end, Hooper and Johnson (1991) have stressed that our challenge will be to educate the clinician or clinical observer to be a geriatric thinker—one who adapts perceptions and expectations during the assessment of the older adult: "Four main procedural changes in assessment of the older adult will make the results more valid and meaningful. Adjusting the 'test' and the instructions; adjusting the examiner's expectations; adjusting the goals of the assessment; and adjusting the listening, speaking, and observing skills of the examiner will all lend more meaning to the results" (p. 308).

Framing Functional Assessment Within the WHO Model

An interesting approach to the concept of rehabilitation is to start from the premise that we are all disabled. We are, for example, unable to drill a hole in the wall with a finger or lift a car to change a tire. We overcome these disabilities (challenges) by finding the right "assistive device" to do the job—a drill or a car jack. Similarly, I may want to become a professional basketball player, but my 5'8" height makes me vertically challenged. In other words, all humans have limitations. The integrated role for rehabilitation and gerontology is to work with older adults along a continuum of ability to disability, removing barriers to independence along the way. A model for conceptualizing this process was presented in "Rehabilitation: Closing The Gap" (National Rehabilitation Hospital [NRH]; 1986) and is shown in Figure 9.1. Although the model focuses on physical disability, it is easy to consider the individual older adult as falling somewhere along the functional ability continuum, and requiring varying levels and intensities

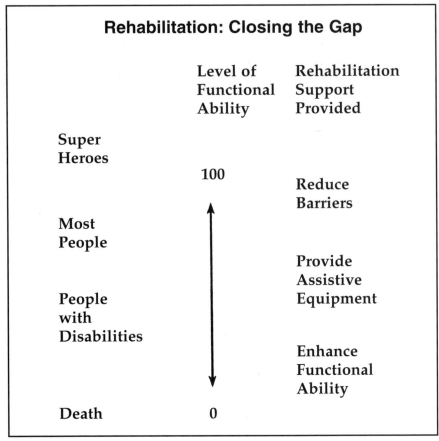

Figure 9.1. The functional ability continuum. From "Rehabilitation: Closing the Gap," by the National Rehabilitation Hospital, 1986, *NRH Today*, p. 1. Copyright 1986 by the National Rehabilitation Hospital. Reprinted with permission.

of rehabilitation support designed to reduce barriers (the demands and challenges of the environment), provide assistive equipment, and enhance functional ability.

The WHO (1980) *International Classification of Impairments, Disabilities, and Handicaps* is particularly helpful in framing the assessment of the elderly along a disability continuum and helping clinicians and clients conceptualize where the elderly person is experiencing the most difficulty in his or her daily activities. This system categorizes a wide range of disease consequences and suggests points of intervention or assistance to help individuals cope with their difficulties. *Impairment,* the first WHO level, refers to damage to or dysfunction of an organ or part of the body (e.g., poststroke, an aphasic language impairment). *Disability* refers to the way in which an impairment affects the functions of an individual (e.g., poststroke, the person with aphasia can no longer communicate on the telephone). *Handicap* refers to the way in which impairment and disability influence a person's reintegration into the community (e.g., poststroke, the person with aphasia must drop her responsibilities as president of a local woman's club, leading to increased social isolation).

Much of the appeal of the WHO classification system lies in the fact that it already enjoys worldwide acceptance, promoting a comprehensive approach for helping persons with disabilities and for preventing new problems and the deterioration of functions. The system also holds promise as a means of achieving a common vocabulary for research; it can assist clinicians in the systematic organization of concepts to facilitate data collection and assessment. Thus we can talk about functional interventions that are designed specifically to prevent diseases that cause impairments, that measure disability and outcomes, and that reduce handicap in the elderly. Wilkerson (1994) has expanded on the WHO model, describing micro-, meso-, and macrolevels of function that parallel closely the concepts of impairment, disability, and handicap. She emphasized the need to demonstrate linkages between microlevel treatment and macrolevel goals and outcomes.

The ultimate question is, Does what we do make a difference in the lives of our clients? Batavia (1991) stressed that "with appropriate rehabilitative interventions, an impairment does not necessarily result in a disability. Similarly, with appropriate social and environmental interventions, a disability does not necessarily result in a handicap" (p. 3). When the WHO framework is applied to evaluating a person with a suspected communication disorder, the role each type of measure plays in a comprehensive assessment becomes clear (see Table 9.2 for an illustration of the model applied to hearing loss in the elderly). According to Frattali (1991), each level requires a different approach to measurement: "Our traditional diagnostic tools are known to measure impairment. They are useful for differential diagnosis and identification of specific speech, language, swallowing, hearing deficits and strengths. Functional assessment tools measure ability to communicate in natural environments. Quality of life scales or handicap inventories measure handicaps. Measures of handicap capture physical, psychosocial, technologic, and economic barriers that create dependency or suppress quality of life" (p. 12). For older clients, disability

Table 9.2
WHO Model Applied to Hearing Loss in the Elderly

Classification Level	Disease	Impairment	Disability	Handicap
Definition	Medical illness	→ Abnormality of structure or function at the organ level ↓	→ Functional consequences of an impairment ↓	→ Social consequences of impairment or disability ↓
Example	Presbycusis	Hearing impairment ↓	Problems listening to conversation ↓	Avoids social opportunities ↓
Outcome		Audiometric evaluation	Functional status measures	Handicap inventory

and handicap may be influenced strongly by age-related factors apart from the specific speech–language–hearing impairment. Speech–language pathologists and audiologists must be aware that assessment of handicap completed by other professional disciplines may contain information critical to our planning for treatment outcomes.

Functional Communication Assessment

Functional Communication Defined

Functional communication has been defined by an American Speech–Language–Hearing Association (ASHA) panel (1990) as "the ability to receive or to convey a message, regardless of the mode, to communicate effectively and independently in a given [natural] environment" (p. 1). This simple but powerful definition relates to functional assessment in a number of ways. First, the ASHA definition views communication as an integrated process in the context of human behavior, rather than as a set of communication components of voice, speech, language, fluency, and resonance. Second, the definition accepts any mode of communication; the older adult can get his or her message across via speech, tone of voice, gesture, drawing, or any other vehicle. Implicit in the definition as well is the concept of burden of care; the more assistance one needs to get a message across, the more dependent one is, and consequently, the more demands are placed on the partner. Thus functional independence is valued inherently as a goal in communicating a message—not just independently but effectively. The assessment of the effective communicator, therefore, must take into consideration how accurate, appropriate, responsive, prompt, and efficient the messenger is.

It has been clear for many years that there is a discrepancy between language and communication (Rao, 1994c). Spoken language usually serves as the primary means for communication, but the communication process also makes use of a variety of other tools, such as intonation, facial expression, eye movements, and body gestures. When the adult with language impairment attempts to communicate, the differences between language and communication become clear. The person with severe aphasia may score poorly on a test that measures impairment but well on a functional assessment tool that measures disability. Conversely, a person with a dementia may score well on a test that measures impairment but poorly on a functional assessment tool that measures disability. The bottom line is the need to assess skills in naturally occurring environments and activities.

The Nature and Roles of Functional Assessment

The difference between the "clinical" and "functional" assessment of the elderly boils down to what the person *cannot* do in the clinic and what he or she *can* do in context (Rao, 1990). Thus, the functional communication assessment of older adults must, by definition, focus on communication in context and strive to determine the impact of primary or secondary aging on natural communication in as many environments as necessary to reflect the client's premorbid functioning.

Consonant with the above definition of functional communication, the ASHA (1990) advisory group defined functional assessment this way: "Functional assessment of communication assesses the extent of the ability to communicate with others in a variety of contexts, considering environmental modifications, adaptive equipment, time required to communicate, and listener familiarity with the client. Special accommodations of the communication partner to either receive or enhance the reception of messages must be considered"

(p. 2). Clearly, this definition of functional assessment goes considerably beyond traditional comprehensive communication assessment (see Rao, 1994a, p. 297, and the ASHA "Preferred Practice Patterns for the Professions of Speech–Language Pathology," 1993, pp. 77–78, for a review of what constitutes a comprehensive communication assessment in speech–language pathology). Functional communication assessment cannot replace the traditional assessment batteries, but together, these measures can accurately profile impairment and disability. For example, how does an aphasic individual's problem following commands affect that individual in naturally occurring activities such as ordering a Big Mac or writing a check?

The focus of functional communication assessment is on *ability* rather than disability or deficit (Frattali, 1992). Once abilities/disabilities are established within the broad spectrum of giving and getting a message, more personalized assessments can be undertaken to answer questions related to handicap (Frattali, Thompson, Holland, Wohl, & Ferketic, 1995). Aten (1986, p. 270) elaborated: "One must consider the severity of the communicative disturbances, the pre-morbid life-style of the patient, and the setting in which the person will ultimately reside." If a disability can be termed a "limitation of choice" (Rao, 1994c), then the functional assessment of the older adult with a disability can be geared toward determining what increased communication opportunities realistically can be realized to maximize the person's options.

One further point must be made before proceeding to an examination of specific functional communication assessment approaches. Issues of functionality are not unique to the communication disorders professions. Our clinicians want our functional assessment tools to be sensitive to functional changes and to cultural differences. Gerontologists desire measures that do not ceiling out with return to the community. Consumers want assessments to be relevant to their daily living needs and to be more individualized and reliable.

At the same time, there is rapid growth and competition in both the rehabilitation and gerontology markets. The sheer number of options and levels of care requires providers to document outcomes and to do so in an integrated and systems-wide approach. Hosek et al. (1986) studied relationships among the cost of rehabilitative care, functional status, and diagnostic classification; he found that functional status, rather than classification, is a better predictor of costs. Not surprisingly, third-party payers want all players to use functional measures;

institutions are being approved prospectively on cost, quality, and outcomes. Functional measures are being used increasingly as a means to set reimbursement rates for rehabilitation care. Most program evaluation procedures are being linked to functional assessment and outcomes. In other words, not only is functional communication a preferred practice pattern, but it is also being mandated by workplace pressures.

Preassessment Measures

The assessment of functional communication involves a series of tasks, including but not limited to the actual administration of some type of functional communication scale or test. Prior to the administration of a formal scale or test, a number of prerequisite evaluative tasks should be accomplished by the clinician, the significant other (SO), and, if possible, by the person served:

- preinterview questionnaire
- interview and case history
- attitude scales
- natural observation
- communication questionnaire

Unfortunately, in the current managed care health care environment, there is less time than ever before to conduct preliminary "intelligence gathering" (Freda & Rao, 1995). In most service delivery settings, the average time between admission of the person served and the completion of *both* the traditional evaluation and the functional assessment is 72 hours. Despite the pressures for efficiency, the early involvement of the SO, in the assessment and treatment process may pay dividends in terms of resource conservation once the person served is discharged. Thus, a brief discussion of SO opportunities for collaboration in the assessment process will be presented prior to the discussion of the functional assessment tools that are currently available.

Preinterview Questionnaire. The purpose of administering a preinterview questionnaire to patients and SOs is to obtain a thorough case history that will provide the basis for follow-up questioning in the interview prior to actual testing. Use of such questionnaires varies considerably in practice, from setting to setting, and within and across professions.

Interview and Case History. Communication patterns of the elderly client can be observed during an interview as well as during testing. During the interview, observation of the client's interaction with family members or caregivers may provide valuable information on the level of functional communication between the patient and the environment. Behaviors that can be observed during an interview with a person with suspected dementia include word-finding difficulties, circumlocutions and substitutions, irrelevant comments and digressions, and inability to follow conversations appropriately (Obler & Albert, 1984). Groher (1988) summarized medical and social queries appropriate for the evaluation of communication disorders in the elderly. The intent is to identify important clues to etiology and other limitations that will aid in designing the assessment protocol. A case history should also explore (a) the subjective complaint of the communication problem, (b) the concerns of the SO, (c) the willingness and ability of the patient and partner to collaborate in solving the problem, and (d) financial considerations.

Attitude Scales. The *Self-Assessment of Communication* scale (Schow & Nerbonne, 1982) and its correlate version for SOs consists of 10 questions probing experiences in various communication settings as well as feelings about communication. Felix (1977) has developed the *Subjective Communication Report,* which is an attempt to obtain a communication history using a *yes/no* format. The patient can complete the form or the examiner can read it aloud. Administration of either of these attitudinal surveys is quick and easy and, with the caveat of response bias, may supply useful information regarding the patient's predisposition toward using a prosthetic device, modifying the environment, or changing his or her behavior.

Natural Observation. According to Davis and Wilcox (1985), natural observation, like conversational samples, constitutes an excellent pragmatic assessment. Of all pragmatic procedures, natural observation has the potential for yielding the most representative information, and therefore is probably the most useful for planning and conducting treatment (Rao, 1990). Holland (1982) described a system for observing persons with aphasia in their natural environment that includes observations of verbal and nonverbal output, reading, writing, and math, as well as other behaviors such as singing, responding to household sounds, and speaking in a foreign language.

More recently, Hartley (1992) developed the *Behavioral Observation and Informal Assessment Form*. This instrument was designed for use with persons recovering from traumatic brain injury (TBI) but can be easily adapted for use with the elderly. The clinician is asked to rate five major behavioral areas under four categories: within normal limits, unable to judge, problem area, and comments. The form has five major macro-categories, including orientation/recall (e.g., biographical information, orientation to place); attention; executive functioning (awareness of deficit, self-correction of errors); rate of processing/responding (impulsivity, motor slowing); and emotional control/affect. Hartley also developed the *Environmental Needs Assessment* for persons with TBI; it, too, can be easily used with the elderly population. The clinician is asked to rate current and projected status for home and general community environment. A sample of the needs assessment is as follows:

Living/family environment:

- type of setting (e.g., nursing home, group home, or supported living)

- activities applicable to individual (e.g., self-care, housework, or home repairs)

- social roles expected of individual (e.g., spouse, neighbor, or parent)

- individual with regular contact in living/family environment

General community environment:

- applicable activities/settings (e.g., church, mall, banking, post office, and movies)

- roles expected of individual (e.g., consumer, citizen, friend, and companion)

- individual with whom regular contact is made

The code for rating level of independence in activities is consonant with functional assessment: NA = *not applicable;* I = *totally independent;*

S = *needs occasional supervision;* P = *needs minimal physical assistance;* D = *totally dependent;* V = *can do but needs verbal cues.* Hartley's assessment tools are remarkably appropriate and easily adaptable for use with the elderly client as a precursor to a formal assessment.

Communication Questionnaire. The identical benefits and caveats noted regarding the use of attitudinal scales with communicatively impaired older adults also apply to the use of questionnaires. An informal measure of communication efficiency particularly well suited for use with the elderly was developed by Swindell, Pashek, and Holland (1982). Designed primarily as a prognostic tool, it asks the informant to rate the patient's background and communicative and personal style on a 1 to 5 scale.

The NRH SLP Service (1995) developed the Patient Information Questionnaire, which solicits not only routine demographic information about the patient, but also personal preference information that may prove useful in future interventions. Information is gathered concerning (a) biographical facts; (b) family members' names; (c) friends' names and relationships; (d) hobbies; (e) favorites (e.g., foods, TV shows, sports teams); (f) dislikes (e.g., household tasks, animals, movies, foods); and (g) additional information the family wishes to share. Clinicians are encouraged to solicit as much information as possible from the client and SO prior to the assessment in order to target those testing tools and treatment tasks that are both individualized and appropriate for the person served. The clear intent of SLP and audiology interventions is to meet the customer's expectations by delivering services that the client not only needs, but wants.

General Rehabilitation Measures

Functional assessment tools have been in use since the late 1970s (Harvey & Jellinek, 1979). Rao (1990) reviewed the status of functional assessment in rehabilitation during the 1980s, noting that the field was developing rapidly because of accreditation pressures and competition. He indicated that there were a plethora of measures currently available, with no industry standard as yet established. Further, there was still a need for a communication-specific functional assessment tool that would provide a capsule profile of the person's disability in a valid, reliable, and efficient manner. The perfect functional assessment tool is not yet available (Adamovich, 1994). Frattali et al. (1995) provided an excellent, state-of-the-art review of the most popular functional assessment tools on the market that include communication as an assessment component. The interested reader is referred to this publication for more detail.

According to Frattali et al. (1995), these measures, which use rating scales as the primary means of evaluating various aspects of communication, were developed to provide a relatively quick estimate of functional status. Some measures concentrate on communication more than others. For example, of the three most popular global functional assessment tools in the industry, the *Patient Evaluation and Conference System* (PECS; Harvey & Jellinek, 1979) rates 11 aspects of communicative behavior, from hearing to the use of gesture; the *Rehabilitation Institute of Chicago Functional Assessment Scale* (RIC-FAS; Cichowski, 1995) rates 9; and the *Functional Independence Measure* (FIM; State University of New York at Buffalo Research Foundation, 1993), which is by far the most widely used functional assessment tool, rates only 7 aspects of communicative behavior. The PECS was designed as a comprehensive data set, including almost all behaviors that might be limited as a result of a disability and that therefore could be rated and reported at a team conference. The FIM was designed as a minimum data set—the least number of functional skills ($n = 18$) that can characterize the level of independence in daily living of a person with a disability. The RIC-FAS was designed to be a supplement to the FIM and can be considered an intermediate data set. Clearly, none of the above global functional assessment tools were designed to be used exclusively with the elderly; therefore, none are instruments of choice when clinicians are charged with conducting a functional assessment in the elderly. All available global assessment tools are rehabilitation measures, designed to assess functional ability following injury or illness.

Brown, Gordon, and Diller (1984) developed Rehabilitation Indicators, which refer to a cluster of functional assessment instruments. The constituents of these instruments can be used separately or in tandem, as dictated by the needs of the users. The component relevant to this discussion is the Skill Indicators (SKIs), which corresponds most directly to traditional approaches to functional assessment. The SKIs document the client's behavioral strengths and weaknesses in diverse areas of functioning (e.g., self-care, mobility, and communication). It is the most extensive list of skills in the business, covering more than 40 broad categories and over 100 items. Each user can select the subset of skills that is relevant to the setting's program and sense of accountability. In addition, the rater may employ a rating scale that is suitable for the setting (e.g., plus/minus or 0–3). According to Rao (1990), the SKIs are particularly well suited to the functional assessment of the elderly. The following case study illustrates the use of SKIs in an elderly person with stroke. The case is designed to illustrate how to involve consumers in addressing goals that are individualized and appropriate to their needs at a given time and setting. The client and clinician can literally select from a functional menu and decide what the functional goals of the therapy regime might be. In addition, the SKIs are an excellent clinical tool for clinician observation of the client functioning in a natural setting and subsequent rate of the presence or absence of a given skill.

Case Report

B.H., a 69-year-old male who had a left cerebrovascular accident (CVA) with severe Broca's aphasia and apraxia of speech, was enrolled in an interdisciplinary rehabilitation program involving physical, occupational, and speech therapies. The initial team workup revealed an extremely supportive, intuitive, and involved spouse who was prepared to become a cotherapist. Although B.H. had a severe communication impairment and a marked right hemiplegia that limited ambulation completion of his own activities of daily living, the team agreed with B.H. to involve his spouse in all aspects of his treatment. The spouse became the common denominator of all three therapies, carrying over each interdisciplinary goal to each session and practicing each of the day's activities with B.H. in the evenings and on weekends. The patient and spouse were encouraged at the outset to complete the entire SKIs by indicating what he could do (+), what he couldn't do (–), what he didn't care to do (0), and finally what he wanted to do (Δ). In short, the team agreed to treat the "skill areas" that the patient/SO elected. Under the language category is the subcategory of reading skills. B.H. and his SO rated the SKIs at the beginning of the program and monthly thereafter. Below is a pre–post comparison of their SKI ratings.

	Item	Pre	Post
20.01	Reads signs	+	+
20.02	Reads safety words/symbols	+	+
20.03	Reads basic instructions	Δ	+
20.04	Reads package instructions	0	0
20.05	Reads newspaper	Δ	+
20.06	Alphabetizes words/names	0	0
20.07	Telephone directory	Δ	+

(Continues)

Item		Pre	Post
20.08	Dictionary	Δ	+
20.09	Braille	N/A	N/A
20.10	Braille	N/A	N/A
20.11	Uses tape recorder for reading	Δ	+
20.12	Reads talking books	Δ	+

Of the six skills B.H. and his SO wished to improve in the area of reading, all six were rated as "can do" at the conclusion of the SLP treatment regime. In summary, the aggressive interdisciplinary cotherapy paid off, with the patient achieving the selected goals that permitted him and his spouse to enjoy a quality of life after stroke that empowered them to do for each other what they both knew they were capable of as a team. They indeed were able to "add life to years" by becoming actively involved in making life skill choices.

Functional Communication Measures

At least seven measures have been developed explicitly for evaluating functional communication in adults, one for adults with voice disorders, and two for adults with hearing loss (see Frattali et al., 1995, for an excellent summary). Among those tools measuring functional communication in adults are the following: the *Functional Communication Profile* (FCP; Sarno, 1969), the *Communicative Abilities of Daily Living* (CADL; Holland, 1980), the *ASHA Functional Communication Measures* (ASHA FCM; Larkins, 1987), the *Communicative Effectiveness Index* (CETI; Lomas et al., 1989), the *Revised Edinburg Functional Communication Profile* (EFCP; Wirz, Skinner, & Dean, 1990), the *Communication Profile: A Functional Skills Survey* (FSS; Payne, 1994), and the *ASHA Functional Assessment of Communication Skills for Adults* (ASHA FACS; Frattali et al., 1995).

Of the seven tools, only the CADL (Holland, 1980) requires the patient's cooperation. The CADL was developed to provide a formal aphasia assessment tool that samples such real-life communication situations as making a doctor's appointment and buying a soda. With the FCP (Sarno, 1969), the SO provides information regarding the patient's communicative behaviors, and then the SLP rates the patient on 45 examples taken from daily communication situations subsumed under five major headings (movement, speaking, understanding, reading, and other). The CETI (Lomas et al., 1989) is a 16-item paper-and-pencil survey rated by the SO on a continuum from *not at all able* to *as able as before the stroke*. The CETI focuses on four aspects of communication, those involving basic needs (e.g., eating and grooming), health threat (e.g., giving or receiving information about one's medical condition), life skills (e.g., shopping and use of the telephone), and social needs (e.g., coffee klatch and writing letters). Although the CETI was designed for persons with aphasia, Rao (1994b) has reported success in using this instrument with persons suspected of being in early stage dementia and also with persons with right-hemisphere communication impairments. In addition, Rao (in press) has reported on the use of the CETI by both the SO and the patient not only to obtain both parties' impressions on functional communication, but also to serve as a framework for functional counseling. In instances where the patient possesses sufficient reading skills to complete the 16-item survey, it can be very instructive for both the patient and the SO to complete the CETI separately. The completed CETI often provides clear instances of lack of correlation and thus probable miscommunication on the part of both parties. If the patient feels that he or she participates in conversations with strangers just as well as before the stroke, and the SO rates the patient as not at all able to do so, an opportunity can be provided to discuss with the family unit concepts such as pragmatics, initiative, and/or self-awareness that, once clarified and understood, should result in better communication awareness and consequent family adjustment.

A similar and more recent communication survey, the FSS (Payne, 1994), is divided into five sections and includes 26 items rated by an adult client on a 5-point scale of levels of communication importance (not communication performance). The FSS is a culturally sensitive survey for determining how important everyday communication skills are to an individual. The FSS sections and examples of each are as follows: survival skills (e.g., reading signs like "exit" and "push"), reading for information (e.g., reading the Bible or Koran), orientation to date and time (e.g., reading the time on a clock), religious activity (e.g., talking to your minister/rabbi/priest), and interpersonal communication (e.g., asking for assistance or help). The FSS is particularly conducive to developing an individual care plan for elderly clients, because the client weights how important each activity is in his or her life.

In their review, Frattali et al. (1995, p. 24) noted that available functional communication measures often have limitations in one or more of the following areas:

- scope of assessment;

- conceptual design (i.e., assessment at the level of impairment rather than disability);

- sensitivity to capturing degrees of functional communication ability;

- psychometric properties (i.e., reliability and validity);

- time requirements for administration; and

- use with a range of populations with communication disorders.

The ASHA FACS (Frattali et al., 1995) is the most recent and most comprehensive functional communication tool in the business. It was developed to overcome many of the limitations in available measures of functional communication. However, Frattali et al. do stress that no tool can overcome all limitations and suit all purposes. The ASHA FACS offers a means for assessing functional communication behaviors at the level of disability in a valid, reliable, and sensitive yet efficient manner. The FACS has four assessment domains: social communication (e.g., understands TV/radio); communication of basic needs (e.g., responds in an emergency); reading, writing, and number concepts (e.g., makes money transactions); and daily planning (e.g., uses a calendar). The ASHA FACS utilizes two ordinal scales. The first is the 7-point Scale of Communication Independence, which measures functional communication performance along a continuum of independence similar to that of the FIM. The second is the 5-point Scale of Qualitative Dimensions of Communication, which measures a range of response dimensions that characterize the client's communication abilities for each domain addressed. Although the ASHA FACS takes longer to administer and rate (about 20 minutes) than most functional assessment tools, it has received extremely favorable peer reviews because

- it describes outcomes that are relevant to payers;

- it can be completed in a relatively short period of time;

- the qualitative dimensions add important information, scoring examples are helpful, and score summaries and profiles are useful;

- its design is comprehensive yet streamlined;
- the format of the measure is outstanding;
- the observation format is a strength; and
- the ASHA FACS is appropriate for a culturally diverse population.

The ASHA FACS is so recent that there is no postpilot data to document its use with the elderly. However, based on its comprehensive scope and qualitative nature, it clearly is the gold standard for functional communication assessment in adults.

Conclusion

By way of summary, the chapter will conclude with a case study (Rao, 1994a, 1995) of an elderly person with stroke who made significant functional gains more than 5 years postonset as measured by the ASHA FCM (Larkins, 1987).

Case Report

R.J., a 72-year-old dextral male, had suffered a left CVA with global aphasia 5 years earlier. He received several years of unproductive treatment and, for the past 3 years, lived at home in Florida with a housekeeper and received no rehabilitation. At his daughter's request, R.J. was evaluated and found to be a candidate for a short-term intensive rehabilitation stay (2 weeks) to be followed by a 1-month outpatient regime. As a result of the joint planning of the team, daughter, and patient, the major interdisciplinary goal was identified: R.J. would convey activity of daily living (ADL) needs via gesture, drawing, or both in all therapy contexts. R.J. quickly developed a repertoire of 30 gestural signals. This repertoire was listed on a name tag that R.J. wore, so that each person encountering him would be aware of what gestures might be elicited, such as "eat and drink" at lunch and "shave and wash" in the morning. The daughter became actively involved in the treatment program, watching the day's SLP session (captured on video) with her father in the evening and practicing the signals and drawings with him. In only 2 weeks, the main interdisciplinary goal was accomplished; in addition, R.J. acquired 30 gestures, a facility for drawing a host of basic needs, and attained 90% accuracy on a standardized aphasia reading and *yes/no* battery. R. J. returned home with the ability to get his needs met and, importantly, the power of initiative in developing his own ADL plan, in "adding life to years." (Rao, 1994a, p. 304)

R.J.'s initial and final functional communication status was measured using the ASHA FCM (Larkins, 1987) (1 = *totally dependent;* 7 = *totally independent*). The results are shown in Table 9.3. In addition to the above-mentioned outcomes and those noted in Table 9.3, customer satisfaction feedback was also provided by R.J.'s daughter in a letter after R.J.'s return home at 3 months following discharge:

> This is to keep you abreast of how dad has sustained his progress since working with you. He has initiated "letters" to his son in California who writes to him every week. He has also written to me several times and enclosed a bird's-eye view drawing of his neighborhood with the streets labeled correctly and the route of his daily walk marked in red. His salutation and signature are correct, but the words in the text of the letter are copied randomly from books. Nevertheless, they are extremely heart warming to receive and make us feel more connected to him. He is able to negotiate his medication with housekeepers and relatives now. As you know, most of his medication was withdrawn while at the hospital and so now he feels pain from arthritis. Previously he would have panic attacks, if he noticed any change of medication routine. Now he is able to trust that he is communicating, both sending and receiving accurately enough to adjust his own pain medication. At his son's wedding in Chicago, his brothers and sisters-in-law noted that he seemed more relaxed, happy, and healthy. He indeed gestured and drew pictures for them and clearly indicated that he was happy with the results of his hospitalization. I gave him a VCR when he left here. He now indicates to his housekeeper through drawing that he wants *National Geographic,* opera or drama video rented for him. He also communicated with drawing to my aunt that he needed a razor. Sincerely, B.J. (Rao, 1995, pp. 54–55)

This case illustrates many aspects of the critical points in this chapter. There is a significant difference between language and communication and between traditional and functional assessment tools; although one may have a significant impairment, the handicap may actually be minor. Family support is often the keystone of an elderly person's aging well with a disability. Ageism is a threat to seniors who may warrant "another chance at rehab"; when the SLP is able to change the environment and behavior while providing assistive devices, the person with a disability is indeed able to "close the rehab gap" and increase his or her options, thereby reducing handicap. Finally, the person served is the prime focus of our interventions, and customer

Table 9.3
R.J.'s Functional Communication Status

Functional Skills	Admit Status	Goal	Discharge Status
Comprehension of spoken language	3	5	4
Comprehension of written language	2	4	4
Comprehension of nonspoken language	4	6	6
Production of spoken language	2	4	3
Production of written language	2	4	3
Production of nonspoken language	4	6	5

Note. From "Drawing and Gesture as Communication Options in a Person with Severe Aphasia" by P. Rao, 1995, *Topics in Stroke Rehabilitation, 2*, p. 54. Copyright 1995 by Aspen. Reprinted with permission.

satisfaction feedback is a crucial ingredient in evaluating our programs. R.J.'s drawing, shown in Figure 9.2, clearly illustrates the dictum that "a picture is worth a thousand words." Here he clearly conveys the message that he no longer uses a quad cane and that he now uses a single-point cane for his daily walk through the neighborhood. This is truly functional communication.

Author's Note

This chapter is dedicated to my "old" mentor and friend, retiree and audiologist extraordinaire, Dr. David M. Resnick. He taught me to never say never and to follow Yogi's advice: "When you come to a fork in the road, take it."

References

Adamovich, B. (1994). Measurement of functional outcomes. *Special Interest Division 2 Newsletter, 4*, 2–4.

American Speech-Language-Hearing Association. (1990, May). *Advisory report, Functional Communication Measures Project*. Rockville, MD: Author.

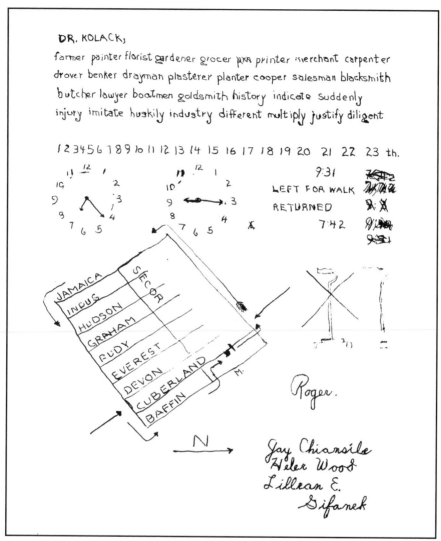

Figure 9.2. R.J.'s drawing.

American Speech-Language-Hearing Association. (1993). Preferred practice patterns for the professions of speech–language pathology. *Asha, 25,* 77–78.

Aten, J. L. (1986). Functional communication treatment. In R. Chapey (Ed.), *Language intervention strategies in adult aphasia* (2nd. ed, pp. 266–276). Baltimore: Williams & Wilkins.

Batavia, A. (1991, May). *Assessing the function of functional assessment*. Paper presented at a session of the National Health Policy Forum, Washington, DC.

Brown, M., Gordon, W. A., & Diller, L. (1984). Rehabilitation indicators. In A. S. Halpern & M. J. Fuhrer (Eds.), *Functional assessment in rehabilitation* (pp. 187–203). Baltimore: Brookes.

Brummel-Smith, K. (1990). Introduction. In B. Kemp, K. Brummel-Smith, & J. Ramsdell (Eds.), *Geriatric rehabilitation* (pp. 3–21). Boston: College-Hill.

Cichowski, K. (1995). *Rehabilitation Institute of Chicago: Functional Assessment Scale–Revised*. Chicago: Rehabilitation Institute of Chicago.

Davis, G. A., & Wilcox, M. J. (1985). *Adult aphasia rehabilitation: Applied pragmatics*. San Diego: College-Hill.

DeCrow, K. (1993, November 23). Harassing the elderly. *USA Today*, p. 11A.

DeJong, G. (1987). Medical rehabilitation outcome measurement in a changing health care market. In M. Fuhrer (Ed.), *Rehabilitation outcomes: Analysis and measurement* (pp. 261–271). Baltimore: Brookes.

Felix, N. (1977). *Subjective communication report*. Puyallup, WA: Good Samaritan Hospital.

Frattali, C. M. (1991). Professional practices: Perspectives and clinical outcomes. *Asha, 33,* 12.

Frattali, C. M. (1992). Functional assessment of communication: Merging public policy with clinical views. *Aphasiology, 6,* 63–83.

Frattali, C., Thompson, C. K., Holland, A. L., Wohl, C. B., & Ferketic, M. M. (1995). *Functional assessment of communication skills for adults*. Rockville, MD: American Speech-Language-Hearing Association.

Freda, M., & Rao, P. (1995, October/November). Rehab's sea change. *Rehab Management*, pp. 62–67.

Friedan, B. (1993). *The fountain of age*. New York: Simon & Shuster.

Granger, C. (1984). A conceptual model for functional assessment. In C. Granger & G. Gresham (Eds.), *Functional assessment in rehabilitation medicine* (pp. 14–25). Baltimore: Williams & Wilkins.

Groher, M. (1988). Modifications in speech–language assessment procedures for the older adult. In B. B. Shadden (Ed.), *Communication behavior and aging: A sourcebook for clinicians* (pp. 248–260). Baltimore: Williams & Wilkins.

Hartley, L. L. (1992). Assessment of functional communication. *Seminars in Speech and Language, 13,* 264–279.

Harvey, R. F., & Jellinek, H. M. (1979). *Patient Evaluation and Conference System: PECS.* Wheaton, IL: Marianjoy Rehabilitation Center.

Holland, A. L. (1980). *Communicative Abilities of Daily Living.* Baltimore: University Park Press.

Holland, A. L. (1982). Observing functional communication of aphasic adults. *Journal of Speech and Hearing Disorders, 47,* 50–56.

Hooper, C., & Johnson, A. (1991). Assessment and intervention issues. In D. N. Ripich (Ed.), *Handbook of geriatric communication disorders* (pp. 307–331). Austin, TX: PRO-ED.

Hosek, S., Kane, R., Carney, M., Hartman, J., Reboussin, D., Serrato, C., & Melvin, J. (1986). *Charges and outcome for rehabilitative care: Implications for the prospective payment system.* Santa Monica, CA: Rand Corp.

Joint Commission on Accreditation of Health Care Organizations. (1995). *Standards manual for hospitals.* Chicago: Author.

Larkins, P. (1987). *Program Evaluation System.* Rockville, MD: American Speech-Language-Hearing Association.

Lezak, M. (1983). *Neuropsychological assessment* (2nd. ed.). New York: Oxford University Press.

Lomas, J., Pickard, L., Bester, S., Elbard, H., Finlayson, A., & Zoghaib, C. (1989). The Communicative Effectiveness Index: Development and psychometric evaluation of a functional communication measure for adults. *Journal of Speech and Hearing Disorders, 54,* 113–124.

National Rehabilitation Hospital. (1986, Spring). Rehabilitation: Closing the gap. *NRH Today,* pp. 1–4.

National Rehabilitation Hospital. (1995). *Patient information form.* Washington, DC: Author.

Obler, L., & Albert, M. (1984). Language in aging. In M. M. Albert (Ed.), *Clinical neurology of aging* (pp. 245–253). New York: Oxford University Press.

Payne, J. (1994). *Communication Profile: A Functional Skills Survey.* Tucson, AZ: Communication Skill Builders.

Rao, P. (1990). Functional communication assessment of the elderly. In E. Cherow (Ed.), *Proceedings of Research Symposium on Communication Sciences and Disorders and Aging* (ASHA Status Report 19, pp. 28–39). Rockville, MD: American Speech-Language-Hearing Association.

Rao, P. (1994a). Communication disorders. In M. Ozer, R. Materson, & L. R. Caplan (Eds.), *Management of persons with stroke* (pp. 281–310). St. Louis: Mosby.

Rao, P. (1994b). *An SLP overview of aging in the '90s.* Address to the 16th Annual G. Paul Moore Symposium, University of Florida, Gainesville.

Rao, P. (1994c). Use of Amer-Ind Code by persons with aphasia. In R. Chapey (Ed.), *Language intervention strategies in adult aphasia* (3rd ed., pp. 358–367). Baltimore: Williams & Wilkins.

Rao, P. (1995). Drawing and gesture as communication options in a person with severe aphasia. *Topics in Stroke Rehabilitation, 2,* 49–56.

Rao, P. (in press). Counseling considerations in managing persons with adult neurogenic communication disorders. In T. A. Crowe (Ed.), *Applications of counseling in speech–language pathology and audiology.* Baltimore: Williams & Wilkins.

Rubenfield, P. (1986). Ageism and disabilityism: Double jeopardy. In S. J. Brody & G. E. Ruff (Eds.), *Aging and rehabilitation: Advances in the state of the art* (pp. 323–328). New York: Springer.

Rubinstein, E. A. (1991, October 7).The not so golden years. *Newsweek,* p. 3.

Sarno, M. T. (1969). *The Functional Communication Profile: Manual of directions.* New York: Institute of Rehabilitation Medicine.

Schow, R. L., & Nerbonne, M. A. (1982). Communication Screening Profile: Use with elderly clients. *The Ear and Hearing, 3,* 135–148.

State University of New York at Buffalo Research Foundation. (1993). *Guide for the use of the uniform data set for medical rehabilitation: Functional independence measure.* Buffalo: Author.

Swindell, D. S., Pashek, G. V., & Holland, A. L. (1982). A questionnaire for surveying personal and communicative style. In R. Brookshire (Ed.), *Clinical Aphasiology Conference Proceedings* (pp. 50–63). Minneapolis, MN: BRK.

U.S. Bureau of the Census. (1990). *U.S. Census report: 1990.* Washington, DC: Government Printing Office.

Weg, R. (1986, December). Lecture on aging. Ida Bean Visiting Professor Class, *The University of Iowa Spectator,* p. 3.

Wilkerson, D. (1994, June). *Measuring and managing clinical outcomes.* Paper presented at the ASHA Directors' Conference, Rye, NY.

Williams, T. F. (1990). Introduction to rehabilitation and aging. In S. J. Brody & L. G. Pawls (Eds.), *Aging and rehabilitation II: The state of the practice* (pp. 3–8). New York: Springer.

Wirz, S., Skinner, C., & Dean, E. (1990). *Revised Edinburg Functional Communication Profile.* Tucson, AZ: Communication Skill Builders.

World Health Organization. (1980). *International classification of impairments, disabilities, and handicaps.* Geneva, Switzerland: Author.

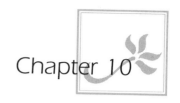

Chapter 10

Families Caring for Elders at Home: Caregiver Training

Michelle S. Bourgeois

Caregiver interventions are addressed in Chapters 10 and 11. In Chapter 10, Bourgeois focuses primarily on the family caregiver as intervention agent for individuals with chronic illness, particularly Alzheimer's disease. Caregiver characteristics and experiences are identified, and approaches to caregiver interventions are reviewed. Techniques used in a current pilot program are presented and outcomes are discussed.

1. *What are the characteristics of individuals serving as primary caregivers to older persons? Where are most older persons with disability cared for, and what types of environmental adaptations may be required to accommodate different disabilities and problem behaviors?*

2. *What are some of the problems in supporting caregivers through available resources?*

3. *Many caregiving intervention models exist. List four of these general models and describe benefits and potential limitations or barriers to implementation.*

4. *Bourgeois describes the Caregiver Intervention Program at the University of Pittsburgh, which was designed to compare two skills training approaches. What are the basic differences between these two approaches? To date, what are the outcomes of this project, and what are the specific positive effects of each approach?*

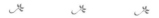

O ne of the most important prognostic indicators for positive outcomes in chronic illness may well be the caregiving situation. Because of the often gradual transformation of family members into caregivers and the home into a therapeutic environment, medical professionals and family alike may be slow to acknowledge the need to expand the radius of their attention beyond the patient's immediate medical needs. Yet, successful medical management of the patient is often inextricably related to the skills and abilities of caregivers and to the constraints of the specific environment in which care is provided. Because current political and policy agendas mandate reducing the costs of caring for the elderly, provision of care in the home or other noninstitutional settings has become a priority area of the National Institute on Aging (NIA) and the Administration on Aging (AoA; Ory & Duncker, 1992). As a result, within the past few years, some progress has been made in learning more about how care is delivered in the home and how families cope with their increased responsibilities. The home environment is becoming less of a "black hole" into which a range of medical services and conditions can be transferred (Gubrium & Sankar, 1990). Increased attention to this area, however, has highlighted the problems and complex issues inherent in the provision of care in homes by nonprofessionals. This chapter focuses on primary family caregivers as intervention agents: Who are they? What are their needs? How well are they managing?

Elder and Caregiver Characteristics

According to data from a national health interview survey, approximately 37.5% of individuals over 65 years have activity restrictions due to chronic conditions such as heart disease and stroke, cancer, Alzheimer's disease, and mental illness (National Center for Health Statistics, 1989). Many, if not most, of these individuals require significant amounts of assistance with the activities of daily living (ADLs), as well as the provision of social supports from caregivers. *Caregivers* have been defined as individuals who provide someone with hands-on assistance with the activities of daily living, such as eating, dressing, bathing, and toileting, or with instrumental activities of daily living (IADLs), such as using the telephone, preparing meals, and taking medications (Schulz & O'Brien, 1994). Surprisingly, it is often difficult for family members to acknowledge their role as caregiver for a close relative. They may not be able to pinpoint the exact time when the usual household tasks and activities rendered to an impaired family member exceeded the bounds of normal or usual care. Nevertheless, Van Nostrand, Furner, and Suzman (1993) reported that approximately 10% of the elderly population (2.97 million persons) reported receiving help from another person in performing ADLs, and that 23.2% (6.26 million persons) reported requiring help with IADLs. Taking into account the fact that some disabled elderly may have multiple caregivers and that some caregivers continue to accept caregiving responsibilities after institutional placement, Schulz and O'Brien (1994) have estimated that there are approximately 5 to 9 million caregivers in the United States.

The results from two national surveys regarding caregiving to older adults indicate that caregivers are predominantly female and married. More than one third are adult children; less than one third are spouses. One quarter are other relatives and nonrelatives, and almost three quarters of them live with the person with a disability (American Association of Retired Persons [AARP] & The Travelers Companies Foundation, 1988; Stone, Cafferata, & Sangl, 1987). Caregiving can be a solitary experience, as most caregivers have sole responsibility for the person with a disability, with little to no help from other care providers or resources. Most caregivers provide care more than 3 hours per day, 7 days a week. Caregiving often creates conflicts with other competing demands, such as caring for children in the household and work schedules. It is no surprise that, as a group, caregivers report lower incomes and lower self-reported health than the population at large (Stone et al., 1987). Caregivers with the increased burdens of caring for elders with cognitive impairments may be at additional risk for psychological distress and burden, as well as psychiatric and physical illness (Schulz, O'Brien, Bookwala, & Fleissner, 1995).

Factors Related to the Caregiving Experience

Much research has been devoted to investigations of caregiver characteristics and demographic variables thought to have an impact on the caregiving experience. One major factor influencing caregiving experiences is the relationship of the caregiver to the elder with a disability. Caregivers who are the spouse, son or daughter, sibling, or friend of the patient have been shown to have different expectations and stresses related to their caregiving responsibilities. Spousal caregivers have been found to be more depressed than nonspousal caregivers (Pruchno & Potashnik, 1989) and to have greater risks for physical illness and financial strain (Baumgarten et al., 1992; Cantor, 1983). Caregiving daughters often report sibling conflict as the most important source of stress when caring for a parent with a disability (Suitor & Pillemer, 1993); however, the multiple role responsibilities of "women in the middle" (Brody, 1981; e.g., wife, mother, grandmother, employee) contribute to the burden and health risks of this group (Wright, Clipp, & George, 1993). In his discussion of the impact of different caregiving relationships for patients with dementia, Morycz (1994) enumerated factors such as gender, age, race, education, and relationship to the elder with a disability as significant sources of variability in caregiving. Additionally, the health and financial resources of the caregiver, the composition of the family network, the coping skills of the caregiver, the quality of the previous relationship between the caregiver and care recipient, and ethnic and cultural traditions and expectations complicate the picture.

In his review of caregiving issues in culturally diverse populations, Henderson (1994) pointed out that cultural differences in health beliefs also serve as barriers to available medical and social support resources. For example, ethnic minority caregivers may tolerate certain disease symptoms differently, have communication difficulties when their native language is not English, and be perceived to need fewer outside sources of help because of tightly knit social networks of multigenerational families and churches. The impact of the chronic illness itself has been shown to influence caregiving, particularly with regard to the onset of the disease (gradual or acute), the course of the disease (progressive, constant, or episodic), the outcome (fatal, life shortening, or nonfatal), and the degree of incapacitation (due to problems of cognition, social stigma, movement, or demands of the treatment regimen; Rolland, 1988).

The Home as the Care Setting: Environmental and Psychological Issues

It has been shown that the household is the key element in the organization of care of the disabled elderly, with families providing 80% to 90% of their medical and personal care (Brody, 1981). In order to provide satisfactory care to the person at home, modifications of the physical and social environment are often required. Whether the elder expects to live alone or to move in with other family members, health care professionals should be consulted to determine the extent of care required and the types of setting changes needed to facilitate maximum independence of the elder (Trocchio, 1981). Much of the research on optimizing environments for the elderly with disability identifies environmental attributes, such as safety, security, accessibility, and legibility, as attainable goals leading to person–environment congruence (Lawton, 1987). Many of these attributes represent physical features of the environment, such as safety hazards; mobility and transport barriers; and familiar, understandable, and predictable objects. Careful analysis is required to determine the demands of the environment, which may pose further barriers to successful functioning. These include the physical health and cognitive level of the patient, the expectations for independence in activities of daily living, appropriate time use, and potential for social interaction. Researchers are finding that interventions designed to teach caregivers ways to manipulate the environment, both physically and socially, are not only enhancing the competence of elderly adults but also reducing the frequency and severity of problem behaviors that can arise (Corcoran & Gitlin, 1991, 1992; Pynoos & Ohta, 1991; Rogers, Marcus, & Snow, 1987). For example, Corcoran and Gitlin (1992) developed an occupational therapy-based intervention designed to help caregivers implement environmental strategies to modify the secondary symptoms of dementia, usually related to self-care activities. During five home visits over a 3-month period, therapists helped 17 caregivers identify problematic behaviors, elements in the environment that might be exacerbating the symptoms, and a plan for changing those disruptive elements. Review of the plan's effect on the problem behavior, as well as refinement of the environmental strategies, was conducted at each visit. Caregivers were found to implement a variety of effective solutions such as graded assistance, encouragement of simple work and leisure tasks, use of formal supports, and preparation of the area with needed objects. The long-term benefits of this intervention were established when caregivers reported the continued use after the study of strategies with the original problems and with newly emergent problem behaviors.

Notwithstanding the financial ramifications of providing care in the home, the psychological and symbolic meanings of the term *home* may contribute to the strength of the commitment to care for impaired elders at home. For many, home means control, security, family development, independence, comfort, protection, feelings, and the presence of people; for others, keeping a sick person at home means that the person is not fully "sick" (Rubinstein, 1990). In fact, one explanation for the fact that use of formal support systems (such as nursing, homemaking, and counseling services) is usually delayed until family resources have been stretched as far as possible may be that families are reluctant to acknowledge the disruptiveness of the illness on the household regimen (Albert, 1990). Alternatively, the adoption of particular adaptation strategies for effective caregiving may evolve over time without overt awareness and decision making on the part of caregivers. Two strategies Albert observed in families dealing with the overwhelming demands of caregiving were the use of routines for caregiving tasks and the redefinition of parent–child roles. But not all families discover successful caregiving strategies; in fact, some households never achieve a satisfactory level of routinization of care tasks, and instead are found to be in constant crisis management. The need for intervention becomes obvious not only to professionals, but also to the caregivers themselves.

Resources for Maintaining Elders at Home

Resources and services for caregivers have proliferated in recent years. The abundance of guidebooks for caregivers underscores the need for information about caregiving resources (e.g., Lustbader & Hooyman, 1994; Mace & Rabins, 1981; Rob, 1991; Smith, 1992). Each book has at least one chapter outlining the specific types of formal and informal sources of caregiving support to be found in most communities. Formal support services encompass government and community services, such as the local Area Agency on Aging, senior health and/or recreation centers, local senior advocacy groups, the United Way, the Veteran's Administration, the Social Security Administration, the Public Health Department, and city and county hospitals, to name but a few. Informal support networks include family members, other relatives, neighbors, and friends. Some communities have made caregiving assistance a priority within community and church-related groups, and social and self-help organizations. Telephone help lines manned by knowledgeable volunteers are popular venues for locating needed services and support groups. The types of services routinely available include transportation to medical appointments, chore and housekeeping services, companion services, personal care assistance, home-delivered meals, and adult day-care. If families have the financial resources, private-pay services can be solicited through geriatric care managers listed in the Yellow Pages.

Although there appear to be adequate resources in the public domain for caregivers to obtain some information about caregiving issues, researchers find that a common reason for not utilizing services continues to be lack of knowledge of the existence of such services (Fortinsky & Hathaway, 1990; Weinberger et al., 1993). In addition to problems of underutilization, dissatisfaction with services designed specifically to relieve caregiving stresses has been observed (Lawton, Brody, & Saperstein, 1989; Zarit, 1990). Conflict between caregivers and service providers involving differences in beliefs about the focus and intensity of caregiving tasks is commonplace (Corcoran, 1993; Hasselkus, 1988). Corcoran (1994) has suggested that understanding the life-style, values, and goals of the caregiver is necessary to provide effective services; her research in caregiving styles shows that different caregiver approaches influence day-to-day management decisions and reflect differences in service choices. Gender differences in caregiving style have also been reported, with men preferring a task-oriented approach (Pruchno & Resch, 1989) and women using a parental model that emphasizes the physical and emotional health of the care recipient (Corcoran, 1994). Researchers are addressing this access problem in programs designed to teach caregivers how not only to locate appropriate resources, but also to persevere and navigate through the often less than "user friendly" domain of social service agencies.

Because caregivers need to rely on both formal and informal support networks, coordinating the care of an elderly person can be particularly challenging. Case management has been defined as planning, obtaining, coordinating, monitoring, and terminating services on behalf of an elderly relative (Simmons, Ivry, & Seltzer, 1985). Case management interventions have shown that caregivers can be trained to perform case management tasks without increasing the level of their subjective or objective caregiving burden. For example, Seltzer, Litchfield, Kapust, and Mayer (1992) provided families with knowledge, information, and skills regarding accessing the services needed by their elderly relative. Family members who received systematic training in performing case management tasks performed significantly more management tasks on behalf of their elderly relatives than did family members who received only information about services.

Caregiving Interventions: A Mixed Bag

If there is only one thing about which caregivers, clinicians, and researchers can all agree, it is that the stresses of caregiving can adversely affect family members. The unrelenting social, emotional, and financial burdens of caregiving place caregivers at risk for psychiatric and sometimes physical illness (Schulz et al., 1995). When social supports and pharmacological intervention aimed at improving cognitive performance prove to be inadequate for dealing with behavioral disturbances, patients are at risk for institutionalization and chemical restraints (Pruchno, Kleban, Michaels, & Dempsey, 1990). The professional response to these risks has been to design, implement, and evaluate interventions aimed at improving caregiver and patient outcomes. Yet, robust and longlasting outcomes have been difficult to achieve because of the variability in theoretical approaches to intervention, methodology, and populations studied.

Range of Interventions

Caregiving interventions reflect a wide diversity of approaches, ranging from general educational programs to support groups to individualized counseling to multicomponent outpatient or home-based approaches (Bourgeois, Schulz, & Burgio, 1996). Table 10.1 presents some benefits and limitations of a variety of caregiving intervention models.

Home-based interventions for caregivers that have been designed across disciplines (e.g., nursing, occupational therapy, psychology) have many commonalities. The focus of most intervention is to improve caregivers' psychological health by teaching them skills for identifying and solving specific caregiving challenges, resulting in improved day-to-day management of the patient and increased satisfaction with and utilization of outside resources (e.g., formal and informal services).

In the past, professionals felt that caregivers simply required more knowledge about the disease process in order to better manage the

Table 10.1

Benefits and Limitations of Caregiving Interventions

Intervention Models	Benefits	Limitations/Barriers
Educational programs	Increased knowledge	Individual caregiving needs not addressed
Support groups	Increased knowledge Sharing of common feelings and experiences Improved practical problem solving	Individual, personal needs not addressed Group setting not appropriate for resolving individual's feelings of guilt, anger, fear of future
Individual family counseling	Increased knowledge Personal needs addressed Ancillary psychiatric, social, and nursing services offered	Social stigma associated with seeking psychological help
Case management	Coordination of informal and formal support services Increased service use	Dissatisfaction with services Conflict between caregivers and service providers
Multicomponent outpatient and home care services	Large menu of services offered Reductions in negative caregiver outcomes Delayed patient institutionalization	Overwhelming array of choices Cost of multiple services
Respite care Day-care In-home care Short-stay institutional	Caregiver has time away from patient Patient benefits from structured program of cognitive and social stimulation	Caregiver reluctance to use due to fear of cost, patient refusal to attend, transportation problems, patient problem behaviors

(Continues)

Table 10.1 *(Continued)*

Intervention Models	Benefits	Limitations/Barriers
Skills training	Caregiver learns new techniques for managing problem behaviors, problem-solving skills, and coping skills	Skills trained may not reflect caregiver needs
		Skills trained may not apply to other future problems
	Skills apply to new behaviors and problems in the future	
	Reductions in negative caregiver and patient outcomes	

patient; educational programs, workshops, and telephone hotlines proliferated. As specific diseases became better understood in terms of how problem behaviors and caregiving responses changed over the course of the illness, thoughts about what might be helpful to caregivers expanded. Support groups arose out of the perceived need of caregivers to express and share common feelings, experiences, and practical problem-solving strategies. Research has documented the value of the information sharing and peer support gained from support groups, but often the personal needs of individual caregivers with unresolved feelings of guilt, anger, and fear of their future relationship with the patient were not addressed adequately in a group setting (Gonyea, 1989).

Individual and family counseling programs available through outpatient clinics have been the traditional vehicle for providing information and ancillary psychiatric, social, and nursing services to individuals and family caregivers of elderly patients residing in the community. Unfortunately, the social stigma associated with seeking psychological help is a major barrier to effective use of these services. Programs that attract families for their medical and diagnostic service components claim to increase the likelihood of enrollment in other counseling services once a trusting relationship has formed between agency personnel and family members (Gwyther, Ballard, & Hinman-Smith, 1990). The counseling literature provides several examples of efficacious treatments for narrowly defined problems when therapy is conducted with individual caregivers (e.g., Kaplan & Gallagher-Thompson, 1995; Toseland, Rossiter, Peak, & Smith, 1990; Toseland & Smith, 1990).

In addition to individual counseling programs, outpatient clinics often offer comprehensive, multifaceted intervention programs that address the changing needs of caregivers throughout their caregiving careers. These programs largely blanket caregivers with a diversity of services in the hope that a combination of components will have an impact on a caregiver's unique needs at the appropriate time. Although there is some evidence to support the "more is better" approach, what is lacking is a clear understanding of the relationship of various single components of the program to specific needs of individual caregivers. For example, Ferris, Steinberg, Shulman, Kahn, and Reisberg (1987) provided intensive individualized attention to caregivers, referrals to appropriate agencies, family meetings, home visits, telephone consultations, and support groups. They found significant reductions in caregiver depression, anger, insomnia, and anxiety, and patient institutionalizations. However, in this age of diminishing resources, it would be helpful to know which component, or combination of components, would be most effective for the least cost. In addition, there is some evidence to suggest that "more" may not always be better; caregivers who are offered too much at once may become overwhelmed and unable to decide where to direct their efforts (see, e.g., Gray, 1983).

Another treatment approach is based on the premise that caregiving crises might be more manageable if the caregiver had periods of relief from caregiving. Respite care, in the form of day-care, in-home care, and short-stay institutional care, is beneficial not only to the caregiver, who can use the time away from the patient to do pleasurable activities, take a vacation, or get caught up on household chores, but also to the patient, who has an opportunity to participate in social and recreational activities. In light of the many positive effects of respite care, it is surprising that this service has been found to be underutilized (Lawton et al., 1989). Fears that the patient might not accept the care situation or that the care might be inferior to their own care have contributed to the observation that caregivers often wait too long or until a crisis occurs before utilizing services offered (Montgomery & Borgatta, 1989). In an effort to prevent caregiving crises, Brodaty and Gresham (1989) provided an intensive 10-day residential training program designed to relieve the psychological distress of caregiving.

While patients were cared for by institutional staff, caregivers participated in group psychotherapy sessions and received didactic instruction about medical, legal, financial, physical, welfare, dietary, and nursing aspects of dementia. This program resulted in increased patient survival at home and decreased psychological morbidity in caregivers. Researchers are currently investigating the barriers to respite use; if respite services are expected to have prevention effects, caregivers may require additional education about the nature and acceptability of available services in the early months and across the entire span of their caregiving careers.

An ideal time to intervene with caregivers may be at the point of patient discharge from the hospital, when they may be particularly receptive to medical and management suggestions. A variety of nursing interventions have been successful in mediating positive patient and caregiver outcomes (Bergner et al., 1988; Hughes, Manheim, Edelman, & Conrad, 1987; Mohide et al., 1990; Oktay & Volland, 1990; Zimmer, Groth-Juncker, & McCusker, 1985). For example, Archbold et al. (1995) designed a multifaceted program in which nurses collaborated with family members in developing individualized plans to resolve specific patient care problems, to increase pleasurable or meaningful activities for the care recipient and caregiver, and to increase the predictability of the caregiving situation by evaluating daily caregiving patterns and identifying ways to prevent potential problems.

Skills Training Interventions

In spite of the apparent plethora of available services and interventions, service providers and researchers are often frustrated that their "good advice" about patient management and service utilization is not always embraced and acted upon by caregivers, even when caregivers agree that the recommendations are necessary and acceptable. One possible reason for caregiver failure to implement management plans successfully may be that caregivers do not have all of the skills needed to carry out the plans. For example, when advised to enroll the patient in respite services, caregivers may not know whom to call, what to ask, and how to arrange transportation; they may not believe the patient would find this service acceptable, or that the service would accept patients who wander or are incontinent. These unresolved questions and concerns often overwhelm caregivers, to the extent that they find it easier to continue dealing with the difficult situation than to act on the professional's advice.

Fortunately, interventions designed to teach specific caregiving skills have evolved. One of the most popular skills taught is problem solving. Interventions that teach problem-solving skills have shown that caregivers can overcome their reluctance to follow professionals' advice when taught procedures that break down an overwhelming task into a series of smaller, more manageable steps (D'Zurilla, 1986; Lovett & Gallagher, 1988). Similarly, other skills training interventions are designed to teach caregivers specific behavior management skills that go beyond the simple advice to "try doing this the next time your husband does that." For example, Pinkston and her colleagues used a variety of procedures, including didactic instruction, role playing, corrective feedback, and data collection, to teach caregivers how to reduce the problem behaviors of their elderly family member (Pinkston & Linsk, 1984; Pinkston, Linsk, & Young, 1988). In addition to significant changes in 76% of the targeted patient behaviors, 78% of which maintained for 6 months posttreatment, Pinkston and her colleagues reported collateral changes in standard measures of patient mental status, independent functioning, and caregiver burden as a result of learning new skills.

Evidence of long-term effects of skills training interventions has also been reported in the literature. For example, Greene and Monahan (1987, 1989) found significant decreases in caregiver anxiety and depression that were still evident 4 months following a relaxation training program. Haley (1989) reported stability in a variety of caregiver outcome measures up to 29 months after a combined educational and skills training program; and Quayhagen and Quayhagen (1989) continued to see improvements in patients up to 8 months after their caregivers were trained to implement a home-based program of cognitive stimulation. Not all caregivers, however, find it easy to maintain positive changes in their own skills when the patient's disease progresses and the problem behaviors worsen. Others have expressed disappointment in interventions in which their own problems and stress were the focus of intervention instead of the problems of the patient (Zarit, Anthony, & Boutselis, 1987). Although not all skills training interventions have reported positive findings (e.g., Zarit et al., 1987) and/or changes in all desired areas (e.g., Greene & Monahan, 1987, 1989), this approach has provided us with the most robust and rigorously evaluated treatments to date. Continued research and evaluation about which components of skills training are most effective is still needed; one such evaluative effort, the Caregiver Intervention Program, funded by the National Institute on Aging (Bourgeois, Burgio, & Schulz, 1994), is described below.

The Caregiver Intervention Program: A Comparison of Two Skills Training Approaches

The Caregiver Intervention Program at the University of Pittsburgh was developed to evaluate two skills training approaches, one in which caregivers are taught behavior management skills to change the problem behaviors of the patient with Alzheimer's disease (AD; patient-change group), and another in which caregivers are taught to change their own caregiving behaviors and affective responses to caregiving challenges (caregiver-change group). The intervention program is targeted to caregivers whose spouse with AD is living at home and exhibits active behavior problems (middle stage, or moderate dementia symptoms). After completing a battery of psychosocial assessments, caregivers are randomly assigned to either one of the two treatment groups or a control group. The intervention program spans 12 weeks; caregivers are visited in their homes for 1 hour weekly for 11 weeks, and during Week 2 of the program they attend a 3-hour workshop at the university. Another battery of psychosocial assessments is completed at the end of the 12-week intervention period and at subsequent 3- and 6-month intervals after program completion.

One important component of this intervention approach is the identification and monitoring of patient problem behaviors. Caregivers identify the three most stressful problem behaviors of the patient and learn how to use a daily data recording sheet to keep track of how often these three problems occur. The data collected by caregivers are useful to both the caregivers and the researchers. Caregivers become more objective and accurate about a problem behavior after they have been counting it; instead of complaining about a behavior happening "all of the time," they report it happening "just two or three times in the morning" or "only when the grandkids visit." Data recording helps caregivers achieve more realistic views about the impact of the problem behavior on their own level of stress and coping; they begin to feel more in control of the situation when they can plan for difficult days and relax on others. Researchers are learning that some of the most stressful behaviors are not necessarily the most frequently occurring, and patterns of behavior are emerging. Clinicians might not think to recommend data recording to their already overburdened caregivers; however, in the past 4 years, 72 caregivers in the project have learned how to use the data recording sheets and over 90% of them continued to use them every day for 9 months. In fact, some of the caregivers found them so useful that they continued to use them after the 9 months, recording the frequency of up to six different behaviors in some instances. It seems feasible that data recording gives caregivers an alternative to their usual interaction pattern with the patient. For example, instead of responding to each repetitive request of the patient, some caregivers walk into the other room to record the behavior, thereby reducing the attention the patient gets for that behavior and the probability that it will occur again.

The next important component of the intervention program is the skills training provided in one 3-hour group workshop and ten 1-hour individualized home visits. Caregivers in the patient-change group learn about basic behavioral principles, antecedents and consequences of behavior, and how to apply those principles when designing behavior management programs for specific behaviors. A behavior management program is written for the most frequently occurring patient problem, and caregivers are taught to implement it consistently at every appropriate opportunity. Caregivers commonly report problems with repetitive verbal and physical behavior, sundowning and related memory deficits, and agitation behaviors such as following the caregiver and pacing, all of which contribute to caregiver reports of increased stress and burden. The most frequently occurring problem behavior of patients is verbal repetition; that is, patients ask the same question (e.g., "Where are we going?" "When is Mary coming over?") or make the same verbal demand (e.g., "I want to go home."). Caregivers have successfully reduced the frequency of this repetitive verbal behavior using a memory cuing strategy; caregivers direct the patient to read an index card, memory book page, or memo board on which is written the specific information asked about by the patient (Bourgeois, Burgio, Schulz, Beach, & Palmer, in press).

All behavior management programs are carefully adjusted to the caregiver's specific situation, and each step of the program is written down in sequence. The steps are reviewed, the application of the treatment program is role-played, and all questions are answered before the caregiver is asked to try the program consistently during the week. At the next week's visit, the caregiver reports on use of the program, the patient's acceptance of it, and effects on the frequency of the problem behavior. If necessary, the program is modified to resolve any problems. Bourgeois et al. (in press) reported on the effects of training caregivers to use behavioral programs, such as the graphic cuing technique described above, to 7 caregivers whose spouse exhibited a high rate of verbal repetition. In all cases, the frequency of this behavior declined and stayed at a low rate through the 6 months of follow-up. This approach has been so useful to some caregivers that they have applied similar techniques to problem behaviors that developed after the end of the study. A variety of simple behavioral manipulations have been used by caregivers to reduce behaviors such as refusal to cooperate with dressing, eating, and bathing; talking about dying; and pacing.

Caregivers in the caregiver-change group learn three strategies for changing their own responses to caregiving challenges: increasing the pleasant activities in their lives, problem solving, and physical relaxation techniques. These strategies were chosen on the basis of prior successes with similar populations (Gallagher & Thompson, 1981; Lewinsohn, Munoz, Youngren, & Zeiss, 1986). In this group, caregivers first learn a modified progressive relaxation technique to change their physical response to daily stresses. They are encouraged to practice this four-step procedure several times daily and, once comfortable with it, to apply it during an active crisis situation.

Caregivers are next taught to increase the pleasant activities in their lives. Caregivers identify a range of activities they find pleasant and may have abandoned because of their caregiving responsibilities. Some of the activities may be as simple as enjoying a cup of coffee and reading the newspaper before the patient gets up in the morning, or watching the sunset; others require more active planning to enjoy, such as maintaining bowling league participation or traveling. Sensitizing caregivers to the pleasant events they routinely enjoy and having them record how often they occur result in caregivers feeling more in control of their own lives and reporting improvements in their daily mood. They often decide it is time to find ways to overcome the barriers to other postponed pleasant activities.

The third strategy is a structured six-step problem-solving procedure that complements the other two strategies when caregivers have trouble overcoming barriers to increasing the pleasant activities in their lives and to finding times to relax. Caregivers identify a problem to solve (e.g., sending the patient to adult day-care) and list the reasons interfering with the problem being resolved. Each reason is discussed and solutions are suggested by program staff. The pros and cons of potential solutions are outlined and the most favorable one is chosen for the caregiver to try. Sometimes a list of steps to achieve an objective is written and caregivers report their weekly progress in meeting each step to the visiting staff person. As the caregiver moves toward attaining an objective, program staff reinforce and assist the caregiver in evaluating his or her success.

In addition to practicing different strategies, caregivers record the frequency of using relaxation and problem-solving techniques and the frequency of pleasant activities on another daily data recording sheet. These data sheets are useful vehicles for discussing caregivers' successes or continuing problems at each weekly home visit with program staff.

To date, evaluation of these two skills training interventions has shown that caregivers are learning specific patient-change or self-change skills in order to cope better with the challenges of caregiving. Eighty percent of the behavior management programs implemented by caregivers reduced the frequency of the most stressful problem behaviors of the patient. Caregivers who learned strategies to change their own behaviors have increased their use of the three strategies by 65% during the 12-week program and 95% of caregivers continued to use the strategies in the 6-month follow-up period. Caregivers' new management strategies resulted in impressive changes in the frequency of patient problem behavior. In the patient-change group, the rates of problem behaviors were reduced and remained low through 6 months of follow-up. In the caregiver-change group, there were some reductions in problem behaviors during the 12-week treatment phase, but once the home visits ended, the frequency of behaviors increased again.

The effects of learning new skills are apparent in the changes on a variety of caregiver psychosocial measures, such as self-efficacy, caregiving strain, burden, anger, anxiety, and depression. In particular, caregivers who learn patient-change strategies demonstrate significant improvements on measures during the follow-up period when they appear to apply learned techniques more consistently. These caregivers feel particularly more efficacious with regard to their caregiving skills; they feel more in control of the patient and their own responses to caregiving challenges, and they predict being able to keep the patient home longer.

The success of these skills training interventions is thought to be related to the individualized approach delivered in the home setting. Because the intervention spans 12 weeks in the life of patient and caregiver, there appears to be ample opportunity to develop a trusting relationship between caregiver and professional. In addition, the professional's individualized advice to the caregiver is based partly on observations of the patient in the home setting and is therefore more valid. Also, new behavior management skills can be modeled, practiced, and modified as needed to fit the situation.

Conclusion

In conclusion, the multiplicity of caregivers and their various, ever-changing needs dictate that a continuum of resources should be available from which appropriate choices can be made at relevant times. Research shows, however, that many barriers to service utilization exist, requiring professionals to be sensitive to the underlying problems and issues confronting caregivers who want to care for the patient at home. Seemingly simple solutions may present overwhelming complexities to some well-meaning, but unskilled, caregivers. Skills training appears to be one technique that should be included in the menu of intervention choices for caregivers.

Author's Note

Preparation of this chapter was supported by National Institute on Aging Grant No. 1 R01 AG09291-01A1 to the University of Pittsburgh.

References

AARP & The Travelers Companies Foundation. (1988). *National survey of caregivers: Summary of findings.* Washington, DC: American Association of Retired Persons.

Albert, S. M. (1990). The dependent elderly, home health care, and strategies of household adaptation. In J. F. Gubrium & A. Sankar (Eds.), *The home care experience* (pp. 19–36). Newbury Park, CA: Sage.

Archbold, P. G., Stewart, B. J., Miller, L. L., Harvath, T., Greenlick, M. R., Van Buren, L., Kirschling, J. M., Valanis, B. G., Brody, K. K., Schook, J. E., & Hagan, J. M. (1995). The PREP system of nursing interventions: A pilot test with families caring for older members. *Research in Nursing and Health, 18,* 3–16.

Baumgarten, M., Battista, R. N., Infante-Rivard, C., Hanley, J. A., Becker, R., & Gauthier, S. (1992). The psychological and physical health of family members caring for an elderly person with dementia. *Journal of Clinical Epidemiology, 45,* 61–70.

Bergner, M., Hudson, L. D., Conrad, D. A., Patmont, C. M., McDonald, G. J., Perrin, E. B., & Gilson, B. S. (1988). The cost and efficacy of home care for patients with chronic lung disease. *Medical Care, 26,* 566–579.

Bourgeois, M., Burgio, L. D., & Schulz, R. (1994, November). *Comparison of caregiver skills training approaches in the home.* Paper presented at the Gerontological Society of America Convention, Atlanta.

Bourgeois, M., Burgio, L. D., Schulz, R., Beach, S., & Palmer, B. (in press). Modifying repetitive verbalizations of community dwelling patients with AD. *The Gerontologist.*

Bourgeois, M., Schulz, R., & Burgio, L. (1996). Interventions for caregivers of patients with Alzheimer's disease: A review and analysis of content, process, and outcomes. *International Journal of Aging and Human Development, 43,* 35–92.

Brodaty, H., & Gresham, M. (1989). Effect of a training programme to reduce stress in carers of patients with dementia. *British Medical Journal, 299,* 1375–1379.

Brody, E. M. (1981). Women in the middle and family help to older people. *The Gerontologist, 21,* 471–480.

Cantor, M. H. (1983). Strain among caregivers: A study of experience in the United States. *The Gerontologist, 23,* 597–604.

Corcoran, M. (1993). Collaboration: An ethical approach to effective therapeutic relationships. *Topics in Geriatric Rehabilitation, 9,* 21–29.

Corcoran, M. (1994, November). *Individuals caring for a spouse with Alzheimer's disease: A descriptive study of caregiving styles.* Paper presented at the Gerontological Society of America Convention, New Orleans.

Corcoran, M., & Gitlin, L. (1991). Environmental influences on behavior of the elderly with dementia: Principles for intervention in the home. *Physical and Occupational Therapy in Geriatrics, 9,* 5–22.

Corcoran, M., & Gitlin, L. (1992). Dementia management: An occupational therapy home-based intervention for caregivers. *The American Journal of Occupational Therapy, 46,* 801–808.

D'Zurilla, T. J. (1986). *Problem-solving therapy.* New York: Springer.

Ferris, S., Steinberg, G., Shulman, E., Kahn, R., & Reisberg, B. (1987). Institutionalization of Alzheimer's Disease patients: Reducing precipitating factors through family counseling. *Home Health Care Services Quarterly, 8,* 23–51.

Fortinsky, R. H., & Hathaway, T. J. (1990). Information and service needs among active and former family caregivers of persons with Alzheimer's Disease. *The Gerontologist, 30,* 604–609.

Gallagher, D., & Thompson, L. (1981). *Depression in the elderly: A behavioral treatment manual.* Los Angeles: University of Southern California Press.

Gonyea, J. G. (1989). Alzheimer's disease support groups: An analysis of their structure, format and perceived benefits. *Social Work in Health Care, 14,* 61–72.

Gray, V. K. (1983). Providing support for home caregivers. In M. Smyer & M. Gatz (Eds.), *Mental health and aging* (pp. 197–213). Beverly Hills, CA: Sage.

Greene, V., & Monahan, D. (1987). The effect of professionally guided caregiver support and education groups on institutionalization of care receivers. *The Gerontologist, 27,* 716–721.

Greene, V., & Monahan, D. (1989). The effect of a support and education program on stress and burden among family caregivers to frail elderly persons. *The Gerontologist, 29,* 472–480.

Gubrium, J. F., & Sankar, A. (Eds.). (1990). *The home care experience.* Newbury Park, CA: Sage.

Gwyther, L. P., Ballard, E. L., & Hinman-Smith, E. A. (1990). *Overcoming barriers to appropriate service use: Effective individualized strategies for Alzheimer's care.* Durham, NC: Center for the Study of Aging and Human Development.

Haley, W. E. (1989). Group intervention for dementia family caregivers: A longitudinal perspective. *The Gerontologist, 29,* 481–483

Hasselkus, B. (1988). Meaning in family caregivng: Perspectives on caregiver/professional relationships. *The Gerontologist, 28,* 686–691.

Henderson, J. N. (1994). Caregiving issues in culturally diverse populations. *Seminars in Speech and Language, 15,* 216–224.

Hughes, S. L., Manheim, L. M., Edelman, P. L., & Conrad, K. J. (1987). Impact of long-term home care on hospital and nursing home use and cost. *Health Services Research, 22,* 19–47.

Kaplan, C. P., & Gallagher-Thompson, E. (1995). The treatment of clinical depression in caregivers of spouses with dementia. *Journal of Cognitive Psychotherapy: An International Quarterly, 9,* 35–44.

Lawton, M. P. (1987). Environment and the need satisfaction of the aging. In L. L. Carstensen, & B. A. Edelstein (Eds.), *Handbook of clinical gerontology* (pp. 33–40). New York: Pergamon.

Lawton, M. P., Brody, E. M., & Saperstein, A. R. (1989). A controlled study of respite service for caregivers of Alzheimer's patients. *The Gerontologist, 29,* 8–16.

Lewinsohn, P., Munoz, R., Youngren, M., & Zeiss, A. (1986). *Control your depression.* Englewood Cliffs, NJ: Prentice-Hall.

Lovett, S., & Gallagher, D. (1988). Psychoeducational interventions for family caregivers: Preliminary efficacy data. *Behavior Therapy, 19,* 321–330.

Lustbader, W., & Hooyman, N. R. (1994). *Taking care of aging family members: A practical guide.* New York: Free Press.

Mace, N. L., & Rabins, R. V. (1981). *The 36-hour day.* Baltimore: Johns Hopkins University Press.

Mohide, E. A., Pringle, D. M., Streiner, D. L., Gilbert, J. R., Muir, G., & Tew, M. (1990). A randomized trial of family caregiver support in the home management of dementia. *Journal of the American Geriatrics Society, 38,* 446–454.

Montgomery, R. J., & Borgatta, E. F. (1989). The effects of alternative support strategies on family caregiving. *The Gerontologist, 29,* 457–464.

Morycz, R. K. (1994). Clinical implications of different caregiving relationships for patients with dementia. *Seminars in Speech and Language, 15,* 206–215.

National Center for Health Statistics. (1989). *Health/United States, 1988* (DHHS Publication No. PHS 89-1232). Washington, DC: U.S. Government Printing Office.

Oktay, J. S., & Volland, P. J. (1990). Post-hospital support program for the frail elderly and their caregivers: A quasi-experimental evaluation. *American Journal of Public Health, 80,* 39–46.

Ory, M. G., & Duncker, A. P. (Eds.). (1992). *In-home care for older people: Health and supportive services*. Newbury Park, CA: Sage.

Pinkston, E., & Linsk, N. (1984). Behavioral family intervention with the impaired elderly. *The Gerontologist, 24,* 576–583.

Pinkston, E., Linsk, N., & Young, R. (1988). Home based behavioral family treatment of the impaired elderly. *Behavior Therapy, 19,* 331–344.

Pruchno, R. A., Kleban, M. H., Michales, J. E., & Dempsey, N. P. (1990). Mental and physical health of caregiving spouses: Development of a causal model. *Journal of Gerontology, 45,* P192–199.

Pruchno, R. A., & Potashnik, S. L. (1989). Caregiving spouses: Physical and mental health in perspective. *Journal of the American Geriatrics Society, 37,* 697–705.

Pruchno, R. A., & Resch, N. L. (1989). Husbands and wives as caregivers: Antecedents of depression and burden. *The Gerontologist, 29,* 159–165.

Pynoos, J., & Ohta, R. J. (1991). In-home interventions for persons with Alzheimer's disease and their caregivers. *Physical and Occupational Therapy in Geriatrics, 9,* 83–92.

Quayhagen, M. P., & Quayhagen, M. (1989). Differential effects of family-based strategies on Alzheimer's Disease. *The Gerontologist, 29,* 150–155.

Rob, C. (1991). *The caregiver's guide*. Boston: Houghton Mifflin.

Rogers, J. C., Marcus, C. L., & Snow, T. L. (1987). Maude: A case of sensory deprivation. *American Journal of Occupational Therapy, 41,* 673–676.

Rolland, J. S. (1988). A conceptual model of chronic and life threatening illness and its impact on families. In C. S. Chilman, E. W., Nunnally, & F. W. Cox (Eds.), *Chronic illness and disability*. Newbury Park, CA: Sage.

Rubinstein, R. L. (1990). Culture and disorder in the home care experience: The home as the sickroom. In J. F. Gubrium & A. Sankar (Eds.), *The home care experience* (pp. 37–58). Newbury Park, CA: Sage.

Schulz, R., & O'Brien, A. (1994). Alzheimer's disease caregiving: An overview. *Seminars in Speech and Language, 15,* 185–194.

Schulz, R., O'Brien, A., Bookwala, J., & Fleissner, K. (1995). Psychiatric and physical morbidity effects of dementia caregiving: Prevalence, correlates, and causes. *The Gerontologist, 35,* 771–791.

Seltzer, M. M., Litchfield, L. C., Kapust, L. R., & Mayer, J. B. (1992). Professional and family collaboration in case management: A hospital-based replication of a community-based study. *Social Work in Health Care, 17,* 1–22.

Simmons, K. H., Ivry, J., & Seltzer, M. M. (1985). Agency-family collaboration. *The Gerontologist, 25,* 343–346.

Smith, K. S. (1992). *Caring for your aging parents.* Lakewood, CO: American Source Books.

Stone, R., Cafferata, G. L., & Sangl, J. (1987). Caregivers of the frail elderly: A national profile. *The Gerontologist, 27,* 616–626.

Suitor, J. J., & Pillemer, K. (1993). Support and interpersonal stress in the social networks of married daughters caring for parents with dementia. *Journal of Gerontology, 48,* S1–8.

Toseland, R. W., Rossiter, C. M., Peak, T., & Smith, G. C. (1990). Comparative effectiveness of individual and group interventions to support family caregivers. *Social Work, 35,* 209–217.

Toseland, R. W., & Smith, G. C. (1990). Effectiveness of individual counseling by professional and peer helpers for family caregivers of the elderly. *Psychology and Aging, 5,* 256–263.

Trocchio, J. (1981). *Home care for the elderly.* Boston: CBI.

Van Nostrand, J. F., Furner, S. E., & Suzman, R. (Eds.). (1993). *Health data on older Americans, United States: 1992 (Series 3).* Hyattsville, MD: National Center for Health Statistics.

Weinberger, M., Gold, D., Divine, G., Cowper, P. A., Hodgson, L., Schreiner, P., & George, L. (1993). Social service interventions for caregivers of patients with dementia: Impact on health care utilization and expenditures. *Journal of the American Geriatrics Society, 41,* 153–156.

Wright, L. K., Clipp, E. C., & George, L. K. (1993). Health consequences of caregiver stress. *Medicine, Exercise, Nutrition, and Health, 2,* 181–195.

Zarit, S. (1990). Interventions with frail elders and their families: Are they effective and why? In M. P. Stephens, J. H. Crowther, S. E. Hobfoil, & D. L. Tennenbaum (Eds.), *Stress and coping in later life* (pp. 147–158). Washington, DC: Hemisphere.

Zarit, S., Anthony, C., & Boutselis, M. (1987). Intervention with caregivers of dementia patients: A comparison of two approaches. *Psychology and Aging, 2,* 225–234.

Zimmer, J. G., Groth-Juncker, A., & McCusker, J. (1985). A randomized controlled study of a home health care team. *American Journal of Public Health, 75,* 134–141.

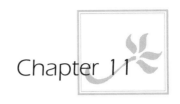

Chapter 11

Communication Intervention for Family Caregivers and Professional Health Care Providers

Lynne W. Clark

Chapter 11 also addresses the topic of caregiver interventions, focusing specifically on communication disorders as a major source of family caregiver stress. A family systems approach is used to identify the nature and causes of communication breakdown due to specific communication disorders. A wide range of family caregiver communication interventions are presented, and the training needs of health care providers are also acknowledged.

1. *How do communication disorders disrupt family homeostasis? How would the impact vary depending upon the type of family structure (according to family systems theory)?*

2. *How do Kobayashi, Masaki, and Noguchi's (1993) stages in adapting for family caregivers of Alzheimer's disease victims compare with the Kubler-Ross (1969) grieving stages?*

3. *What are the four essential components of successful communication interventions with caregivers? Give specific examples of each component as applied to a particular communication disorder.*

4. *How do communication disorders in older adults adversely affect health care providers? What types of communication training programs might be helpful to such providers?*

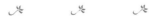

With a large percentage of the population living to an older age, and with the baby boomers about to reach late adulthood, the number of older adults with chronic communication disorders and their family caregivers will continue to increase dramatically. The types of chronic communication disorders seen in older persons include aphasic language disorders, most commonly resulting from stroke; laryngeal cancer; cognitive-communication disorders associated with right-hemispheric involvement, traumatic brain injury (TBI), and the dementias, such as Alzheimer's disease (AD), HIV/AIDS, and Parkinsonism; as well as severe motor speech disorders secondary to static or progressive neuromuscular disorders.

Communication disorders diminish the quality of life, not only for the older adult suffering from the disorder, but also for the family, who must assume a caregiving role and, with it, experience enormous stresses. Speech–language pathologists (SLPs) have traditionally provided direct intervention for adults with communication disorders, but only recently have SLPs begun to implement effective family caregiver intervention programs for reducing the emotional impact of caregiving and for enhancing communication exchanges among caregivers and their relatives. Further, the quality of human communication in the delivery of health care services promotes the physical and mental well-being of older adults, as well as consumer satisfaction. The influence of communication on the quality of health care provided to both normal older adults and those with chronic communication disorders necessitates the provision of effective communication intervention programs for health care providers by the SLP.

As discussed in Chapter 10, successful intervention with family caregivers of older adults suffering communication disorders requires SLPs to have a clear understanding of who the caregivers are, and what their major sources of caregiving burden may be. As a brief guide to the reader, the first section of this chapter focuses on communication intervention for family caregivers, illustrating how a chronic communication disorder serves as a major source of stress. This is followed by information about how a chronic communication disorder disrupts family homeostasis, and how families follow various adapting stages. The reader is then provided with a description of the basic components for implementing a caregiver communication intervention program—education, emotional support, problem solving, and communication strategies. The last section discusses the need for communication intervention with health care providers.

Caregiver Needs and Stresses

Communication Disorders as Major Source of Stress

The bulk of the literature on adult communication disorders and the needs of family caregivers reveals that the inability to communicate adequately and appropriately with relatives suffering chronic communication disorders causes intense emotional stress and burden. This is particularly true for families of AD victims, who are unable to cope effectively on their own with their relatives' communication difficulties (Clark, 1991, 1995). Gurland, Toner, Wilder, Chen, and Lantigua (1994) showed that those AD victims who present with blatantly impaired communications are at increased risk for early institutionalization by their caregivers. O'Brien and Pheifer (1993) demonstrated that caregivers of HIV/AIDS relatives listed the communication problems associated with the infection as one of the eight major physical and psychosocial problems they experienced in caring for their loved one. Similarly, Blood, Simpson, Dineen, Kaufman, and Raimondi (1994) showed that 75% of their caregiving spouses of relatives with laryngeal cancer ranked speech communication difficulties as the major problem causing them moderate to severe strain. Additionally, these caregivers reported the need for pre- and postoperative counseling. Ross and Morris (1988) pointed out that family caregivers of relatives suffering from aphasia are highly vulnerable to developing emotional and psychological problems. Additionally, their caregivers' psychological well-being was directly affected by the inability to communicate with their relative and by their own feelings of loss of independence. These caregivers stated that their perceived degree of strain was as substantial as and comparable to that reported by spouses of AD victims. Finally, Lubinski (1991) alluded to the fact that family caregivers of relatives with severe dysarthria experience strong emotional reactions to the speech disorder.

Disrupted Family Homeostasis

The exact nature of the impact of a communication disorder on the family will vary according to the nature and severity of a relative's disorder, whether its prognosis is favorable for recovery, and whether the onset of the disorder is sudden or gradual. Additionally, the impact will vary according to the family's patterns of functioning prior to the onset of the disorder.

The presence of a chronic communication disorder in an older family member typically becomes a family illness, creating a major family crisis by disrupting the family's homeostasis. Roles, responsibilities, and life-styles of family members become disorganized, especially for those families where communication served as a framework for defining and conferring roles and behaviors, and for dictating social and vocational activities of its members. The SLP needs a working knowledge of family systems therapy to understand fully how families operate when an older member suffers a communication disorder (Kerr, 1981). However, SLPs should not become so engrossed in systems theory that they become less sensitive and empathetic to all those involved.

In systems theory, families are viewed as a complete unit or system with interlocking relationships. Thus, anything that alters the behavior or status of one member of the system, such as a communication disorder, will cause a change in all other members' behaviors. As stated by Norlin (1981), at the core of family systems theory is the belief "that individual actions are embedded in a complex, interdependent tapestry of family dynamics, and what seems like independent, autonomous behavior is, in fact, subtly controlled by the actions of other family members, both past and present" (p. 175).

One function the family performs for its members is to fulfill the goal of equilibrium, seeking to maintain the family's integrity as a stable unit by keeping activities in balance from the demands of the external environment. Systems theory describes family stresses in terms of both vertical stress (i.e., upholding legacies passed on by previous generations on how the family should behave) and horizontal stress (i.e., how the family responds to events that occur during the family's developmental life span). Three types of family functional structures are described by systems theory: closed families, where members' boundaries are fixed, and hierarchical parental authority pervades; open families, where boundaries are flexible with a great sense of democracy and adaptiveness among its members; and random families, where boundaries are unfixed and individuals operate independently of each other. When an older family member suffers a chronic communication disorder, families are placed in a state of disequilibrium. For families to return to a state of functional equilibrium, they must marshal all their internal resources for finding ways to cope, sharing points of view with each other, making role changes, adjusting to changes in their daily routines, and tolerating the tensions and distresses they feel. If the family's internal resources for dealing with these changes and stresses prove insufficient, the entire family enters a period of crisis. Communication normally serves families as an avenue for successfully coping with their member's disability or loss. However, for those families where a member suffers from a communication disorder, an even greater loss is felt because the family is prevented from using communication as a vehicle for coping and sharing feelings. The SLP and other health care professionals can assist the family in restoring its homeostasis or equilibrium.

By having a working knowledge of systems theory, the SLP can effectively assess the family's patterns and values; the members' relationships; styles and content of communication; the role communication serves for the family; the impact of the onset of the communication disorder; members' coping and problem-solving strategies; and the familial sequence of grieving. Assessment occurs through directly observing the family's dynamics and by questioning family members. Formal interview questionnaires for families, for example, *Analysis of Nonlinguistic and Linguistic Behaviors of an Adult Aphasic Patient from His Child's Perspective* (Chapey, 1981) or *The Aphasic Impact Rating Scale for Children and Spouses* (Chwat & Gurland, 1981), can also assist SLPs in obtaining this pertinent information. The SLP should refer families for outside professional counseling if (a) the family homeostasis appears severely disrupted; (b) the presence of the communication disorder serves to feed negatively into the family's previous maladaptive patterns of behavior and interaction; or (c) the SLP reacts by finding fault with certain family members, by trying to rescue family members who appear helpless, or by labeling a situation as resistance when a family member rejects a suggestion from the SLP. The SLP should be aware that, for older caregivers, the onset of a communication disorder may serve as a reminder of the less pleasant aspects of aging rather than the "blissful golden years" of retirement. For the caregiver who is a son or daughter, the onset may constitute the first recognition that their parents are growing older and more frail, and may even serve as a signal of their own mortality.

The Family Process of Adaptation

A natural family response to a loss of communication experienced by an older family member involves the adapting or grieving process.

Regardless of the specific type of communication disorder, some amount of family grieving or mourning will occur. The SLP must be knowledgeable about the grieving process to anticipate, recognize, and support the family effectively as it learns to cope. Additionally, such knowledge serves as a signal for the SLP in determining when the caregiver may benefit from receiving communication intervention and when a referral to a professional for family counseling is warranted (i.e., when grieving is delayed or becomes extended and pathological). Although caregivers go through similar stages of grieving, the length and intensity of the grieving process at any one stage may vary depending on the type, severity, and onset characteristics (sudden or progressive) of the communication disorder. Caregivers typically remain for 1 to 4 months at each of the five grieving stages discussed by Kubler-Ross (1969).

In the first stage, families deny the diagnosis or existence of a communication disorder as a means of controlling their fears, anxieties, and feelings of hopelessness. In particular, caregivers of aphasic, laryngeal cancer, and TBI victims fear that the person will not survive. For TBI caregivers, the stage of denial may exist for many months and even years. In the second stage, the caregiver thinks, "Why me?" and displays feelings of anger, betrayal, and abandonment toward the relative as a normal response to losing control of his or her own life and destiny. The anger, which is often displaced to other family members and even health care providers, results in feelings of guilt. In the third stage, the caregiver bargains in an attempt to delay the loss or reduce its magnitude, thinking, "If I help, he [she] will get better, and may even get back all his [her] communication skills." Improvement may even be fantasized when none has occurred. In an effort to improve their relative's communication skills, caregivers are more accepting of the diagnosis and seek to gather information concerning the nature and prognosis of the communication disorder. In the fourth stage, caregivers may become depressed and self-pitying, actually letting themselves feel the pain of the loss. In the last stage, caregivers display acceptance of the communication disorder and begin restoring order and control over their personal lives.

Kobayashi, Masaki, and Noguchi (1993) studied the stages of adapting for family caregivers of AD victims. These stages are of value to the SLP for they provide insights into the shifts experienced by caregivers in viewing the communication changes associated with AD. These stages may also be applicable for those caregivers whose relatives suffer from other types of gradual and progressive communication disorders. In Stage 1, the caregiver has not yet learned the clinical diagnosis of AD, but expresses concern over the individual's communication abilities and their other behavioral changes. The caregiver misinterprets these changes as intentional and confrontational behavior on the part of the relative. In Stage 2, the caregiver recognizes that these changes are a direct result of disease. However, the caregiver responds to these changes on a trial-and-error basis, not knowing how to adequately cope with such changes on his or her own. For example, the caregiver carries on verbal conversations like he or she did in the past, not knowing whether the relative actually comprehends. During Stage 3, in hopes that the relative's condition will return to normal, the caregiver treats and scolds the individual like a child, in an unsuccessful attempt to regain the type of relationship he or she had with the relative prior to the onset of the disease.

In Stage 4, the caregiver becomes resigned to the clinical diagnosis of AD, adopting a hands-off care policy where no verbal or nonverbal attempts to interact communicatively with their relative are instigated, thinking, "Nothing I say will have any effect, so why talk to him [her]." In Stage 5, the caregiver recognizes that his or her own interactions with the relative can take place through nonverbal avenues, and that his or her own behavior does in fact influence the relative's functional capabilities. In Stage 6, the caregiver expresses empathy for the relative by actively using nonverbal avenues for expressing themselves, and for comprehending the relative's thoughts and needs. By Stage 7, the caregiver has established a successful, warm, nonverbal communicative relationship, accurately perceiving the relative's remaining functional strengths.

Communication Interventions for Caregivers

Intervention Goals

Although compensation may be difficult for older adults with a chronic communication disorder, conversations are enhanced if caregivers learn successfully to shift their role from that of an equal participant to that of a facilitator (Clark, 1995). For the family caregiver, group communication intervention programs are designed to (a) reduce emotional stresses and burdens in caregiving, (b) improve

competency in the delivery of quality care, (c) correct any misconceptions concerning the nature of the communication disorder,
(d) develop realistic expectations regarding the relative's functional
communication abilities, and (e) promote feelings of satisfaction and
of being emotionally connected with the relative through successful
communication exchanges. For older adults with a chronic communication impairment, such intervention is intended to (a) promote the
maximum use of their functional communication skills, (b) provide
them with social communication opportunities, (c) increase their self-
esteem by gaining a sense of control over their communication interactions with others, (d) prevent excess functional disability (i.e., disability over and above the degree of the actual impairment) and
learned helplessness from occurring by promoting a sense of competency as a communicator, and (e) delay the onset of institutionalization.

Initially, general intervention approaches for reducing the stresses
and burdens of caring for older adults developed out of family systems counseling therapy and the gerontological literature. Recently,
SLPs have begun applying these same principles to the design and
implementation of interventions for family caregivers of older adults
suffering from various communication disorders, with more emphasis
on caregiver programs associated with aphasia and the cognitive-
communication disorder of AD (Clark, 1995). Besides understanding
how family homeostasis becomes disrupted and how families learn to
adapt, the following four components are essential to the success of
any communication intervention program: (a) educating the caregiver,
(b) emotionally supporting the caregiver, (c) imparting communication strategies to caregivers for facilitating communication exchanges,
and (d) teaching problem-solving skills for effectively managing difficult communication situations. Each of these is discussed in the following sections.

Types of Programs

Educating the Caregiver. Information is one of the basic needs of
caregivers. Education calls for understanding and acceptance by the
caregiver as to the nature and severity of the communication disorder,
including communication strengths, weaknesses, and prognoses.
Additionally, caregivers need information about those normal aging
changes that may have an impact on communication. Besides verbally

imparting such knowledge, the use of written descriptions with examples and even cartoon illustrations or the use of simulated demonstration videotapes have proven effective (Lesser & Algar, 1995). For example, Ripich, Wykle, and Niles (1995) designed instructional videotape vignettes using actors to role-play persons with communication impairment, illustrating various communication problems. Without factual and experiential knowledge of the disorder, caregivers may develop unrealistic expectations of their relative's communication abilities. Expectations that are too high may result in false hopes that their relative's communication abilities are improving. Expectations that are too low may create premature dependency or learned helplessness when a caregiver speaks for a relative, or may cause an imposed sensory deprivation condition when the caregiver withdraws a relative from familiar communication situations. In addition, inadequate information may lead caregivers to erroneous conclusions regarding the relative's communication ability. For example, they may believe that they can no longer interact communicatively with their relative or that their relative's communication disorder is intentional, rather than a result of the neurological involvement.

Cognitive restructuring is a method that the SLP can use to modify a caregiver's automatic, usually negative, thoughts concerning the communication disorder and the problems it creates. For example, a caregiver may respond to a relative's inability to follow a simple verbal instruction by stating, "He just acts this way to irritate me." A more realistic explanation might be that the relative is too neurologically impaired to understand. If this is true, the caregiver can replace his or her negative, inaccurate thought with a more accurate realistic thought such as, "I get frustrated when he doesn't understand me, but the problem is the result of the neurological impairment and not an attack on me." This more accurate thought generates less negative feelings than the original thought.

As part of the educational process, the SLP needs to assess the caregiver's communication needs and styles of interaction. Besides questioning the caregiver, a number of questionnaires are available to the SLP for obtaining such information, for example: *Communicating with Others: What's My Style or Hidden Feelings that Influence Communication* (Santo Pietro, 1994) or *Questionnaire for Surveying Personal and Communicative Style* (Swindell, Pashek, & Holland, 1982).

Emotionally Supporting the Caregiver. For primary caregivers of relatives with a communication disorder, support groups serve to

(a) assist caregivers in working through the grieving process and accepting the communication disorder; (b) adjust to their new role as communicative facilitator; (c) share their feelings, experiences, and frustrations concerning the disorder in a nonjudgmental atmosphere; (d) mutually assist group members to become better communicators; and (e) enable caregivers to mobilize needed community resources and other social support groups (e.g., Lost Chords Club for spouses of laryngeal cancer victims, Stroke Club for spouses of aphasic victims, or Alzheimer's Disease and Related Disorders Association, Inc. (ADRDA) groups for spouses of Alzheimer's victims). Groups need to be composed of homogeneous participants, either primary or secondary family caregivers of relatives presenting with similar types of communication disorders, and caregivers who are in similar stages of the coping process. The SLP should recognize that older caregivers may initially feel anxious in the group situation because their generation places value upon keeping one's feelings to oneself.

Communication Principles and Strategies for Enhancing Communication Exchanges. Caregivers need to understand the critical value of social communication in allowing their older relatives to remain engaged in human contact and in preventing a premature functional disability from becoming superimposed on the true communication disorder. SLPs must help the caregiver learn how to self-assess and recognize the communication strengths and weaknesses of the family member, as well as the important difference between linguistic and communicative competency skills. The SLP should also teach the caregiver strategies to maintain communication through any modality. Ideally, normal aspects of conversational exchange should be facilitated. This includes turn-taking exchanges during conversation, even if the content of the relative's verbal output is difficult to understand. Too often, caregivers anticipate the needs and wants of a relative. During conversation, turn-taking patterns become asymmetrical, with the caregiver dominating the conversation. As a result, the person with a communication disorder forfeits many of his or her communication turns, occupying a respondent's role. Thus, caregivers need to use fewer communication turns and initiations, reducing control over the conversational exchange so that relatives are given more opportunities to communicate. When verbal interaction is not possible, caregivers need to be taught that they can maintain some level of communication with their relative, if only through nonverbal avenues (e.g., gestures, drawing, pantomime, key written words, symbolic pictures). Caregivers need to accept any communication attempts by their relatives, no matter how simple or primitive (e.g., a smile).

Formal caregiver skills training has proven effective in enhancing communication exchanges with persons suffering from aphasia (Lesser & Algar, 1995), severe motor speech disorders (Light, Dattilo, English, Gutierrez, & Hartz, 1992), AD (Bohling, 1991; Clark, 1995; Clark & Witte, 1995; Shulman & Mandel, 1988), and TBI (Acorn, 1993). The SLP must first assess the effectiveness of the communication strategies spontaneously used by caregivers to determine whether they are facilitative. For caregivers of moderately severe aphasic relatives, Lesser and Algar identified strategies that caregivers can apply successfully to repair the conversational breakdowns, using ethnomethodological techniques of conversational analysis. This type of analysis can be used by the SLP to determine how a relative's communication interactions are positively influenced by the caregiver's facilitative strategies. Besides direct observation and conversational analysis of caregivers' speech during communication exchanges, written questionnaires such as *The Family Interaction Analysis Form* (Florance, 1981), which lists facilitative and nonfacilitative strategies, or *Ineffective Communication Tactics* (Santo Pietro, 1994), which lists those strategies that contribute to communication breakdowns, can also be utilized by the SLP. As illustrated in Table 11.1, Ripich (1993) effectively used the acronym FOCUSED to train and remind caregivers of AD victims of verbal and nonverbal facilitative communication strategies.

Role playing by caregivers in a group situation or viewing videotape vignettes illustrating the strategies are highly effective techniques for skill training. Eventually, strategies should be used by caregivers in real-life situations with their relative, initially under the direct supervision of the SLP. Care must be taken to ensure that caregivers do not perceive any of the strategies as infantilizing or patronizing. Otherwise, such strategies will be doomed to failure. Written materials should provide a description of the nature of and rationale for each strategy along with specific examples (see Lesser and Algar, 1995, for excellent examples). Caregivers should self-evaluate and then discuss their use of strategies with other group members. As well as effecting the use of facilitative strategies, caregivers also need to eliminate those poor and nonfacilitative communication strategies that they may be using habitually and unconsciously.

In recent years, SLPs have started using nonverbal and verbal communication strategies designed by Feil (1992, 1993) with AD caregivers (Benjamin, 1995). For example, if an AD victim at Feil's Level 2

Table 11.1
FOCUSED Program for Alzheimer's Disease Caregivers

F = **Functional and Face** to attract attention
- Face persons directly and check lighting
- Call persons by their name or use gentle touch
- Gain and maintain eye contact at eye level

O = **Orientation** to topic of conversation
- Repeat the topic, key words, and sentences
- Repeat sentences exactly as spoken
- Use specific nouns, names of persons, and places
- Give person time to comprehend what you say

C = **Continuity,** or maintenance of the topic (**Concrete** topics)
- Continue same topic of conversation for as long as possible
- Prepare person for when a new topic is being introduced

U = **Unsticking** for overcoming communication blocks
- Use questions to seek clarification (e.g., "Do you mean . . . ?")
- Repeat the person's sentences using the correct word
- Indirectly suggest the word for which you think the person is searching

S = **Structure** of questions
- Use choice rather than open-ended questions
- Provide only two options at a time

E = **Exchange** ideas, needs, and feelings during conversation and **Encourage** interaction
- Keep the conversational exchange of ideas going
- Begin conversations with pleasant, normal topics
- Give the person clues as to how to answer

D = **Direct** types of verbal messages
- Use simple, short sentences
- Use sentences with the active rather than passive voice
- Use specific, concrete nouns and avoid pronouns
- Communicate verbally and nonverbally in as many modalities as possible

---

Note. From "A Communication Strategies Program for Caregivers of Alzheimer's Disease Patients," by D. Ripich, 1993. In L. Clark (Ed.), *Communication Disorders of the Older Adult: A Practical Handbook for Health Care Professionals.* New York: Hunter/Mt. Sinai Geriatric Education Center.

of disorientation states, "Take me home. I want to go home," the caregiver avoids "why" questions, but asks "who," "what," "where," and "when" questions such as, "What do you miss about home? What do you want to do at home?" and "Does this place remind you at all of home?" If the person at Level 3 disorientation says, "The little ones are turning, learning, turning, learning, turtle, turtle . . . ," the caregiver responds, "You're thinking about your children, and all the work and fun you had as they grew up. Did you like being a mother?" Another therapeutic communication technique used by Feil (1992) for "maloriented" persons is keying into the person's preferred sensory modality. By listening closely to the person's words, caregivers can discover the person's key descriptive "sense," then use it in their own comments. For example, when the AD person states, "I *feel* heavy pressure on my head" (kinesthetic), the caregiver may reply, "How does it *feel*? Is it like a hammer *pounding*?" or "Does it *feel* like a weight *pressing* on your head?" If the person says, "I *heard* a noise last night" (auditory), the caregiver can reply, "How *loud* was it? What did it *sound* like?"

Bohling (1991) demonstrated the importance of the caregivers becoming sensitive listeners in understanding the communication intentions of persons with Alzheimer's disease. Under normal conversational situations, frame shifts occur frequently between participants. Frame marks that control the direction of naturally occurring conversations set the stage for a new direction of thought, but persons with Alzheimer's disease fail to provide these socially expected breaks, causing the listener to become disoriented by the person's frame and unable to comprehend the person's communication attempt. However, Bohling suggested that, if the listener searches for transformational cues in the person's frame and verbally uses such cues before returning to his or her own frame, the AD victim will attempt to verbally repair his or her own frame so the listener can discern the AD speaker's intentions. Examples of transformational cues include temporal cues (e.g., "*When* I was young"), geographic cues (e.g., "Back in *Chicago*"), and physiologic cues (e.g., "I am *starving*").

Problem-Solving Skills for Managing Stressful Communication Situations. "Problem-solving is a vital process by which the caregiver identifies those communication problems or situations that create the most stress, and determines to what extent these problems can be modified" (Clark, 1991, p. 61). Caregivers keep a daily log of when, where, and how often a particular problem behavior has occurred, rating the level of emotional reaction for each communication behavior, as well as listing the antecedent and consequential events surrounding each behavior. The final step in this process involves the caregiver's evaluation of the effectiveness of each solution by determining whether the problem is occurring less frequently. "Active problem-solving leads to cognitive rehearsal where the caregiver mentally carries out steps toward a solution for the problem, thus anticipating and even preventing future communication problems from occurring" (Clark, 1991, p. 61). Overwhelmed caregivers may at first have trouble identifying difficult communication problems or situations on their own. In these instances, use of questionnaires such as *Tough Communication Situations* (Santo Pietro, 1994) should be employed. With assistance from the SLP and other group participants, the caregiver actively assesses the problem and determines alternative solutions, examining the advantages and disadvantages of each. The end goal is the caregiver's independent application of the problem-solving process to other communication problem behaviors.

Group Duration and Intervention Setting

Each of the previous sections describes issues that involve group interventions. An example of a specific programming sequence is described below, but there may be other preferred sequences for addressing all aspects of these issues during group intervention.

As seen with the grieving process, caregivers require education and communication coping strategies when they display the greatest degree of emotional stress, usually at the beginning stages. The SLP should provide the component of emotional support to group participants at the very onset of the communication disorder. It is best to spread the educational component over a number of group sessions, because participants may become overwhelmed when too much information is presented in one session, particularly if caregivers have not yet resolved their own feelings regarding the diagnosis of the communication disorder. Six or seven 2-hour group modules are recommended, divided according to the following organization:

- Module I: Assessing Family Dynamics and Reactions to the Communication Disorder

- Module II: Nature of the Communication Disorder

- Module III: Value of Interpersonal Skills and Assessing Styles of Communication

- Modules IV and V: Promotion of Facilitative Communication Strategies and Evaluation of Communication Strategies

- Module VI: Application of Problem-Solving Process to Difficult Communication Situations

Booster sessions may later be implemented as the needs and concerns of the caregivers shift, or when caregivers request that information from any of the modules be repeated. With the first two modules, the group can consist of 30 caregivers; however, the group should then be subdivided into three groups, each composed of 10 participants for Modules III through VI, so that caregivers' individual concerns can be addressed.

Group programs can be run in a variety of settings: day-care or senior citizen centers, nursing homes, outpatient clinics, rehabilitation centers, or hospitals. They can be run solely by the SLP or in conjunction with other health care professionals. New computer network groups, called "groups without walls," might even be tried for the caregiver who is homebound or physically disabled. Brennan, Moore, and Smyth (1992) used an experimental computer link-electronic network called LINK to promote social support for home-based caregivers of AD relatives. Their communication pathway to peers and a nurse practitioner was available 24 hours a day to provide information and answer caregiving questions.

Communication Management for Health Care Providers

The Need for Intervention

The effectiveness of health care efforts with older adults is directly related to the quality of human communication. Health care providers depend on communication to gather relevant information about health care complaints and to provide services to older adults. The communication styles and strategies employed by health care professionals have an important effect on the communication successes experienced by older adults in their health care encounters, as well as on their satisfaction and compliance with the health care services they receive. Thus, SLPs can ensure the quality of interpersonal communication of health care providers with older adults by providing appropriate education and communication skills training for the care providers. Such training also assists in combating against ageism in health care by recognizing older adults as important health care recipients. In turn, older adults will have communication opportunities to make informed choices and decisions about their own health care, as well as having positive perceptions of themselves, their personal independence, and their control over the health care system.

Ageism and Its Impact on Communication

Marked differences between health care providers and older adult health care recipients may lead to basic communication misunderstandings. One of the major factors contributing to these poor communication interactions is ageism. For other factors that may also have a significant impact, such as gender, ethnicity, education, and socioeconomic factors, see Chapter 10 of this volume.

Age of the care recipient is one of the most important criteria used by health providers in judging social value. In other words, the greater the social value of the care recipient, the greater the health care efforts that will be expended by providers. Ageism, or the system of destructive false societal beliefs about older adults, is also reflected through negative health care providers' attitudes and their general reluctance to deal with older persons. Often, the health care provider does not display blatant ageism, but does respond differently to younger and older adults with regard to the content and style of communications and patterns of communication exchanges.

Many of these communication interactional patterns are described by Shadden in Chapter 7 of this volume. Of particular interest with respect to health care providers is Ryan, Giles, Bartolucci, and Henwood's (1986) discussion of the communication predicament of aging as "a vicious cycle in which the changes of aging (e.g., physical appearance, voice quality, hearing difficulties, slowness of movement, loss of role) elicit [exogenous] interpretations from others of diminished competence; and these inferences then lead to constraining conditions in which the older person has less opportunity to communicate effectively . . . diminished self-esteem and withdrawal from social interactions . . . [and further] physiological, psychological, and social declines" (pp. 16–17). Thus, speech overaccommodation and other forms of "elderspeak" are assumed to be a function of the health care provider's perception that the normal older adult is physically frail, as well as cognitively and linguistically impaired. The terms *secondary baby talk, institutionalized* or *patronizing talk,* and *controlling talk* have been used to describe speech overaccommodations. Secondary baby talk, as described by Caporael and Culbertson (1986), consists of using a high pitch, exaggerated intonation, and encouraging comments with older adults. Controlling talk, or elderspeak, refers to the use of a patronizing speech style with older adults that resembles the speech addressed to children by their parents (Hummert, 1994). It includes slow speaking rate and longer pauses, precise articulation, exaggerated intonation, demeaning emotional tone, increased loudness, simplified syntax, lexical redundancy, reduced use of polysyllables, and use of concrete, familiar words and explicit references (Kemper, 1994; Ryan & Cole, 1990), as well as other controlling nonverbal behaviors.

The use of speech overaccommodation directly affects older adults by (a) constraining their communication opportunities, (b) reinforcing age-stereotyped behavior, (c) reducing their personal control and self-esteem, and (d) lessening their psychological activity and interactions. Speech overaccommodation is typically judged by normal younger and older community dwelling adults and by institutionalized older adults as conveying a negative evaluation of the competency of older adults (i.e., patronizing, demeaning, and disrespectful). However, under certain circumstances, speech overaccommodation has been positively received and has actually facilitated communication. For example, Kemper, Anagnopoulos, Lyons, and Heberlein (1994) showed that speech overaccommodation facilitated the performance of 16 mild to moderately severe AD subjects on a picture barrier description task.

Health care providers also employ speech underaccommodation, using slang terms with unfamiliar persons, speaking more rapidly and in a softer tone of voice than normal, physically distancing themselves from older persons, making exchanges briefer, or talking with a relative as a substitute for directly speaking to an older adult. Examples of linguistic markers that reflect controlling and dependency-inducing speech used with older adults are shown in Table 11.2 (Lanceley, 1985).

SLPs need to caution health care providers regarding how the use of these language devices can be perceived negatively by older adults

Table 11.2

Controlling Language Devices Used with Older Adults

- Use of directives

- Use of tag questions or words like *just* to soften directives (e.g., "You'll have lunch, won't you?" or "I *just* want you to lie down on your side so that I can give you a shot.")

- Use of pet terms (e.g., "Dearie") or use of the person's first name as opposed to his or her title and last name

- Impersonalizing, where care provider uses terms to talk about the person similar to how a parent would discuss his or her child (e.g., Patient: "No, no, I'm not going." Caregiver: "*These* men are miserable. I can't understand *them.*")

- Use of passive objective with the person where the only active agent is the care provider (e.g., While two care providers were helping a patient from the commode, one provider said, "We're just going to stand you up.")

- Use of *must* and *may* words to imply authority (e.g., "John, you *must* eat your lunch now.")

- Placing a reply in a verb tense other than the present tense (e.g., Patient: "I want to go home." Care provider: "That would be difficult. We'll have to see.")

- Use of sarcastic humor

- Ignoring any of the person's verbal/nonverbal requests or comments

- Performing routine daily tasks involving the patient without explaining or commenting about what is being done

- Talking to other persons present while ignoring the patient

- Talking about the person as if he or she where physically absent

---

Note. From "Use of Controlling Language in the Rehabilitation of the Elderly," by A. Lanceley, 1985, *Journal of Advanced Nursing, 10,* 125–133.

as "controlling talk," and how their use reinforces in older adults a sense of helpless dependence, when in fact the explicit goal of interaction should be to foster the confidence and independence of the older adult as part of the rehabilitation process. Health care providers should be cautioned not to modify more aspects of their speech than necessary or appropriate.

Communication Disorder and Its Impact on the Health Care Provider

Health care providers have reported stress and dissatisfaction in caring for older adults with a chronic communication problem (Buckwalter, Cusack, Kruckeberg, & Shoemaker, 1991; Burgio & Burgio, 1990; Clark, 1991; Ripich et al., 1995). Inappropriate verbal behaviors of patients are listed as among the three most stressful behaviors with which health care providers have to deal. Health care providers (a) complain of difficulty understanding what the patient has said, (b) label adults with a communication disorder as "problem" patients, (c) seek fewer interactions with patients, and (d) interact superficially with such patients by centering any conversations around their daily care needs. They find it difficult to establish any rapport or relationships with patients, who are viewed as "empty shells," rather than as human beings who have difficulty communicating their needs.

Researchers have reported, however, that when health care providers participated in communication intervention programs, they reported more positive feelings toward caring for those older adults with a communication disorder; similarly, the older adults reported increased levels of satisfaction in the care they received (Buckwalter, Cusack, Sidles, Wadle, & Beaver, 1989; Clark, 1995; LeDorze, Julien, Brassard, Durocher & Boivin, 1994; Richter, Boltenberg, & Roberto, 1993; Ripich et al., 1995). With intervention, care providers feel that their understanding of the communication disorders has increased, which in turn has altered their attitudes toward older adults with a communication disorder. By using the communication strategies they learned, care providers have reported, they feel a greater sense of self-control during conversational exchanges and when managing patients' difficult behaviors. Rather than patronizing or avoiding communication interactions, care providers have reported more attempts to interact with patients; and they have found that conversational interactions are more satisfying.

To date, care provider communication intervention programs have focused primarily on nurses and nursing assistants in extended health facilities who spend the most time in caring for older adults with a communication disorder (Buckwalter et al., 1989; Ripich et al., 1995). The intervention focus has been primarily on the educational and communication strategies skills training components, as described in the previous section. Although the emotional burdens of caring may be different from those seen for family caregivers, health care providers still experience the stresses of caring, and thus some emphasis on emotionally supporting health care providers should be incorporated into the intervention program. Additionally, the SLP needs to impart relevant information regarding styles of communication, speech accommodation, and intercultural/ethnic considerations (see Waltzman, 1993).

The following suggestions should be considered by the SLP. First, weekly homework assignments, and individual out-of-class contacts with participants to observe their successful use of the communication strategies, serve to decrease the group's participant dropout rates. Second, a sense of accomplishment can be fostered by offering continuing education credits where applicable, and holding a reception to award certificates at the conclusion of the program. Finally, the intervention groups should consist of participants who share similar educational levels and occupational backgrounds (e.g., nurse assistants, medical personnel, rehabilitation therapists, maintenance employees, etc.), because group heterogeneity may serve to threaten some participants, reducing active group involvement.

Conclusion

As discussed in this chapter, family caregiver communication intervention is designed to reduce the emotional impact of caregiving and to enhance communication exchanges among caregivers and their relatives. Additionally, communication intervention with health care providers is essential in order to combat ageism, which has a significant negative impact on care providers' communication interactions with older care recipients, and consequently on health care providers' quality of care to the older care recipient. With more older adults at risk for acquiring communication disorders, and as changes in the delivery of health care services to older adults are effected, the SLP will witness a major shift in treatment paradigms. This shift will be from the provision of more traditional or direct intervention approaches to approaches involving indirect intervention with family caregivers and health care providers of older adults with chronic communication disorders. In order to ensure reimbursement of services for these indirect intervention approaches, more efficacy studies of the merits of family caregiver and health care provider communication intervention programs are warranted.

References

Acorn, S. (1993). Head-injured survivors: Caregiver and support groups. *Journal of Advanced Nursing, 18,* 39–51.

Benjamin, B. (1995). Validation therapy: An intervention for disoriented patients with Alzheimer's disease. *Topics in Language Disorders, 15,* 66–74.

Blood, G., Simpson, K., Dineen, M., Kaufman, S., & Raimondi, S. (1994). Spouses of individuals with laryngeal cancer: Caregiver strain and burden. *Journal of Communication Disorders, 27,* 19–35.

Bohling, H. (1991). Communication with Alzheimer's patients: An analysis of caregiver listening patterns. *International Journal of Aging and Human Development, 33,* 249–267.

Brennan, P., Moore, S., & Smyth, K. (1992). Alzheimer's disease caregiver's uses of a computer network. *Western Journal of Nursing Research, 14,* 662–673.

Buckwalter, K., Cusack, D., Kruckeberg, T., & Shoemaker, A. (1991). Family involvement with communication-impaired residents in long-term care settings. *Applied Nursing Research, 4,* 77–84.

Buckwalter, K., Cusack, D., Sidles, E., Wadle, K., & Beaver, M. (1989). Increasing communicative ability in aphasia/dysarthric patients. *Western Journal of Nursing Research, 11,* 736–747.

Burgio, L., & Burgio, K. (1990). Institutional staff training and management: A review of the literature and a model for geriatric long-term care facilities. *International Journal of Aging and Human Development, 30,* 287–302.

Caporael, L., & Culbertson, G. (1986). Verbal response modes of baby talk and other speech at institutions for the aged. *Language and Communication, 6,* 99–112.

Chapey, R. (1981). The assessment of language disorders in adults. In R. Chapey (Ed.), *Language intervention strategies in adult aphasia* (pp. 81–140). Baltimore: Williams & Wilkins.

Chwat, S., & Gurland, G. B. (1981). Comparative family perspectives on aphasia: Diagnostic, treatment, and counseling implications. In R. H. Brookshire (Ed.), *Clinical Aphasiology Conference Proceedings* (p. 212). Minneapolis: BRK.

Clark, L. (1991). Caregiver stress and communication management in Alzheimer's disease. In D. Ripich (Ed.), *Handbook of geriatric communication disorders* (pp. 127–142). Austin, TX: PRO-ED.

Clark, L. (1995). Interventions for persons with Alzheimer's disease: Strategies for maintaining and enhancing communicative access. *Topics in Language Disorders, 15,* 50–69.

Clark, L., & Witte, K. (1995). Nature and efficacy of communication management in Alzheimer's disease. In R. Lubinski (Ed.), *Dementia and communication* (pp. 238–256). San Diego: Singular.

Feil, N. (1992). Validation therapy. *Geriatric Nursing, 3,* 129–133.

Feil, N. (1993). *The validation breakthrough: Simple techniques for communicating with people with Alzheimer's-type dementia.* Baltimore: Health Professions Press.

Florance, C. L. (1981). Methods of communication analysis used in family interaction therapy. In R. H. Brookshire (Ed.), *Clinical Aphasiology Conference Proceedings* (p. 204). Minneapolis: BRK.

Gurland, B., Toner, J., Wilder, D., Chen, J., & Lantigua, R. (1994). Impairment of communication and adaptive functioning in community-residing elderly with advanced dementia. *Alzheimer's Disease and Associated Disorders, 8,* 230–241.

Hummert, M. L. (1994). Stereotypes of the elderly and patronizing speech. In M. L. Hummert, J. Wieman, & J. F. Nussbaum (Eds.), *Interpersonal communication in older adulthood* (pp. 162–184). Thousand Oaks, CA: Sage.

Kemper, S. (1994). Elderspeak: Speech accommodations to older adults. *Aging and Cognition, 1,* 17–28.

Kemper, S., Anagnopoulos, C., Lyons, K., & Heberlein, W. (1994). Speech accommodations in dementia. *Journal of Gerontology, 49,* 223–229.

Kerr, M. (1981). Family systems theory and therapy. In A. Gehman & D. Kniskern (Eds.), *Handbook of family therapy* (pp. 75–90). New York: Brunner/Mazel.

Kobayashi, S., Masaki, H., & Noguchi, M. (1993). Developmental process: Family caregivers of demented Japanese. *Journal of Gerontological Nursing, 10,* 7–12.

Kubler-Ross, E. (1969). *On death and dying.* New York: Macmillan.

Lanceley, A. (1985). Use of controlling language in the rehabilitation of the elderly. *Journal of Advanced Nursing, 10,* 125–133.

LeDorze, G., Julien, M., Brassard, C., Durocher, J., & Boivin, G. (1994). An analysis of the communication of adult residents of a long-term care hospital as perceived by their caregivers. *European Journal of Disorders of Communication, 29,* 241–267.

Lesser, R., & Algar, L. (1995). Towards combining cognitive, neuropsychological and pragmatics in aphasia therapy. *Neuropsychological Rehabilitation, 5,* 67–92.

Light, J., Dattilo, J., English, J., Gutierrez, L., & Hartz, J. (1992). Instructing facilitators to support the communication of people who use augmentative communication systems. *Journal of Speech and Hearing Research, 35,* 865–875.

Lubinski, R. (1991). Dysarthria: A breakdown in interpersonal communication. In D. V. Vogel & M. P. Cannito (Eds.), *Treating disordered motor control: For clinicians by clinicians* (pp. 153–181). Austin, TX: PRO-ED.

Norlin, P. F. (1981). Familiar faces, sudden strangers: Helping families cope with the crisis of aphasia. In R. Chapey (Ed.), *Language intervention strategies in adult aphasia* (p. 174). Baltimore: Williams & Wilkins.

O'Brien, M., & Pheifer, W. (1993). Physical and psychosocial nursing care for patients with HIV infection. *Advances in Clinical Nursing Research, 28,* 303–316.

Richter, J., Boltenberg, D., & Roberto, K. (1993). Communication between formal caregivers and individuals with Alzheimer's disease. *The American Journal of Alzheimer's Care and Related Disorders and Research, 9,* 20–27.

Ripich, D. (1993). A communication strategies program for caregivers of Alzheimer's disease patients. In L. Clark (Ed.), *Communication disorders of the older adult: A practical handbook for health care professionals* (pp. 61–72). New York: Hunter/Mt. Sinai Geriatric Education Center.

Ripich, D., Wykle, M., & Niles, S. (1995). Alzheimer's disease caregivers: The FOCUSED program. *Geriatric Nursing, 16,* 15–19.

Ross, S., & Morris, R. (1988). Psychological adjustment of the spouses of aphasia stroke patients. *International Journal of Rehabilitation Research, 11,* 383–386.

Ryan, E., Giles, H., Bartolucci, G., & Henwood, K. (1986). Psycholinguistic and social psychological components of communication by and with the elderly. *Language and Communication, 6,* 1–24.

Ryan, E., & Cole, R. (1990). Evaluative perceptions of interpersonal communication with elders. In H. Giles, N. Coupland, & J. Wieman (Eds.), *Communication health and the elderly* (pp. 172–190). Manchester, UK: Manchester University Press.

Santo Pietro, M. (1994). Assessing the communicating styles of caregivers of patients with Alzheimer's disease. *Seminars in Speech and Language, 15,* 236–246.

Shulman, M., & Mandel, E. (1988). Communication training of relatives and friends of institutionalized elderly persons. *The Gerontologist, 28,* 797–799.

Swindell, C. S., Pashek, G. V., & Holland, A. H. (1982). A questionnaire for surveying personal and communicative style. In R. H. Brookshire (Ed.), *Clinical Aphasiology Conference Proceedings* (p. 50). Minneapolis: BRK.

Waltzman, D. (1993). Understanding and respecting cultural and linguistic diversity in older adults. In L. Clark (Ed.), *Communication disorders of the older adult: A practical handbook for health care professionals* (pp. 173–186). New York: Hunter/Mt. Sinai Geriatric Education Center.

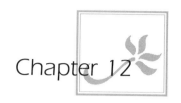

Chapter 12

Innovative Communication Programming in Retirement Communities

Patricia J. Dukes

Chapters 12 through 14 address innovative strategies for enhancing and/or maintaining communication skills. In Chapter 12, Dukes uses a series of "problem" scenarios to identify the manner in which Quality Assurance Committees in long-term care and retirement facilities can address a wide range of communication-based concerns. Examples of communication management issues include posttreatment communication maintenance, generalization of communication skills, effective management of hearing aids, monitoring of appropriate diet levels in dysphagic residents, dementia interventions, and aural rehabilitation. Dukes highlights the importance of team input and participation in developing programs.

1. *How do Omnibus Budget Reconciliation Act of 1987 (OBRA) guidelines provide opportunities for speech–language pathologists to develop innovative transdisciplinary programs in retirement and long-term care facilities? What does Dukes recommend as the primary vehicle for team problem solving and program development within the context of OBRA mandates?*

2. *Pick two of the problems used by Dukes to illustrate problem resolution in long-term care settings. For each problem area, identify the precipitating problem, the solution (specific activities and professionals involved), and the desired outcome(s). What funding issues were raised for each problem area?*

❧ ❧ ❧

As we move into the 21st century, the need for rehabilitation professionals to respond effectively to both current and projected health care delivery issues has changed, probably forever, traditional approaches to rehabilitation services. Health care reform (including managed care), reductions in the Medicare program, a rapidly aging population, the need to target functional outcomes, and government-mandated accountability have dictated a multitude of interdependent changes in the delivery of rehabilitation services. Many of the changes are viewed positively and have already led to needed reform. Others require more intensive problem solving by transdisciplinary teams. Quality Assurance (QA) Committees, mandated by the Omnibus Budget Reconciliation Act of 1987 (OBRA), have been established in long-term care (LTC) facilities, but few function well enough to be pivotal for facility-wide change. Well-functioning QA teams have become the principle instrument of change and are based on the philosophy of total quality management (TQM) and the methods and procedures of continuous quality improvement (CQI; Hodgetts, 1995).

Innovation in speech–language pathology services to residents of LTC facilities has been largely a result of compliance with OBRA mandates. OBRA guidelines dictate that transdisciplinary care be provided to residents to prevent unnecessary loss of function; if loss of function does occur (particularly as the result of illness or injury), reasonable efforts must be made toward restoration. OBRA also requires that efforts be made to assist residents in maintaining newly restored functions subsequent to discharge from treatment. A dilemma exists because Medicare reimburses practitioners only for the provision of restorative services, not for prevention or maintenance. Other restrictions imposed on reimbursement relate to criteria for eligibility of service and number of allowable treatments.

The purpose of this chapter is to assist speech–language pathologists (SLPs), audiologists, and other rehabilitation professionals working in LTC facilities to learn how a well-functioning Quality Assurance team implements a transdisciplinary problem-solving approach leading to innovative solutions as professionals collaborate across disciplines. The examples provided, though representative of some of the most common problems reported by SLPs, are taken from the writer's personal experiences (Dukes, 1991a, 1991b). Each example is presented as an exercise in team problem solving through the mechanism of the Quality Assurance committees in place in LTC facilities. It is hoped that the described instances of problem resolution will demonstrate how LTC Quality Assurance committees work to provide quality care that is reimbursable under the Medicare system.

Innovative problem resolution is demonstrated through the following examples: (a) identifying the need to shift to assisted level of care, (b) failure to maintain communication skills upon discharge, (c) creating a communication-rich environment, (d) lost/nonfunctioning hearing aids, (e) establishing aural rehabilitation services, (f) fine-tuning a transdisciplinary dysphagia program, and (g) lack of SLP involvement in treating communication disorders in residents with dementia.

Problem 1: Identifying the Need to Shift to Assisted Level of Care

Problem

The social services director of a continuum of care retirement community noted that residents living in independent housing often were not recognized as needing to move to an assisted level of care until a crisis developed. She brought this problem to the attention of the QA Committee.

Solution

After considerable brainstorming, it was suggested that a quarterly transdisciplinary screening of functional level be performed on "at-risk" residents with results reported to a yet-to-be created "Level of Living" Committee. The functional assessment would be created by a transdisciplinary team based on a combination of medical, social, physical, and emotional variables. The SLP would oversee a functional communication assessment, which would include speech, language, and hearing screening.

Results

When pre–post audits were compared 6 months after the program was implemented, only one resident required a level of care change due to deterioration unknown to facility staff. (These figures excluded residents who changed levels due to sudden illness or injury.)

Interestingly, this resident had not participated in the screening. Although Medicare would not reimburse the SLP for time spent creating the assessment tool or screening residents, the process resulted in the addition of 3 residents to the SLP's caseload after the first screening, with the anticipation that this trend would continue.

Problem 2: Failure to Maintain Communication Skills Upon Discharge

Problem

The director of the rehabilitation department, who in this facility was an SLP, reported to her QA Committee that follow-up studies indicated that several residents had not maintained their communication skills 6 months after discharge from treatment. The director of nursing (DON) agreed that this seemed to be a problem. She reported her observation of a resident, recently discharged from speech therapy with a communication notebook, who had not initiated use of the notebook with staff since his discharge. Subsequent QA monitors completed by the rehabilitation department revealed that the problem was not isolated to residents being discharged to any particular section of the retirement community, but appeared to be rather universal.

Solution

Because of the global nature of this problem, it was decided to directly involve staff from other departments to assist residents in the maintenance of communication skills following discharge from treatment. Staff from housekeeping, dietary, laundry, maintenance, administration, social services, and nursing were provided individualized departmental inservices designed to heighten awareness of each department's unique opportunities to facilitate communication during interaction with residents. Seven different procedural approaches targeting communication maintenance were developed and implemented.

Procedure 1. In the nursing unit, one nurse was designated the "rehab" nurse, and one certified nurse assistant (CNA) became the "rehab" aide. The physical therapist (PT), occupational therapist (OT), and SLP worked directly with the rehab nurse, teaching her how to instruct nursing staff to assist residents in maintaining discharge goals. Either the rehab nurse or the rehab aide was present during each resident's treatment sessions the week prior to discharge and was involved in writing the resident's discharge plan, so that it was functional and realistic for both the resident and the staff. In this way, the nursing department was represented in planning maintenance programs and would, hopefully, feel some ownership of the program. The rehab nurse was responsible for writing the documentation for all Medicare Part A residents with input from the therapists, and the rehab aide was active in hands-on interventions required during maintenance and prevention phases of care.

Procedure 2. The SLP established communication support groups led by the rehab aide for residents discharged from treatment. Staff CNAs took turns attending the group to receive instruction by the rehab aide along with the residents. The groups met for two 1-hour sessions weekly. During the last 2 weeks prior to discharge, the SLP accompanied the resident to the communication group. Prior to each group session, the SLP suggested thematic activities believed to be of interest to the resident and strategies known to facilitate the resident's comprehension and expression. The SLP taught the rehab aide how to manipulate the environment to create more opportunities for communication and how to use specific language and communication strategies to maximize functional communication for that resident. In this way, the SLP was reimbursed for significant amounts of time spent training staff members to carry out maintenance programs tailored individually to each resident's needs. (Some facilities set up communication support groups targeting residents in need of preventive interventions, as well as residents placed on maintenance programs.) Medicare Part B paid the SLP for establishing programs for these residents, as well as for time spent teaching staff to implement the programs.

Procedure 3. The QA Committee was aware that functional communication is maximized in real-life settings and with people in the resident's natural environment. Therefore, the committee decided to use its exceptional activities department to help solve the problem of maintenance of treatment goals following discharge in the assisted living section of the retirement community. During the 2 weeks prior to discharge, the SLP accompanied the resident to an activity of the resident's choice and encouraged him or her to use newly learned oral or nonverbal communication skills. Both prior to and following the activity, the SLP consulted with the activities staff and volunteers, offering strategies to increase the number of communication opportunities and to facilitate the resident's maximum communication potential. The activities were ones routinely scheduled by the activities department, as well as those jointly contrived by the SLP and activities director to meet the needs of a particular resident.

Procedure 4. It was also suggested that the SLP do more of her therapy in the resident's natural environment. The committee agreed that it was difficult, at best, to implement a treatment program whose primary focus of care was to achieve "functional" communication when working in an isolated room with the SLP creating artificial situations and requiring the resident to respond to contrived stimuli. This suggestion actually led the entire therapy department to become more creative in designing functional treatment tasks. A Main Street concept similar to that used in large rehabilitation hospitals was instituted. On Main Street, PTs, OTs, and SLPs work together to take the resident through a hierarchy of functional tasks simulating real-life experiences in a variety of artificial environments.

By simply changing her assumptions about how therapy should be conducted, this SLP did not need to look far to find settings within which to practice functional communication. In this particular facility, a Main Street concept did not need to be simulated. The facility actually had a post office, variety store, soda fountain, card room, library, exercise room, swimming pool, sauna, and a miniature golf course. Staff and volunteers were trained in these settings to respond to each resident's communication needs, so that the highest possible form of communicative interaction was facilitated. As each resident was discharged from treatment, the SLP directly monitored them in these settings. The SLP took advantage of these opportunities to reinstruct staff (and to instruct new staff) as they interacted with residents. In this way, the SLP's efforts to establish functional communication outside the therapy room were billable to Medicare, as she monitored residents previously discharged from treatment and directed the staff's attention to the resident being discharged.

Procedure 5. Training family members to become more effective communication partners became an integral part of therapy. For example, if the resident's spouse lived in an independent unit while the resident was cared for in the skilled nursing section of a continuum of care facility (as frequently happens during poststroke rehabilitation), the SLP took the resident "home" to be with the spouse during treatment. Motivation was high in this environment of meaningful communication. As the couple worked through difficult but important topics or issues of concern, the SLP facilitated communication. The SLP modeled communication behaviors known to facilitate both comprehension and expression and pointed out behaviors that were likely to interfere with the resident's ability to communicate. If memory, verbal problem solving, sequencing, or spatial and temporal relations were problematic, the SLP demonstrated compensatory techniques or memory aids that were directly applicable to the couple's needs. Other family members were involved in treatment from the beginning, as they were able. The last few sessions were scheduled at times convenient for working families, in order to monitor how they performed in their roles as communication partners. The SLP videotaped these sessions, then pointed out behaviors that facilitated and impeded communication.

Procedure 6. Another procedure established to promote maintenance of communication skills in residents living independently was to videotape conversations between the resident and key staff members with whom the resident communicated on a regular basis (e.g., maintenance, housekeeping, activities, dietary, and business office staff). Staff were then provided an inservice during which they viewed the videotapes. Most staff readily identified conversational behaviors that facilitated or impeded communication with a particular resident. Often, the techniques a staff member learned for facilitating communication with one resident generalized to others, so instructional time was reported to be greatest with new, untrained staff.

Procedure 7. While establishing the maintenance program, the SLP helped the resident (and family) to develop a hierarchy of communication settings ranked from easiest to most challenging. To keep the focus on functional communication, the resident, spouse (if applicable), and SLP worked in each of these settings, beginning with the setting in which the resident felt most comfortable as a communicator. For example, SLPs reported working in the beauty or barber shop, the post office, the "general store," the soda fountain, and the dining room. SLPs also reported accompanying the resident outside the facility to hearing aid and eyeglass appointments, the dry cleaner, the grocery store, and a local restaurant. Again, family members were encouraged to be present so that the SLP could demonstrate effective verbal and nonverbal methods to support the resident's communication. If a communication notebook was used, the SLP, resident, spouse, and family members worked together to select words and phrases appropriate to the resident's needs and level of cognitive/linguistic function (including reading ability).

Results

CNA training provided by the rehab nurse made a significant impact. A follow-up questionnaire revealed an increase in the CNAs' knowledge of communication in general, specific conversational repair strategies, and techniques that facilitate comprehension and expression. Unsolicited comments indicated that the CNAs were often very excited when the strategies they learned actually did facilitate communication with residents. The effect was circular. The CNA now communicated more with the resident, which enhanced the resident's communication skills, thereby causing the resident to initiate more conversations with the CNA. The final result was increased meaningful communicative interactions across settings and communication partners.

The SLP reported that she often saw trained staff informally teaching new staff some of the more common methods to facilitate comprehension (e.g., get eye contact before speaking; speak loud enough but don't yell; paraphrase rather than repeat if the resident does not comprehend; increase the use of meaningful gestures and body language; include contextual references, etc.). Trained staff were also overheard informally teaching new staff ways to facilitate expressive language (e.g., see if they can write the word; have them find the word in their communication notebook; give them a starter phrase and see if they can fill in the word; ask them to point, show, or demonstrate the word with gestures; ask if they can draw the event or action, etc.).

Problem 3: Creating a Communication-Rich Environment

Problem

The QA Committee of the facility described above believed many of their problems stemmed from a communication-impaired environment (Lubinski, 1981). For example, the SLP reported her concern over a communicative interaction she had observed between a CNA and a resident the preceding day. The SLP had recorded the interaction verbatim and read it aloud to the committee members. All present agreed that the CNA spoke as though she were talking to a very young child. She asked rhetorical questions in rapid succession, speaking to the resident with her back turned, while she arranged clothes in the resident's closet. Her language structure was much less complex than appropriate for speech directed to an adult, even though the resident had only mild comprehension problems accompanying a moderate to severe hearing loss. There was also evidence that the CNA did not anticipate communication breakdowns and, once they occurred, did not know how to repair them. For instance, when the resident did not understand (because the CNA spoke with her back turned), the CNA repeated the message verbatim several times in rapid succession with increasing volume (with her back still turned). Very little auditory processing time was allowed. Further, when the resident became anxious because of her inability to comprehend, the CNA made no effort to help her remain calm so that she could access her linguistic knowledge efficiently. Rather, once the resident became upset and started to cry, the CNA proceeded to talk to her as she would to an infant, resulting in the resident's response turning from frustration to anger.

The activities director then reported that she seldom saw residents in the nursing unit carrying on meaningful conversations among themselves or with the staff, an observation consistent with the research literature (e.g., Kaakinen, 1995; Lubinski, 1995). She was certain that many of these residents were highly verbal and enjoyed engaging in conversation because they did so routinely with her at a weekly coffee hour.

Solution

A second hierarchy was generated. This hierarchy focused on communication partners rather than communication settings. It ranked the resident's most frequent conversational partners from easiest to most challenging. For example, the soft-spoken cashier in the business office, who tended to speak with only fleeting eye contact, was high on the difficulty list, even before the conversational context of confusing finances due to Medicare rejections was considered. In any communication dyad, conversational partners share the burden of communicating meaning and must be equally diligent to prevent communication breakdowns and to repair breakdowns when they occur. Although therapy is performed directly with the resident to increase his or her ability to prevent and repair conversational breakdowns, it is often more effective and efficient to change the communication behaviors of the resident's normal speaking partners as well. Therefore, the SLP began working with communication dyads between the resident and each person listed on the hierarchy, going from easiest to most challenging. During an inservice on supporting communication, the SLP and staff members also role-played communication dyads, demonstrating both facilitating and interfering behaviors. Posters were displayed to remind staff and residents to use the communication behaviors they had been taught.

Results

This inservice was extremely well received. In fact, it was voted the best all-staff inservice of the year. After watching the videotapes, staff indicated that they had never realized how their communication "bad habits" had such a devastating effect on communication. Interestingly, the topic of discussion at all shifts eventually turned to communication breakdowns with a spouse, children, or significant others. It seems the inservice had a more widespread effect than planned. The pay-off was greatest as work was done with partners at the top of the hierarchy. If they could be shown how to change the verbal and/or nonverbal behaviors that impaired communications with one resident, these newly learned behaviors were believed to transfer to their communications with others as well.

Problem 4: Lost/Nonfunctioning Hearing Aids

Problem

At another facility's monthly QA meeting, the social services director reported that three residents in the nursing unit had lost hearing aids during the previous quarter. He asked for input from the committee to help him plan a monitor targeting the nature and magnitude of the problem. The housekeeping supervisor reported that a hearing aid had recently been found in a washing machine. The assistant administrator reminded the committee of the facility's policy to pay for a replacement hearing aid under these conditions and told the committee that this was the third hearing aid to be ruined by going through the laundry in the last 6 months. Because of the high cost of hearing aids, the problem was deemed to be significant for both quality of life and financial reasons.

It was decided that a practicum student in the social services department would conduct an audit on one floor of the nursing unit. She began by verifying an inventory list of known hearing aid users and their hearing aids with chart notations written by the SLP. She checked each resident to determine whether the hearing aid was in the resident's possession, whether the hearing aid was clean and in good working condition, and whether a cerumen management program had been established.

Results of the audit revealed that, out of 18 hearing aid users on the floor sampled, 3 residents were in possession of their hearing aids, but the aids were in their bedside tables. Four residents were wearing their hearing aids, but either the aid was not working or the battery was dead. Two other residents were apparently not in possession of their hearing aids; a search of residents' rooms was done with no success. Cerumen management programs had been established for all residents.

Solution

Results of the audit indicated that the original problem of hearing aids going through the laundry was only a small part of a much larger problem. The committee brainstormed potential solutions and agreed to implement the following procedures on a trial basis.

Procedure 1. For cognitively or physically challenged residents, hearing aids were kept on the medicine carts and dispensed each morning by the nurse. Prior to dispensing, the nurse checked the aid for cleanliness of the tubing, positive battery charge, and general working condition. Tubing was cleaned and/or the battery replaced as needed. A system for maintaining a supply of batteries was established. If the aid was determined to be in need of repair, it would be sent to the rehab aide to determine the nature of the needed repair. If minor, the rehab aide, who had been trained to troubleshoot and make minor repairs, made the repair and sent the aid back to the nursing unit. If the aid needed major repairs, it was returned to the audiologist.

Procedure 2. For cognitively impaired residents, the manufacturer put a small plastic loop on the hearing aid case so that fish line could be used to secure the aid to the resident's clothing. This ensured that the aid stayed in the resident's possession if the resident removed it from his or her ear.

Procedure 3. For cognitively impaired residents who often removed their hearing aids and whose aids had no plastic loops, the CNA providing care checked regularly to see that the hearing aid was present. Some nursing units put a symbol of an ear on the chart, the bed, and/or the door frame under the resident's name to designate that the resident was a hearing aid user.

Procedure 4. Finally, it was decided that the CNA who took the soiled sheets off the bed and the laundry staff who put the sheets into the washer would be "on the lookout" for hearing aids. Finding an aid was rewarded with a dinner for two at a local restaurant.

Results

A follow-up audit, conducted 3 months after the plan was implemented, revealed that all 18 residents on the floor sampled were found to be wearing clean, working hearing aids.

Problem 5: Establishing Aural Rehabilitation Services

Problem

The DON in another facility reported that even with clean, properly fitted, working hearing aids, some residents continued to demonstrate nonfunctional hearing. He was also concerned that some previously outgoing residents with hearing loss still had to be coaxed to attend activities, even though they had recently purchased a hearing aid.

Solution

The SLP explained the need to address the issues of auditory perception and the functional use of residual hearing, as well as auditory acuity. She explained that many residents with new hearing aids never adjust to wearing them and cannot be convinced to even put them on. She felt that the problem was partly one of expectation level (i.e., the belief that, like eyeglasses, things become clearer the moment you put them on). She explained that residents must learn to use a number of strategies to maximize residual hearing in the presence of amplification. With this in mind, the following procedures were implemented.

Procedure 1. The SLP began providing communication therapy targeting receptive and expressive conversational strategies to both aided and nonaided residents with hearing impairment. Residents were taught (a) to use their residual hearing more effectively; (b) to use assertive strategies to create an environment conducive to listening; (c) to seat themselves away from noise sources; (d) to maximize speechreading ability by sitting where there was light on the speaker's face; (e) to use metalinguistic skills (i.e., knowledge of language) to help fill in the gaps for words they could neither hear nor speechread; and (f) to clean, maintain, and make minor repairs on their hearing aids.

Procedure 2. The SLP began coordinating hearing services for residents at all levels of living throughout the retirement community. As a result of staff, family, or physician referral, the rehabilitation department secretary scheduled an appointment for the resident with the audiologist or hearing aid dealer. In this facility, these professionals worked as a team to provide services through a written contract with the facility. Evaluations were provided at no cost to any resident requesting this service. (Note: Some insurance policies require that the evaluation be performed by an audiologist.) A hearing aid assessment occurred at a follow-up visit for residents considering amplification.

Procedure 3. Subsequent to evaluation, the audiologist made a recommendation that often included amplification with, or without, additional aural rehabilitation services. At this point, the resident (or the resident's family) made the decision to purchase a hearing aid and/or to undergo further aural rehabilitation. If the family purchased the aid from the audiologist serving the facility, all financial transactions were between the resident (or the resident's family) and the audiologist.

Procedure 4. The hearing aid dealer scheduled weekly office hours at the facility for both scheduled appointments and walk-in visits. Some residents who lived independently or in assisted living sections had difficulty cleaning and adjusting their hearing aids because of physical impairments. These residents had standing appointments during which their hearing aids were cleaned and the batteries replaced. All services were free to the resident. The resident was billed only one time for the purchase of the hearing aid. Hearing aid insurance was included for an additional charge for residents at risk of losing their aids. (The facility decided to provide this insurance for residents in the skilled nursing section, because it was more cost-effective than replacing lost hearing aids.)

Procedure 5. New hearing aid users were evaluated jointly by the SLP and audiologist to determine the benefit of further intervention. As a result of this evaluation, most new hearing aid users residing in independent or assistive living sections were seen by the SLP on an outpatient basis for a six-session (individual or small group) hearing aid orientation. This orientation covered anatomy and physiology of the ear, types of hearing loss, care and maintenance of the aid, assistive listening devices, how to maximize use of residual hearing (including environmental manipulations), suggestions for optimizing speechreading performance, conversational strategies (i.e., anticipatory and repair), assertiveness training, coping strategies, and community resources. Residents needing more intensive intervention received treatment twice weekly for 12 weeks in a combined group–individual format. Each week, the resident received an individual session targeting speechreading and auditory training and a group session targeting functional communication. Families were involved in this treatment on a regular basis.

Cognitively alert residents with hearing impairment from the nursing section typically attended a group with residents from other sections of the retirement community. Residents from the nursing section who exhibited memory loss typically received individual therapy initially; then they were accompanied by the SLP to activities in the nursing unit in order to establish a functional maintenance program. (See solution to Problem 2.)

Speechreading materials were drawn from various sources, including The New York League for the Hard of Hearing's (1988) video set, *I See What You Are Saying,* which has entertaining vignettes on various topics done in humorous fashion by Gene Wilder. *Speechreading: A Way to Improve Understanding* (Kaplan, Bally, &

Garretson, 1987) provided material easily modified for this population. It was found to be particularly useful for its sections on teaching conversational anticipatory and repair strategies. Numerous additional references were found to be of help to the SLP providing programming (Clark & Martin, 1994; Erber, 1982, 1988, 1993; Spitzer, Leder, & Giolas, 1993).

Clinician-produced conversational sequences based on familiar contexts (e.g., bakery, gas station, football game, etc.) were used to practice the following anticipatory strategies: predicting dialogue, using constellations, controlling the situation, and asking specific questions. Receptive repair strategies taught included asking the conversational partner to repeat, paraphrase, or shorten the message; giving only a key word; or writing the message, depending upon the difficulty of the communication. Expressive repair strategies included asking both general and specific questions, making educated guesses using linguistic context clues, and confirming a message.

Nonimpaired conversational partners (i.e., spouses, family members, and friends) often attended these groups and were taught the techniques along with the resident. Lessons were provided in an informal atmosphere, often in the format of popular TV game shows. Grandchildren living nearby were particularly encouraged to be involved in treatment. They were often found at the very top of a resident's hierarchy as the most difficult communication partners, because of their rapid speech, high pitch, low volume, and lack of awareness of listener requirements. Children tend to use run-on, poorly sequenced sentences so that "sense of story" is hard to follow. They also frequently fail to make eye contact, talk while walking away from the listener, or speak to the listener from another room.

Residents kept a notebook with materials from each lesson to assist recall and review. Between sessions, residents watched videotapes providing additional speechreading practice. Other videotapes covered assorted topics, including care and maintenance of a hearing aid, assistive listening devices, using a text telephone, preferential seating, reducing signal-to-noise ratio in the communication environment, and preventing and repairing communication breakdowns. Assertive listening strategies applicable to listening in group situations were also taught (e.g., asking the speaker to move into a position that is more conducive to speechreading or asking the speaker to use a microphone if one is available). Many of the videotapes were made by the SLP with assistance from the rehab aide. Commercially developed tapes were purchased, rented, or checked out from a library serving persons with hearing impairment (e.g., a Gallaudet Regional Center Library).

Videotapes were also played through closed-circuit TV channels in some facilities, so that residents needed only to "tune in" to watch the tapes and practice listening and speechreading skills in the comfort of their living rooms. Closed-captioned videos were also aired on a number of topics. Dates and times of closed-circuit programming were published weekly in the resident newsletter.

Procedure 6. The last 2 weeks of treatment targeted functional tasks across the resident's hierarchies of communication settings and partners. Subsequent to discharge, residents joined "alumnae" in a monthly social/review support group. As the result of one support group's efforts, an FM sound system was installed in areas of the facility where residents experienced difficulty hearing, such as the chapel, social hall, and dining room.

Results

All residents in the aural rehabilitation program showed improvement from pre- to posttest on measures of functional communication ability. Residents who did poorly speechreading when the subject matter was unknown and no voicing was given performed considerably better speechreading conversation when the context was known, the topic was familiar, and residual hearing was utilized. Residents who learned to speechread each other formed a bond that promoted continued growth following treatment. In fact, the rehab aide, who conducted the monthly support groups, boasted an attendance of almost 100% at each session. (He admitted this might have been due to the delicious home baked "goodies" residents brought to share!) One unexpected positive outcome was that a spouse or friend often watched the videotapes with the resident, thus learning to be an effective communication partner.

Interestingly, it was difficult to make prognostic statements based on pretest scores, age, related diagnostic conditions (with the exception of dementia), or skepticism that the program would make a significant difference in ability to communicate. Some residents who were very skeptical and approached the initial tasks with a negative attitude exhibited noticeable increases in functional communication. The resident's age was also not a reliable predictor of success in the aural rehabilitation program. Some very elderly residents were found to outperform those who were considerably younger and in better physical health. (One very "young" 90-year-old woman reported that, since being discharged from the aural rehabilitation group, she checks out the videotapes periodically just to keep her "skills sharp.") This, and other unsolicited comments, confirmed the SLP's feeling that the ability to communicate is highly valued by elderly residents who are physically limited in their choice of social outlets. For these reasons, a trial period of diagnostic therapy may be the best indicator of progress in treatment. Perhaps the best finding of all was that the billing history of paid Medicare claims revealed no denials from this aural rehabilitation program.

Problem 6: Fine-Tuning a Transdisciplinary Dysphagia Program

Problem

A state audit resulted in a citation issued to an LTC facility for failure to evaluate a resident for a diet upgrade. The resident was receiving a diet of pureed food after a single choking episode 6 months earlier, with no record of a swallow study. A subsequent QA monitor revealed three residents whose diets had been downgraded after single choking episodes, with no referral to speech pathology for a swallow study. The DON asked for help from the committee in brainstorming possible solutions.

Solution

It was decided that the transdisciplinary dysphagia team (i.e., nursing, SLP, OT, dietary) would staff residents on a bimonthly basis, with the following changes being implemented on a trial basis.

Procedure 1. Physician orders for a diet change were written on multiple copy order pads, with each team member receiving a copy and the original going to the resident's chart. The dietary department agreed that, although a diet would be downgraded immediately upon receiving the physician's order, the diet change would not go into effect officially until all team members had evaluated the resident and had met to develop a care plan.

Procedure 2. Previously, because of difficulty transporting residents to the hospital for a modified barium swallow study, the only means of evaluating some residents had been a mealtime swallow study. The team wanted to provide better care; they decided to use Fiberoptic Endoscopic Evaluation of Swallowing (FEES; Langmore, Shatz, & Olson, 1988). The FEES procedure has several advantages: The equipment is mobile, provides an objective means of evaluating the swallow, and assesses the risk of residue build-up and the effects of rapid feeding (both common problems in the nursing facility).

Results

A follow-up audit indicated that the system was working well. Diet changes were being made on the basis of objective data and the team was sharing responsibility for establishing and implementing formal swallowing and feeding programs.

Problem 7: SLP Involvement in Programming for Residents with Dementia

Problem

The director of a large memory loss unit in one LTC facility was concerned that the SLP had very little involvement with the residents on her unit. The only involvement noted in the charts was with a resident who had suffered a stroke. That resident had been seen once for evaluation, followed by a notation in the chart that the resident was a poor candidate for rehabilitation because of her dementia. In fact, the SLP had informed the director that she could not work directly with any of the residents on the unit because of difficulties with Medicare reimbursement. She also expressed her personal belief that treatment was likely to be ineffective.

The director of this unit had recently attended a conference at which SLPs reported good results obtaining Medicare reimbursement for residents of a similar unit. The director wanted to know if any other QA Committee members knew of such programs. After some discussion, the committee decided that it needed more information and recommended that members from the memory loss unit, the nursing department, and the rehabilitation department attend an upcoming conference on communication and dementia and table the brainstorming of potential solutions until they had further information. After attending the conference, consulting with professionals at a nearby university, and doing suggested readings on the topic (Clark, 1995; Glickstein & Neustadt, 1992, 1993; Orange, Ryan, Meredith, & MacLean, 1995), the SLP changed her assumptions about treating this population and suggested the following solution.

Solution

The SLP and activities director cofacilitated communication groups that incorporated approaches from validation therapy (Feil, 1982, 1992) and reminiscence therapy and life review (Lewis & Butler, 1974). Validation therapy was used with residents struggling to maintain contact with the environment because it confirmed the resident's internal emotional state rather than attempting to force the reality of the external environment on the resident. The committee liked this approach because it seemed more humane than previous ineffective efforts at "reality orientation."

The SLP showed staff how to promote the use of residents' residual communication skills through use of the FOCUSED program for caregivers (Ripich, 1993). Techniques to increase opportunities for both verbal and nonverbal exchanges were also demonstrated. (For specific approaches, see Clark, 1995; Kaakinen, 1995; Lubinski, 1993; and Orange et al., 1995). Staff and residents were taught how external communication and memory aids might be used to facilitate conversation. Thematically based activities (e.g., gardening, holiday decorating, planning, preparing and serving a special meal related to the theme, planning a shopping trip, etc.) were used as a basis for communication. Residents were taught to apply adaptive and facilitative communication strategies (Clark & Witte, 1991) as they engaged in conversations centered around these themes.

Group goals (based on Clark & Witte, 1991) were (a) to help prevent premature excess functional communication disability and "learned helplessness," (b) to facilitate use of residual abilities to compensate for those lost, (c) to increase self-esteem through the ability to control at least parts of the conversation, and (d) to reduce emotional stress and anxiety caused by increasing communication difficulty. Groups were also taught to predict communication breakdowns and were instructed to use repair strategies when breakdowns occurred. Specific intervention strategies followed Benjamin's (1995) guidelines. After each session, staff were provided activities to extend learning. These activities targeted specific goals in each week's lesson (e.g., auditory comprehension, verbal memory, verbal problem solving, and/or expressive language).

Services provided to the resident targeted for treatment were billed to Medicare Part B at the facility's group rate. Charges were assessed for establishing a written preventive maintenance plan for communication abilities and for teaching staff to implement it. Shadden (1995) has suggested using discourse analysis for documenting pre–post treatment effects because it is directly related to functional outcome and is sensitive to targeted communication changes. Data that may be extrapolated for comparison purposes might include turn taking, topic maintenance, topic initiation, communication efficiency, number of irrelevant/redundant informational units, and balance in conversational turns (number and length). Other measures might include number of opportunities for communication (an outcome of staff training) and number of communicative interactions with staff and peers.

Results

The SLP reported that it was difficult initially to change her intervention focus from working directly with the resident to training staff and caregivers to promoting successful communication with each resident. (Interestingly, this therapist had received her degree from a university program that taught from a strictly medical model.) Once she had made the shift, however, she thoroughly enjoyed her new role and began spending her spare time in this unit. She stated her belief that university programs need to require more coursework in the area of communication and aging, with special attention given to providing direct and indirect treatment to residents with Alzheimer's disease.

Summary

Effective Quality Assurance Committees in "cutting-edge" long-term care facilities have provided a format for innovative thinking and transdisciplinary problem solving. Rehabilitation professionals face challenges requiring continued innovation as they move into the 21st century. Challenges include health care reform, a rapidly aging population, the need to target functional outcomes of treatment, and government-mandated accountability. Speech–language pathologists and audiologists must be prepared with the knowledge and skills needed to take the lead in developing innovative transdisciplinary programs to meet the needs of the next generation of elders with communication impairment. To do so, communication disorders specialists need to adopt a wider perspective and a more holistic view of the communication needs of the elderly. It is time to move away from traditional models of speech–language pathology and look through a wider lens—one that is focused on improving the quality of life of all residents by helping them to express their opinions, beliefs, and feelings in the most effective way they possibly can. A well-functioning Quality Assurance team is the LTC facility's key to the successful development of transdisciplinary systems. Speech–language pathologists and audiologists must prepare themselves not only for collaborative participation on QA teams but also for leadership roles in the development of systems that deliver quality care to elderly residents with communication disorders.

References

Benjamin, B. (1995). Validation therapy: An intervention for disoriented patients with Alzheimer's disease. *Topics in Language Disorders, 15,* 66–74.

Clark, L. W. (1995). Interventions for persons with Alzheimer's disease: Strategies for maintaining and enhancing communicative success. *Topics in Language Disorders, 15,* 47–65.

Clark, J. G., & Martin, F. N. (1994). *Effective counseling in audiology: Perspectives and practice.* Englewood Cliffs, NJ: Prentice-Hall.

Clark, L. W., & Witte, K. (1991). Nature and efficacy of communication management in Alzheimer's disease. In R. Lubinski (Ed.), *Dementia and communication* (pp. 238–256). Philadelphia: Decker.

Dukes, P. J. (1991a, May). *Hearing conservation/aural rehabilitation programming in long-term care facilities.* Poster session presented at the annual meeting of the Michigan Speech and Hearing Association, Traverse City.

Dukes, P. J. (1991b, May). *Life after speech therapy: Maintenance programs following discharge from treatment.* Poster session presented at the annual meeting of the Michigan Speech and Hearing Association, Traverse City.

Erber, N. P. (1982). *Auditory training.* Washington, DC: A. G. Bell Association for the Deaf.

Erber, N. P. (1988). *Communication therapy for hearing-impaired adults.* Melbourne, Australia: Clavis.

Erber, N. P. (1993). *Communication and adult hearing loss.* Melbourne, Australia: Clavis.

Feil, N. (1982). *V/F validation: The Feil method.* Cleveland, OH: Edward Feil Productions.

Feil, N. (1992). Validation therapy. *Geriatric Nursing, 13,* 129–133.

Glickstein, J. K., & Neustadt, G. K. (1992). *Reimbursable geriatric service delivery: A functional maintenance therapy system.* Gaithersburg, MD: Aspen.

Glickstein, J. K., & Neustadt, G. K. (1993). Speech–language interventions in Alzheimer's disease: A functional communication approach. *Clinics in Communication Disorders, 3,* 15–30.

Hodgetts, R. M. (1995). *Implementing TQM in small and medium sized organizations: A step by step guide.* New York: American Management Association.

Kaakinen, J. (1995). Talking among elderly nursing home residents. *Topics in Language Disorders, 15,* 36–46.

Kaplan, H. K., Bally, S. J., & Garretson, C. (1987). *Speechreading: A way to improve understanding* (2nd ed.). Washington, DC: Gallaudet College Press.

Langmore, S. E., Shatz, M. A., & Olson, N. (1988). Fiberoptic endoscopic examination of swallowing safety: A new procedure. *Dysphagia, 2,* 216–219.

Lewis, M. J., & Butler, R. N. (1974). Life review therapy: Putting memories to work in individual and group psychotherapy. *Geriatrics, 29,* 165–174.

Lubinski, R. L. (1981). Environmental language intervention. In R. Chapey (Ed.), *Language intervention strategies in adult aphasia* (pp. 223–245). Baltimore: Williams & Wilkins.

Lubinski, R. (1995). State-of-the-art perspectives on communication in nursing homes. *Topics in Language Disorders, 15,* 1–19.

New York League for the Hard of Hearing. (1988). *I see what you are saying* [videotape]. New York: Author.

Omnibus Budget Reconciliation Act of 1987, Public Law 100-203.

Orange, J. B., Ryan, E. B., Meredith, S. D., & MacLean, M. J. (1995). Application of the communication enhancement model for long-term care residents with Alzheimer's disease. *Topics in Language Disorders, 15,* 20–35.

Ripich, D. N. (1993). A communication strategies program for caregivers of Alzheimer's disease patients. In L. Clark (Ed.), *Communication disorders of the older adult: A practical handbook for healthcare professionals* (pp. 61–70). New York: Hunter/Mount Sinai Geriatric Education Center.

Shadden, B. B. (1995). The use of discourse analyses and procedures for communication programming in long-term care facilities. *Topics in Language Disorders, 15,* 75–86.

Spitzer, J. B., Leder, S. B., & Giolas, T. G. (1993). *Rehabilitation of late-deafened adults: Modular program manual.* St. Louis, MO: Mosby.

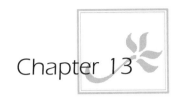

Chapter 13

Volunteers and Partners: Moving Intervention Outside the Treatment Room

Jon Lyon

In Chapter 13, Lyon takes the reader beyond the treatment room and traditional treatment time frame to explore the use of volunteer partners in working with aphasic older adults. The Communication Partners program is designed to help aphasic individuals maximize their communicative interactions and opportunities within the community, as illustrated by an extended case example. Lyon also discusses potential applications of this model to working with communicatively at-risk older adults.

1. *Lyon contends that the therapeutic role of speech–language pathologists should not be restricted to "repairing" disordered communication in clinical settings. What role(s) does he suggest, and how will changing roles influence treatment approaches?*

2. *What is the cornerstone of the Communication Partners program for restoring participation in daily activities? Why are community volunteers considered preferable to family members or professionals?*

3. *The Communication Partners program for adults with aphasia has two primary phases. What are these phases and how do their objectives differ?*

4. *Lyon suggests that the Communication Partners approach might be expanded to work with older adults who are at risk for communication breakdown, despite the absence of a specific communication disorder. Examine Table 13.4 carefully, and describe at least two different circumstances in which an older adult might benefit from this intervention.*

꙳   ꙳   ꙳

For the last 50 years in America, a single model has prevailed for the delivery of clinical services to adults with acquired communication disorders: the repair or circumvention of dysfunction within medical or clinical settings. This form of rehabilitating speech and language disorders gained prominence during World War II when young soldiers who sustained head injuries came home from combat zones (Goldstein, 1942; Wepman, 1951). Favorable brain plasticity and intensive rehabilitative care resulted in many of these GIs returning to everyday lives as functional verbal communicators. These clinical successes and their methodologies laid the foundation for how adults with acquired communication disorders in later life would be approached and treated in the decades that followed.

Nearly a half-century later, a medical or clinical model continues to dominate the delivery of services in this country. Despite this model, as practicing clinicians, we are fully cognizant that our clientele and their projected outcomes have changed over the years. Speech–language pathologists in today's medical centers encounter a much more aged population—one whose etiologies are often less forgiving in the resumption of lost or impaired communication. With people in the United States living longer and having greater awareness of preventing debilitating diseases associated with aging, the trend toward clients who are older and less capable of being habilitated is only apt to increase in the years ahead. In addition, we live in an age of health care reform. Even a decade ago, adults with aphasia experienced the relative luxury of months of rehabilitative care within a medical setting; today these services are substantially reduced in form, in site of service delivery, or in the manner in which they are rendered.

It is this combination of an aging populace, questionable immediate return from acute rehabilitative services, and an era of shrinking health care dollars that signals forthcoming change in service delivery to aging adults. Speech–language pathologists are being challenged, as never before, to provide more and better proof that our services do make a difference. Whatever may evolve from this current debate and reform, the simple truth is that our services to aged adults with communication breakdowns are no less valuable or warranted than they were a half-century ago. To offset what health care providers may judge as less worthy, practicing clinicians need to reshape therapy to include targets that stand to enhance communication and well-being in everyday life—targets previously unmet and largely unattended to in a medical treatment model.

Redefining Our Role in Treatment

Contrary to what health care providers often assume, the therapeutic role and value of speech–language pathologists are *not* bound solely to "fixing" or "repairing" disordered communication in clinical settings. Whether communicative disruption in later life results from insult, disease, or the normal aging process, we must be prepared to demonstrate convincingly that we are the professionals of choice to ensure that our clients are not robbed of a meaningful, purposeful, and rewarding daily existence. In fact, in today's managed health care system, it is far more important and better rewarded to validate that our treatments are not just restorative of language or communication, but are also "life-enabling" and "life-sustaining."

Making our treatments restorative of quality of life requires fundamental shifts in emphasis. First, we need to foster models and methods that promote our role as mediators or facilitators in optimizing communication in natural settings, and not restrict our management to the confines of a clinic or treatment room. Second, and more important, our treatment must target life enhancement from its outset, rather than simply promote adequate communication in everyday life. Ecologically speaking, our therapy is only as good as it blends with, and actively improves, life's chosen pursuits. Just as treatment of impaired communication, when confined to a clinic, may lack relevance in the home or community, so too treatment of impaired communication at home or in the community may lack relevance in furthering one's desires and wishes in daily life.

Thus, "what we do" and "how we do it" require careful reconsideration and revamping. As clinicians, we need to search out other delivery models that satisfactorily address the totality of our clients' needs and desires, those both directly and indirectly related to their communicative difficulties. By fulfilling this obligation, we more than justify our continued presence in treating those who, later in life and for many unexplainable reasons, find a most cherished resource, their communication, impaired.

Communication Partners: Treating a Different Way

This chapter offers an overview of an alternative model for treating adults with communication disorders—one outside a medical or clinical setting. It is called Communication Partners. In accordance with the philosophy above, it espouses restoring a sense of one's self in daily life—that is, reestablishing participation in activities of choice for the adult who is communicatively impaired. Whether or not this restored participation is directly facilitative of communication, communication is not the prime target of this treatment. Instead, Communication Partners strives to develop an operative means whereby adults who are communicatively impaired are able to resume responsibility, control, and direction over the daily happenings in their lives. By promoting a renewed assertion of being, this model focuses on the ultimate aim of our communicative treatments—enhancing the well-being of our clientele in daily life.

The cornerstone of accomplishing these real-life objectives in this alternative model is the assistance of community volunteers. Typically, such volunteers are people previously unknown to and unfamiliar with the adult who is communicatively impaired. They are nonetheless willing to serve as an adjunct or liaison in moving treatment from clinical to natural settings. The use of volunteers to aid in the transference of clinical gains is not untried. Kagan (1995) has detailed a treatment model with volunteers providing "conversational ramps" for adults with aphasia whose verbal competencies are often misunderstood or misjudged. Her contention is that the adult's disordered communication, when left unaided in everyday conversations, does not permit an accurate representation of that person's capabilities. With Communication Partners, volunteers assume an extended role beyond those discussed by Kagan. Not only do they learn and promote interpersonal communication, but they also serve as a liaison in introducing and carrying out activities of choice in daily life at home or in the community.

To date, this treatment method has been refined primarily with adults having aphasia (Lyon, 1989, 1992; Lyon et al., in press). However, the worth and application of Communication Partners are by no means restricted to this communicatively impaired group. Any acquired disorder of communication in later life that alters the effectiveness of communication while sparing the abilities to think, reason, and remember is equally amenable to the clinical protocols that follow. Even when integrity of the mind or thought is altered (e.g., in dementing diseases or when other aspects of aging have a negative impact on daily communication), Communication Partners offers therapeutic advantages not attainable within the confines of the clinic room.

Although these latter applications are less studied, the fundamental constructs in implementing treatment are not. Thus, a later section of this chapter contains a preliminary view of how volunteers might be used with elders suffering from communication breakdowns associated with normal aging.

Using a Community Volunteer?

Why select a community volunteer in the first place? Why not make use of a family member or close friend—someone more familiar, more available, and more committed to long-term improvements in the affected adult? The fact is that the community volunteer adds a therapy ingredient not otherwise available, and an ingredient that is critical in gaining access to treatment's ultimate objective.

The prime objective of Communication Partners is to reinvolve the impaired communicator in as much of life as the person desires and as much as residual skills allow. To accomplish this end, it is essential to legitimize the current status of the impaired communicator—how he or she "is" at this moment. For many family members and friends, the person's changed status is often as difficult to reconcile and integrate into daily life as it is for the afflicted adult. Try as they might, they find the transition awkward and often difficult to accept. They cannot help but reflect on how the impaired communicator was before, and how different he or she is now. Perhaps most influential is an unspoken desire for the person of the past to return.

A volunteer brings no past referent; such a person knows the communicator only as he or she is now. The volunteer who elects to be with, and foster the growth of, the impaired communicator as he or she is today brings a form of validation not attainable through spouse, friend, or even clinician. It takes an unobligated, and seemingly unbiased, other person to bridge critical aspects of one's new and old selves. There is no more humanly unique or bonding way to accomplish this than through communication with a novel and caring "other."

Building a Communicative Bond

As part of a medical model, clinicians have come to view the treatment of communication as a twofold process: (a) repairing or circumventing disordered language components and (b) fostering an improved exchange of content between prime interactants. In defining "what we do" and "how we treat," Communication Partners sets a distinctly different course and projected outcome.

Simmons-Mackie and Damico (1995) have made several important observations pertaining to the role and use of communication with adults having aphasia. As part of a carefully constructed and executed ethnographic study, these two investigators found that communication at home and in other natural settings serves dual purposes: (a) to transact or exchange content and (b) to interact or remain personally tied to others. More significantly, these adults relied on the "personal connecting" function of communication far more than on the "transacting of information." That is, when they did engage in a communicative exchange, it was to bond with people and not necessarily to convey or request information. As these investigators noted, such an emphasis on the interactional aspects of communication is not surprising. After all, normal interactants commonly spend a majority of their time and efforts connecting with others, rather than exchanging facts.

In light of the Simmons-Mackie and Damico (1995) finding, it may seem unwarranted that speech–language pathologists have targeted, almost obsessively, the repair of transactional aspects of communiqués. This preoccupation with "fixing" the exchange of content, however, makes perfect sense at a basic operational level. Transactional communiqués between normal interactants give way quickly to interactional aspects because of the ease of exchanging information whenever necessary. However, when the system for exchanging content becomes impaired in such a way that either participant struggles to discern the other's intended message, communication in all forms, whether transactional or interactional, abruptly halts. For example, the first reaction of an untrained volunteer to a neologistic utterance of an adult having aphasia is typically, "Whoa . . . what the heck was that?" More importantly, the reaction actually means, "Whoa . . . what the heck did that mean?" Thus, it is neither strange nor uncalled-for that clinicians have come to single out the repair of transactional parts of communiqués as the first step in making communication viable.

What may have eluded consideration in our treatment is the degree to which transactional aspects must be repaired for communication to work again. With adults having aphasia, it is not necessary to restore much of the past skill of transacting information in order to gain access to and enjoyment of interactional aspects. Clinicians have always known that establishing an effective communication bond between the impaired communicator and the volunteer is essential in the beginning. However, we now know that the overall treatment equation must emphasize resuming "connecting" as much as "transferring content." The forms selected for interacting, and their use, determine the effectiveness of treatment. Far less important in this equation is how efficient, complete, or even accurate the content will be. As long as there exists a viable means to exchange information, it provides a way of interacting and connecting. As clinicians, we need to devote as much time to finding a successful means of interacting as we do to repairing the means of transacting information.

When a volunteer from the community is first paired with an adult having aphasia, the prime goal is not to make that normal interactant an expert "encoder" and "decoder" of content to and from their aphasic partner. The treatment goal is to establish a way for these two adults to begin to interact effectively. During their interactions, the qualities that permit equal turn taking to evolve and to dominate the exchange are crucial. Quite secondarily is how much, or how well, content is conveyed. It is the give and take between the interactants, irrespective of their status or communicative proficiency, that is the true objective of this first treatment phase.

Treating Adults with Aphasia: Phase 1

Putting treatment into motion is the heart and soul of therapy for most clinicians. To ensure that this practical transition can emerge from the above theoretical rhetoric, Table 13.1 provides a step-by-step overview of the key components of Phase 1 of Communication Partners, along with their intended purpose and applications.

Untreated transactional communication skills are initially baselined between the adult with aphasia and the communication partner using a series of contrived PACE-like scenarios (Davis & Wilcox, 1981). Five scenarios of increasing semantic complexity make up this baseline sample. Level 1, for example, contains a single content unit and involves going to a familiar local site (e.g., eating lunch at Ovens of Brittany, a local restaurant). Level 3 contains two content units, a personal happening, and a related fact (e.g., you went for a walk last week and found yourself in a thunderstorm with lots of lightning).

Table 13.1

Treatment Chronology for Instructing Communication Partner in
How to Interact Effectively and Freely with Adult with Aphasia During Phase 1

Component	Purpose	Application
Baselining transactional communication skills	To establish how effectively CP and AA can exchange content prior to treatment	One at a time, five scenarios of increasing semantic difficulty are explained to AA by C; AA attempts to convey content of scenarios to CP through any means possible; 10-minute allotment per scenario; performance assessed on an 8-point *Communication Effectiveness Index* (Lyon et al., in press).
Part 1: Between CP and AA		
Baselining transactional communication skills	To establish transactional treatment target for CP	Same application as above except that the uninformed interactant with AA is C.
Part 2: Between C and AA		
Explaining the purpose of communication treatment	To differentiate and define the critical parts of communicating, i.e., both transactional and interactional aspects	C explains to CP that transacting of content will happen, that until CP gets the hang of how to do this, it will likely dominate his or her concerns; the truth is, though, it's *not* the most important part of the exchange; rather it's how and why people interact; C gives CP permission to *not* understand the totality of what's being conveyed, instead, to work as much on coming to feel comfortable in the presence of AA and sharing equally.

Reviewing strategies for establishing communication	To instruct CP in how best to optimize an effective and mutual exchange of content with AA	C explains, item by item, a written account of strategies for permitting information to move "to and from" AA; C provides list of strategies chronologically ordered (i.e., they begin with "what" the CP should do from the moment the interaction begins, through the completion of the communiqué).
Modeling of communication strategies	To show CP how communication exchange with AA should look, feel, and proceed	CP provides AA with plausible scenarios to convey to C; C assumes role of uninformed interactant with AA; demonstrates how informational exchange should look, feel, and proceed; as much emphasis placed on connecting as on exchanging content.
Practicing communication strategies	To permit CP and AA to practice using communication strategies with ongoing assistance from C	C provides AA with scenarios and CP assumes interactive role; as difficulties arise, C prompts and further demonstrates to CP the implementation of strategies.
Verifying transactional communication bond	To determine whether CP has become an effective transactor of content	Reassessment using the types of communicative exchanges presented initially; new scenarios of comparable semantic difficulty are used.
Terminating communication phase of treatment	To determine whether CP and AA adequately interact in order to move to the next treatment phase	Although ability to "exchange" content is important, the key to terminating the communicative phase of treatment is whether CP and AA comfortably and mutually interact and whether they feel confident that they could figure out whatever may befall them while undertaking activities of choice in the real world.

Note. C = clinician; CP = communication partner; AA = adult with aphasia.

Level 5 contains two content units of increased length and complexity involving a national or international news item (e.g., there has been a recent eruption of a volcano in the Philippines and a huge cloud of ash is expected to cover much of the southwest United States by week's end). Lyon et al. (in press) have provided further examples of scenario levels, as well as the 8-point ordinal scoring index used to quantify such exchanges.

In the next treatment session, the above protocol is replicated. This time the adult with aphasia interacts with the clinician using different and novel scenarios. This second baselining procedure provides a treatment target for the communication partner and the aphasic adult.

After baselining transactional skills, training the communication partner in how to interact with his or her aphasic partner begins. The prime steps include reviewing transactional and interactional aspects of communicating, teaching specific ways of enhancing communication, modeling and practicing these strategies, verifying treatment effects, and preparing to enter the second phase of treatment. To move these treatment constructs another step closer to practical reality, a case example follows involving a volunteer named Bonnie, and Jack, an adult with aphasia.

Bonnie and Jack: Phase 1

Bonnie was a 26-year-old, TV station employee with little prior knowledge or awareness of aphasia. Her partner, Jack, was a 75-year-old adult who, 11 years prior, was nearing retirement from a 30-year position as an office manager for a local IBM branch. Suddenly, he was left totally incapacitated by a cerebral vascular accident to his dominant hemisphere. Jack had recouped many facets of function during his early years of rehabilitation, most notably integrity of mind and memory, receptive language skills, and a personal zest for life and others. However, a fluent aphasia with totally neologistic speech and a pronounced right hemiparesis continued to inhibit a life-style that had once contained a diverse assortment of personal interests.

In their first encounter, Jack was prompted to try to convey a number of brief, contrived scenarios to Bonnie. One of these was:

> Jack owned a lawnmower that would start but wouldn't continue. After 5 to 10 seconds, it suddenly stopped. He could restart it as before, but once again it quickly failed. He needed to get the mower repaired!

Bonnie attended to all of the nuances of Jack's communication as he attempted to vocally and gesturally imitate a mower starting, running briefly, and stopping. Although adequate to those of us who knew Jack's message, his spoken and gestured signals lacked specificity. As a result, one could sense an initial state of surprise, bordering on alarm, as Bonnie tried to figure out what Jack's barrage of meaningless words, variety of vocal tones and inflections, and assortment of accompanying gestures might mean. Although Bonnie did not panic and was able to discern the main intent of his message after 4 or 5 minutes, one could sense a total loss as to "what to do" and "how to proceed" at different times in this initial exchange.

Over the next 6 weeks, Bonnie, Jack, and a clinician met twice weekly for hour-long treatment sessions. During that time, they worked on refining the use of a set of communication strategies tailored specifically for Jack. Table 13.2 contains an abbreviated accounting of these suggestions. Notice that the strategies offered Bonnie are ordered chronologically from what she should do at the outset of her communiqué until it ends. Initially, she simply allows Jack to finish his explanation in full. If she has any notions about his message, Bonnie attempts to approach them with general, rather than specific, questions. If Jack's message is still unclear, then she asks him to "write" or "draw" a main part. If he is unable to do that, Bonnie begins drawing as much of the message as she knows or might infer. Even if her drawing isn't accurate of Jack's true intent, it provides a context in which Jack can respond and add or subtract information freely. Through this form of turn taking, they stand to further their interactive skills with time and practice.

By the end of Phase 1 of treatment, Bonnie and Jack were exchanging content as effectively as Jack and the clinician. To better gauge this change, another description follows of a posttreatment interaction. The scenario involved then was as follows:

Last week, Jack found an old baseball card of a famous player in his attic. He thought it might be worth some money in today's market. He and his wife took it to a card shop where a dealer told him it was worth $1500!!! He was astounded, but chose not to sell it.

From the moment of initiation, Bonnie and Jack's communication proceeded on an entirely different plane. Bonnie began by allowing Jack to convey his message in full before reacting. He began with a combination of spoken, written, gestured, and drawn cues. When she

Table 13.2

Communicative Strategies Used with Bonnie and Jack

Strategy	Implementation
Allowing time to respond	• Let Jack complete his message in full before attempting to respond
	• Pay particular attention to his vocal inflection, hand and facial gestures, and nonverbal imitations of sounds for cues about his message.
	• Always have pen and paper at hand while he's communicating
Questioning	• If something from his initial communiqué seems recognizable, begin by asking general questions. For example, "Oh, it seems like your doing something with your hand, is that right?" (Not, "Oh, you must be hammering a nail?")
	• Move from general questions that are confirmed to more specific possibilities. For example, "Oh, you're using your hand . . . are you holding something?"
Facilitating the writing and drawing of key concepts	• If you're unable to move closer to Jack's intended target through questioning, ask if he might write or draw the most important part of his message.
	• Again, allow him time to finish his graphic attempt before interacting.
	• If he writes or draws something you can't discern, start broadly with your questioning and from there try to zero in on its intent.
	• Reverify frequently what you think you know about his message as you go along.
	• With drawing, it may be helpful to have him point to the key element in his representation and enlarge just that portion (i.e., redraw it but make it bigger).
Providing a model and communicative referent	• If you still don't know Jack's message or a portion of it, try drawing your own version of what you think he's trying to convey.

(Continues)

Table 13.2 (*Continued*)

Strategy	Implementation
	• Don't be concerned about the accuracy of your guess or your ability to draw; it's only a reference from which Jack can respond.
	• Don't be surprised if Jack simply takes the pen from your hand once you begin and corrects or adds to your effort.
Arranging a mutual conclusion to the exchange	• If you are still unclear about his message, either in full or a portion of it, and you've carefully attended to all of the above suggestions, ask Jack how important it is to determine the missing part *now*, at this very moment.
	• If it is not crucial to him, which it often isn't, ask if you might return to it a later time or date.
	• If it is crucial, search for the part that is most urgent and typically different from the more general intent of his messsage.
	• If you do postpone the exchange to a later time or date, be sure you return to it.
	• Often returning to a topic, be it minutes or hours later, will prompt something new communicatively that hadn't been present before.

did respond, Bonnie did so through the same ways of "connecting" that Jack had used. Even though Bonnie could have said everything in her message much more quickly and easily, by augmenting important points with drawn and written cues, she set the stage for Jack's being able to respond more freely and easily. Within a minute's time, Bonnie knew that Jack had found something in his attic. She thought, at first, that it was money. Jack quickly indicated differently by starting to draw a baseball player on the found object. While doing so, he suddenly stopped half-way in his drawn figure and wrote, "basebael." Bonnie followed with, "Oh, it's something with a baseball player on it?" She wrote out, "baseball card." Jack excitedly acknowledged the correctness of this. They continued with more drawing, writing, and gesturing until several minutes later, Bonnie learned of the card dealer, the card's value, and Jack's unwillingness to sell it.

Bonnie and Jack became effective communicators during this initial phase of treatment. Of equal importance was the fact that they became friends. Anyone unfamiliar with them, and observing them interact, would instantly see and sense their enjoyment of each other. A lightness and humor prevailed in their exchanges that was not there when they first met. Occasionally, Jack still experienced the frustration of a momentary impasse when neither gesture, written word, drawing, nor vocal inflection was enough to capture his intent. However, there was minimal despair; it was more a timely desire to make his point understood more quickly. These moments of breakdown were quite permissible and manageable. Bonnie and Jack were ready to undertake the second phase of treatment, venturing out in the community together in some chosen pursuits.

Establishing Chosen Activities in Daily Life

Csikszentmihalyi (1990, 1993) has written extensively about the merits of becoming so engaged in the "doing" of an activity that one loses an awareness of self. He speaks of the merging of action with actor as creating a state of enhanced well-being, called "flow." When flow exists, neither self nor any potential reward from participating compares to the pleasure and moments of just "doing." Flow emerges when, in the pursuit of a chosen desire or interest, challenge and skill align. For adults with communication disorders, finding and establishing flow may seem like something from the past; it may appear to these adults that active participation in life is neither possible nor advisable. However, communication deficits alone seldom eliminate one's ability to act. It is not a case of "can" flow resume, but of "how"—what must be brought into alignment to permit interest, challenge, and skill to merge. It is toward this very pursuit that the second phase of treatment is directed.

Treating Adults with Aphasia: Phase 2

As treatment in the second phase commences, the role of the communication partner shifts. Now the volunteer's role moves from interactant to catalyst in promoting and ensuring increased client participation in chosen activities of daily life. With this shift in emphasis, the volunteer's role is more of enabling or empowering the adult with aphasia to be able to act in his or her own behalf. The sequence of this second phase of treatment is detailed in Table 13.3. Treatment commences by searching out plausible activities, selecting from a list those that stand to enhance participation in life the most, carefully examining the operative parts of those chosen activities, planning their implementation, carrying them out, reviewing and refining what did and did not work, and working to make those activities self-sustaining. To illustrate this phase of treatment, the case of Bonnie and Jack is reintroduced. Bonnie's role is now to aid Jack in becoming more of his own agent in determining what constitutes his daily life.

Bonnie and Jack: Phase 2

By the time Bonnie entered the second phase of treatment with Jack, he had worked with several other communication partners. Through these encounters, Jack had become an independent volunteer at a local day-care center. He was affectionately known as "Grandpa Jack," and his role was quite varied. He typically spent the first 15 or 20 minutes with the cook in the kitchen at this center; they had independently developed their own friendship, interacting through the sharing of a doughnut and glass of milk, and Jack responding with a lightness, warmth, and humor in his voice, facial expressions, and gestures. Following his stop at the kitchen, Jack went down to a classroom with four to eight preschool children, aged 3 to 5 years. Sometimes there was a specific activity he would select, for example, presenting an audiotaped book to a small group of children or participating in a group sing-along. At other times, he stayed more removed from direct activity with the children but stayed actively engaged by watching and enjoying their company from afar. Jack's wife was amazed at his interest and his dedication to attending. Often, despite bad weather or poor health, he would indicate a desire and willingness to attend.

When Bonnie entered the treatment picture, Jack was interested in pursuing other activities that might make him more independent outside the home. The initial treatment sessions of Phase 2 focused on isolating further activities of Jack's choice. One activity pertained to an earlier interest of Jack's, his close association with youth sports programs. He had helped coach Little League when his son played, and later had umpired baseball games. In seeking some extension of these,

Table 13.3

Treatment Chronology for Establishing Activities of Choice in Daily Life for Adult with Aphasia with the Aid of a Communication Partner

Component	Purpose	Application
Finding activities	To isolate possible activities of choice that AA might wish to undertake at home or in the community	C, CP, and AA sit down together and begin accumulating a list of AA's interests; initial emphasis is on designating areas for potential exploration, *not* so much on their feasibility; most activities of choice are "doable" at some sustainable level; the key is matching skill level with perceived challenge, interest, and motivation; common areas to explore are past interests/hobbies, yet unexplored interests of the past, and volunteerism (helping others while being personally benefited in that process).
Selecting activities	To specify which of the possible activities of choice might be undertaken	C, CP, and AA review list of choices; it is then hierarchically ranked in terms of interest; based on the time required, skill level of AA, and needs and motivation of AA and CP, one or more activities are selected.
Defining activities	To put selected activities into an operative framework where they might be initiated safely and successfully with the CP's assistance; to lay out a general plan for how they might evolve over time into a self-sustaining format	C, CP, and AA meet to define which activities will be pursued, in what form and manner they will be initiated, and where each might lead over time; emphasis placed on AA, CP, and C being comfortable with entry levels; activities self-styled in accordance to desires, needs, and skills of AA; that is *not* a case of trying to find something to do but rather something of inherent worth and choice.

Planning activities	To establish a workable plan for carrying out each activity	C, CP, and AA review each aspect of forthcoming outing, i.e., when, where, transportation to and from designated site, what will happen, who will do what and how it will be done, and what to do if something goes awry or doesn't work; emphasis placed on all parties agreeing about outing ahead of time.
Carrying out activities	To permit AA and CP to undertake the above plan as completely as time and circumstances permit	AA and CP meet at site of activity; they carry out activity as planned; permission is given to abort or modify any aspect of plan, as seems necessary or desired by AA or CP; emphasis placed on keeping AA's experience positive and participation active.
Reviewing and redefining activities	To allow for a thorough review of outings carried out, and from that, to determine if further involvement with that activity is warranted or if the activity needs replacing	C, CP, and AA meet to review outings of CP and AA from the prior week; complete assessment of what happened and whether continued pursuit of chosen activity is justified; if so, all parties return to planning stage for upcoming week; if not, they return to selecting stage to find another activity.
Completing activities	To bring AA's activity of choice to a self-sustaining functional level	C, CP, and AA continue to work toward implementing and refining a weekly activity so it can be sustained either independently (e.g., volunteering in a hospital escort service) or with support within a trained environment (e.g., attending day-care to interact with children; staff and children familiar with AA's communication, and able and desirous of providing necessary support to keep him involved); activities of choice that can't meet the above levels of independence over time are reduced in their form so they can.

Note. C = clinician; CP = communication partner; AA = adult with aphasia.

Bonnie, Jack, and the clinician began to explore his use of a video camcorder. The proposed plan was for Jack to become familiarized with a group of children in a sporting activity, videotape that activity, and then make the recorded tape available to the children for their subsequent viewing.

The second activity involved Jack's attendance at movies. He was a long-time movie buff, whereas his wife never found this activity particularly interesting or rewarding. Bonnie and the clinician's plan was to find three or four other ardent moviegoers in the community and arrange a way that they might meet Jack at the theater and attend a weekly afternoon matinee. By having these newly acquired volunteers alternating their participation, it was thought that Jack could attend an afternoon matinee weekly and acquire several new friendships, while each movie-going volunteer would only need to assist Jack once monthly.

Both activities of Jack's choosing were pursued simultaneously. With regard to the videotaping, Bonnie first familiarized Jack with the technical operations of the camcorder. A tripod was adopted to offset Jack's physical limitations. Bonnie and he practiced filming in a clinical setting. She then accompanied him to the day-care center, where arrangements were made for him to film the children in their regular classroom activities. Concurrently, Bonnie and the clinician began recruiting potential movie enthusiasts from the community by visiting senior centers and running ads in a local newspaper. In preparation for aiding these movie-going volunteers, Bonnie and Jack attended a couple of movies on their own. Her role in these outings was to establish a safe and workable plan that could later be passed on to new recruits.

Over several months of therapy, Bonnie, Jack, and the clinician met weekly to review and plan weekly outings that might move both these selected plans along. A natural evolution has emerged from each.

Videotaping. Once Jack felt comfortable with the basic operational aspects of the camcorder, Bonnie and the clinician began looking for youth sporting activities for Jack to film. Initially, several soccer matches were considered, but they fell on dates when Jack had previous commitments. Next, the clinician contacted the principal at an elementary school in Jack's neighborhood to see if videotaping recreational activities might be possible and beneficial. Such an option seemed workable and desired. Arrangements were made for Jack, Bonnie, and the clinician to meet with school personnel (the principal, the volunteer coordinator, and physical education [PE] teachers). Jack's participation was highly embraced and encouraged by all the school personnel at that meeting, and a tentative plan was devised for how this might be set into motion.

As of this writing, the implementation of that plan has begun. Jack has met the children in four classes and learned which activities the PE teachers would like him to film. It would appear from the initial enthusiasm shown by the school staff that Jack's participation was not only welcomed, but also highly valued, for what he might provide the school and the children. PE teachers have emphasized the instructional benefits of his videotaping. Over the next several months, it seems likely that a schedule and routine can be established in which Bonnie's presence will no longer be required in that environment.

Attending Movies. Initially, several volunteers were found to accompany Jack. Because of outside circumstances, only one of these volunteers remained involved. Through Bonnie's assistance, this young woman has come to a point where she can, and does, accompany Jack to afternoon matinees. Further, Bonnie has commented on her enjoyment of this intermediary role of showing other interactants, people unfamiliar with aphasia, how to relate to Jack and enjoy his company in an activity he thoroughly loves. Over the next month, it seems likely that additional recruits will be sought.

Thus, through Bonnie's presence, it seems reasonable to project that within the next few months, Jack's weekly routine will have expanded from a morning with children in a day-care environment to another activity, videotaping children in PE classes at a nearby elementary school, and also an afternoon attending a weekly matinee with one of several newly acquired friends. Together, these additions make an immeasurable difference in his quality of life, as well as fostering ways of interacting with others in natural settings.

Communication Partners with Adults Experiencing Communication Dysfunction as a Part of Normal Aging

Shadden (1988a, 1988b, this volume) has described the nature and management of communication breakdowns associated with normal aging. She has cited a host of age-related reasons that daily interactions and communiqués may become problematic with elders.

Combined, these consequences of later life may wreak havoc with "a normal societal curve" for exchanging content and staying socially connected. The impact of age-associated changes upon communicative functioning is highly variable from individual to individual. All elements, however, may lead to diminished interactional skills with others, particularly with people unfamiliar with the nature of and reasons for these breakdowns. As described by Lubinski (1988), communicative dysfunction may be less directly attributable to a diminishing of communication skills, and more directly a consequence of modifications in communication effectiveness and opportunities. Central to the latter two domains is access to communication partners—or more broadly, to social contacts that provide a forum for interpersonal interactions.

What may be as important as understanding the nature of communication breakdown in normal aging is knowing that it often escapes recognition or acceptance by the person involved. Slowly, certain cognitive, linguistic, perceptual, motoric, or sensory deficits may accrue. Unlike aphasia, where few sufferers misperceive its typically abrupt arrival, many normally aging adults may fail to see or acknowledge a changed status to their communication. In fact, they may overtly or covertly deny or resist such changes, viewing them, if they are able, merely as confirmation of an age-related decline. In this context, initially making communication repair a prime focus for bringing a volunteer and elder together may prove unwelcome and therapeutically unwise. However, this does not mean that impaired communication tied to normal aging is unapproachable, or that the Communication Partners program cannot be modified.

The most prominent revision of treatment is the subtle merging of Phases 1 and 2 of Communication Partners into a single phase. Because of the complexity of communication breakdowns and their unacknowledged presence, treatment must be approached indirectly in the very real-life contexts where change is sought. Table 13.4 lays out a proposed chronology for engaging communicative partners with adults experiencing communicative disruptions in later life due to aging. No longer is the volunteer designated as a "communication partner," but rather as just a "partner." Simply providing a volunteer partner begins to address the problem of accessibility of communication opportunities for the elder. There is now only one treatment phase, where the volunteer comes to serve as a communicative intermediary in real-life situations, helping to reframe the elder partner's intent when it becomes misunderstood or misconstrued. In this context, communicative effectiveness is served as well (Lubinski, 1988).

Table 13.4

Treatment Chronology for Using Partner with Adult with Normal Aging Communication Deficit

Component	Purpose	Application
Orienting partner	To define therapy and partner's role; also, to overview key aspects of EA's communication and other pertinent skill or deficits related to establishing treatment goal	C and P convene, EA not present; C explains that purpose of therapy is to facilitate and augment EA's participation in daily life; reviews EA's communication difficulties, how they interfere in daily life, strategies to minimize or compensate for them personally and around others; reviews other levels of function (e.g., cognition, memory, perception, sensation, etc.) that might interfere with EA's ability to participate in everyday life.
Identifying activities and modeling of preferred interactive strategies	To isolate activities of choice in daily life that would heighten interest and participation and are no longer deemed possible or successful; also to give P a chance to observe EA's communicative style and how C interactively manages these breakdowns	C, P, and EA meet and begin jointly exploring possibilities that EA might wish to undertake; focus is on finding activities that would stimulate and motivate EA to become more active in daily life; less emphasis on whether such activities are "doable"—just on accumulating a list for consideration; forum also provides P with opportunity to observe and model C's communicative style with EA.
Selecting activities and continued modeling of preferred interactive strategies	To select from list of options which activities would be best to undertake given EA's interests and residual skills	C, P, and EA overview list of possible activities; discuss pros and cons of each; arrive at a mutual beginning point to probe.

(Continues)

Table 13.4 (*Continued*)

Component	Purpose	Application
Observing chosen activities and communication style at designated settings	To determine the precise requisites and demands on EA to make chosen activities in real world functional, acceptable, and pleasurable; also opportunity to better judge effects of communication	P and EA undertake chosen activities in natural setting; purpose is to observe what is and isn't interfering with EA being able to participate independently; P also able to observe EA's communication in chosen environments and its effects.
Reassessing and planning participation at designated settings	To review outing and all aspects of what did or did not work; also, to formulate a plan as to how to minimize future problems and promote increased EA participation	C and P meet alone to begin with; P overviews any perceived difficulties; C discusses possible strategies for dealing with these problems; offers to model strategies in selected site for P; EA joins them; reviews his or her impressions of outing; jointly agree upon adopted plan for next outing.
Modeling treatment strategies at designated settings	To permit P to observe treatment strategies first-hand in designated sites	C, P, and EA undertake chosen activities together; C models treatment strategies for P to observe, whether communicative or otherwise; also, C able to get a much better sense of their operatives.
Transferring treatment strategies to partner at designated settings	To allow P to assume full responsibility of intended treatment role at designated sites	P and EA undertake chosen activities alone; emphasis on establishing a functional state that might, in the future, permit EA to proceed independently or with less support.
Reviewing and completing activities	Comparable to earlier sections in Table 13.2 with AA	

Note. C = clinician; P = partner; EA = elderly adult with difficulties communicating due to normal aging.

Revised to meet the needs of the normal aging, Communication Partners can help to ensure that meaning, purpose, direction, control, and a self-sustaining state of well-being remain an active part of daily life. Thus, a state of "flow" may once again be a part of daily life. There is yet to evolve a sample case of this treatment chronology with a volunteer and an elder exhibiting communication decrements associated with normal aging. The treatment framework here is intended solely to aid clinicians in bridging the obvious needs and challenges unique to this expanding, and often ignored, communicatively at-risk group of older adults. Many of the modifications put forth in this version of treatment would be equally applicable to adults with progressive dementing diseases.

Concluding Remarks

Managed care in America is at our front doors. The loud rapping we all perceive may seem like an unfamiliar knock, but it has been there quietly for decades. It is traceable, in part, to years of confining therapy to medical and clinical settings. Fifty years ago, the target of therapy was not to help World War II GIs become better communicators in a treatment room, but to help them return to productive lives in the real world. Since then, clinicians have learned that what we attain clinically is not automatically or fully transferred to real-life settings or situations. Now, as part of a shift in the emphasis of health care services, we are being held accountable for what we do clinically. That is, we are being asked to demonstrate that clinical gains *do* make a difference in real life, not just communicatively, but also to one's overall well-being. To achieve these ends, it seems imperative that we look to alternative treatments that target real-life communication at the outset of management, rather than indirectly and obscurely at its termination.

Communication Partners is one such model. Numerous other models, and variations of this one, await exploration. The purpose of this chapter has been to provide a therapeutic framework from which to start. Hopefully, from here, readers can construct and implement their own versions of how to move treatment effectively from clinical to natural settings. In this way, we not only justify what we do, but also better serve the needs of those we treat.

Author's Note

The author is thankful to the adults with aphasia, community volunteers, and clinicians who have participated in and furthered Communication Partners over the past decade. He is especially grateful to Marge Blanc for her assistance and encouragement in expanding treatment applications of this approach. In addition, he is appreciative of Ms. Blanc's editorial efforts and her careful review of this manuscript.

References

Csikszentmihalyi, M. (1990). *Flow: The psychology of optimal experience.* New York: HarperCollins.

Csikszentmihalyi, M. (1993). *The evolving self.* New York: HarperCollins.

Goldstein, K. (1942). *After-effects of brain injuries in war.* New York: Grune & Stratton.

Davis, G. A., & Wilcox, M. J. (1981). Incorporating parameters of natural conversation in aphasia treatment. In R. Chapey (Ed.), *Language interventions strategies in adult aphasia* (pp. 168–190). Baltimore: Williams & Wilkins.

Kagan, A. (1995). Revealing the competence of aphasic adults through conversation: A challenge to health professionals. *Topics in Stroke Rehabilitation, 2,* 15–28.

Lubinski, R. (1988). A model for intervention: Communication skills, effectiveness, and opportunity. In B. B. Shadden (Ed.), *Communication behavior and aging: A sourcebook for clinicians* (pp. 294–308). Baltimore: Williams & Wilkins.

Lyon, J. G. (1989). Communicative partners: The value in reestablishing communication with aphasic adults. *Clinical Aphasiology, 18,* 11–18.

Lyon, J. G. (1992). Communication use and participation in life for adults with aphasia in natural settings: The scope of the problem. *American Journal of Speech–Language Pathology, 1,* 7–14.

Lyon, J. G. (1996). Optimizing communication and participation in life for aphasic adults and their prime caregivers in natural settings: A use model for treatment. In G. Wallace (Ed.), *Adult aphasia rehabilitation* (pp. 137–160). Newton, MA: Butterworth-Heinemann.

Lyon, J. G., Cariski, D., Keisler, L., Rosenbek, J., Levine, R., Kumpula, J., Ryff, C., Coyne, S., & Blanc, M. (in press). Communication partners: Enhancing participation in life and communication for adults with aphasia in natural settings. *Aphasiology.*

Shadden, B. B. (1988a). Communication and aging: An overview. In B. B. Shadden (Ed.), *Communication behavior and aging: A sourcebook for clinicians* (pp. 1–11). Baltimore: Williams & Wilkins.

Shadden, B. B. (1988b). Interpersonal communication patterns and strategies in the elderly. In B. B. Shadden (Ed.), *Communication behavior and aging: A sourcebook for clinicians* (pp. 182–196). Baltimore: Williams & Wilkins.

Simmons-Mackie, N., & Damico, J. S. (1995). Communicative competency in aphasia: Evidence from compensatory strategies. *Clinical Aphasiology, 23,* 95–105.

Wepman, J. M. (1951). *Recovery from aphasia.* New York: Ronald Press.

Chapter 14

Augmentative and Alternative Communication for Older Populations: A Unique Perspective

Sheela Stuart

Stuart suggests that augmentative and alternative communication (AAC) interventions for older adults with communication disorders could be significantly enhanced if systems allowed clients to maximize their communicative strengths. After reviewing the types of adult speech–language disorders potentially requiring AAC, Stuart identifies some common age-related considerations in the assessment and design of augmentative communication systems for older individuals. The primary focus of the chapter is upon the unique role of story telling in the communications of older adults, and upon ways to incorporate story-telling functions within AAC systems.

1. What are the four categories of adults who have a need for augmentative communication? For each group, list some of the unique needs and challenges involved in attempting to design an effective AAC system.

2. What are some of the social, cognitive, emotional, and physical aspects of aging that may influence selection of appropriate AAC systems for older adults and effective use of such systems?

3. What aspects of normal older adults' communications may be useful to consider in developing AAC systems for individuals with communication disorders? In particular, what is unique about story-telling abilities in the elderly and how can opportunities for natural story-telling be incorporated into AAC?

4. Describe at least one low-tech approach to AAC that may facilitate communication between individuals with communication disorders and their partners.

number of communication disorders seen in older adults may warrant exploration of augmentative and alternative communication (AAC) interventions. In considering AAC for older populations, three perspectives should be addressed. First, effective AAC service delivery to older clients must consider the unique cognitive, linguistic, and motor challenges and deficits of the specific communication disorder. Second, aspects of normal aging discussed in Chapters 2 through 7 of this text may influence many aspects of AAC service delivery to older persons. For example, the design of individual AAC systems may have to be modified to accommodate sensory and motor limitations apart from the specific communication disorder. General health status can affect levels of fatigue and consequently energies available for learning a new system and using it on a daily basis. Financial considerations are also unique in the older population. Because speech has been the primary communication modality for many years, issues of acceptance and motivation of the older client and significant others must be addressed.

The third perspective addresses the unique communicative content and strategies employed by many older adults and the needs served by communicative exchanges involving the elderly. Ideally, for those older clients with speech–language disorders who possess the necessary linguistic and cognitive skills, AAC systems should allow them to participate in the types of communication events and discuss content enjoyed prior to the onset of the communication disorder. In particular, a means to promote topic variations and story-telling strategies must be considered.

This chapter focuses on the third perspective, maximizing communicative options; the ideas presented here are consistent with the general heading of "communication enhancement" that links the preceding chapters by Dukes and Lyon. Information concerning the AAC challenges of specific communication disorders can be found elsewhere (e.g., Beukelman & Mirenda, 1992; Blackstone, 1988, 1991; Yorkston, 1992). The effects of aging on design and implementation of AAC systems for older users are addressed in Lubinski and Higginbotham (in press). Only a brief discussion of clinical populations and aging considerations is presented as a backdrop to the unique content and style needs of older adults.

AAC Service Delivery to Older Adults: General Considerations

AAC Systems and Service Delivery Models

Although AAC systems may take different forms with varying features, they can be classified as belonging to one of two categories—low technology or high technology. Communication aids that are classified as low technology may be electronic, but they are not microcomputers and do not have printed or speech output. They frequently include booklets or lap trays with overlays of written words or symbols. High-technology communication aids are systems that utilize microcomputers with specialized software to provide a printed output and/or synthesized or digitized speech (Church & Glennen, 1992). Many persons vary their use of low and high technology depending on the situation, combining a number of techniques and strategies.

Early AAC interventions tended to focus narrowly on compensation for identified weak areas of communicative performance, seeking to determine "candidacy" for AAC assistance. Over the years, AAC assessment and intervention efforts have become more sophisticated. The first shift occurred when greater attention began to be paid to "communication needs." The most widely used assessment model today is Beukelman and Mirenda's (1992) Participation Model. This model broadens the concept of communication needs to include the following three elements: (a) identification of participation patterns and communication needs, (b) determination of opportunity barriers, and (c) assessment of access barriers. The model presupposes that the overall goal of successful intervention is more likely to be achieved if we design AAC systems to provide users with a means of participating in activities of personal importance, thereby displaying competence and usefulness. Each of these elements has unique implications for the speech–language disorders seen with some frequency in older adults, and for the specific challenges to AAC interventions presented by the aging process and the reality of being an older person.

Garrett and Beukelman (1992) stated that the augmentative and alternative communication (AAC) field recently has begun focusing on communication as a holistic process. They indicated a need for more sociocommunicative, interactional goals that reflect an understanding of the AAC communicator within the context of his or her life-style, environment, needs, and goals, reflecting "who the AAC user is." The following sections briefly identify the characteristics of the older AAC candidate.

The Older AAC Candidate: Common Communication Disorders

There are at least four categories of adults who have a need for augmentative communication: (a) individuals with acquired static disabilities (including, but not limited to, stroke, traumatic brain injury, spinal cord injury); (b) individuals with degenerative neurological disorders, particularly those affecting neuromotor systems (e.g., amyotrophic lateral sclerosis, multiple sclerosis, Parkinson's disease, Huntington's chorea, AIDS); (c) individuals with developmental disability moving into adulthood and through the life span; and (d) persons with short-term needs for AAC systems resulting from acute medical problems. The first two are of primary interest here.

For stroke patients and individuals suffering traumatic brain injury, the particular combination of cognitive, linguistic, sensory, and motor challenges created by the precipitating event may require a totally different set of assessment and intervention strategies. For example, Garrett and Beukelman (1992) and Garrett (1992) identified five different types of communicators among persons with severe aphasia, pointing out that loss of language functions does not necessarily mean that the pragmatic, perceptual, and experiential skill bases for communication have eroded. Their four communicator types— basic-choice, controlled-situation, comprehensive, specific-need, and augmented-input—each require very different assessments, training, and systems.

For individuals diagnosed with progressive neuromotor disorders, different but equally challenging problems in designing effective AAC systems are presented; a variety of intervention issues are raised. These problems and issues include (a) the evolving nature of deficits and the consequent need to design systems that can be modified over time or that may have built-in expectations of replacement; (b) the timing of the introduction of the topic of planning for AAC; (c) the need for intensive, holistic involvement of family and other caregivers; (d) questions of financial resources for purchase of one or more devices; and (e) the personal resources available for learning a complicated AAC system (Beukelman & Garrett, 1988; Beukelman & Mirenda, 1992; Blackstone, 1988). For example, for clients with amyotrophic lateral sclerosis (ALS), the rapid progression of the disorder mandates early introduction of AAC, and a clear definition of strategies for dealing with the evolving nature of motor deficits over time. Unfortunately, many ALS clients and families are experiencing high levels of stress and may be unwilling to accept the inevitability of decline, making it difficult to obtain full participation in assessment decisions and training. Disease progression may also be more rapid than the assistive technology delivery system can accommodate, in terms of delivery of devices in a timely fashion.

Whether the communication disorder in an older client reflects a static or progressive etiology, one issue is paramount. These individuals have acquired and used normal speech, language, and communication skills and interactions successfully prior to the neurological insult. This prior experience with normal verbal communication sets up unique expectations on the part of the client and family and may define unique constellations of communication needs (Garrett & Beukelman, 1992). For example, one client experiencing moderate aphasia and severe verbal apraxia secondary to a stroke ultimately rejected a sophisticated communication device, despite his ability to access and use the system, because it did not fill in the missing syntactic forms and words that his language system could not supply.

The Older AAC Candidate: Age-Related Design Considerations

As earlier chapters have demonstrated, older adults are not a homogeneous population; even the exact definition of who fits this category varies. Designing an AAC system requires careful consideration of many areas of functioning, including social supports and networks, motor skills, health, sensory and/or perceptual deficits, cognitive shifts, depression, and preexisting language or communicative changes. These aspects of aging exist apart from the effects of a specific communication disorder but require equal attention. A discussion of the impact of aging upon AAC use can be found elsewhere (Lubinski & Higginbotham, in press). Only a few examples are provided here.

Many communication aids have a limited number of vocabulary items and messages that must be organized in some manner and be represented by graphics (pictures, symbols, or words). To use these, the individual must provide a predetermined memorized code to recall, be able to scan the entire contents, or remember what is available and where it is located within the system. This must occur after or during the mental formulation of the intended message. Challenges to working memory may be high, yet working memory resources may be limited in aging (Hasher & Zacks, 1979). Learning such strategies may also take longer (Salthouse, 1985) and may challenge already reduced problem-solving capabilities (e.g., Denney, 1982). Clinicians must customize the organization of messages to support the short-term memory and cognitive demands of new learning in the use of an AAC system.

Visual changes associated with aging may present AAC utilization difficulties for some older adults. Changes include diminished acuity, increased sensitivity to glare, reduced ability to adapt to dark and light, reduced peripheral vision, and increased difficulty distinguishing between cool colors such as blues, greens, grays, and violets. Unfortunately, AAC computer screens are sometimes done in shades of gray, with image disruption due to screen dimness and glare from external light sources. Graphic symbols are often line drawings that require visual acuity and visual closure skills for identification.

Voice output communication aids (VOCAs) utilize either digitized speech or synthesized speech. Although digitized speech is generally more intelligible than synthesized speech, it does not contain the full range of frequencies in human voice output and this element, combined with variations in resonance, makes it hard to understand at times. Synthesized voice output has gone through several generations of development, and intelligibility has improved with each change (originally it was as low as 30% to 40% intelligible output). Most current VOCAs that utilize synthesized speech employ a considerably improved voice output software called DecTalk. Despite improvements, it is logical to assume that difficulties in understanding message output would make using a voice output device less appealing to an older adult. Understanding can be complicated further by hearing loss, a sensory deficit found commonly in older adults (Campbell & Lancaster, 1988). Auditory status in client and caregiver must be considered.

Motor limitations may influence the selection of input modality and design (e.g., a small keyboard may not be used readily by some arthritic older adults). Health problems and generalized fatigue on the part of the client and/or caregiver may limit the energy either or both are able to invest in learning and using an AAC system. AAC interventions are also costly in terms of personal effort, time, and funding for equipment and training. Unfortunately, it is often more difficult to access outside resources for older adults, and they often resist using family resources for this purpose. The list of age-related considerations could go on and on. However, only one other concern will be noted before the primary focus of this chapter is addressed.

In a review of studies of technology and aging, Straker (1992) noted that many older adults feel that technology makes life more complicated and is often dehumanizing. Additionally, older partners may be resistive to using these types of communication tools for interactions with their family members (Beukelman & Mirenda, 1992). Kemp (1993) discussed the importance of motivation in the successful use of technology; motivation involves wants (desires, wishes for, needs, dreams, etc.). Kemp suggested that technology must provide something the older person really wants—often something that will increase functional ability (i.e., allowing maintenance of independence and performance of daily tasks). If the AAC system is designed to perform functions that are rewarding to the older adult, the motivation to overcome some of the above stated concerns will be much greater.

The remainder of this chapter focuses on the unique perspective of the older adult as a communicator first, an individual with a communication disorder second, and an AAC user third. This ordering is supported by our understanding of the nature of successful AAC interventions. In all cases, a successful system reflects an understanding of appropriate communicative functioning for the particular client age group. In addition, effective systems focus on providing some type of increased participation through the use of the AAC system.

The Uniqueness of Older Adult Communications: Implications for AAC

Topics

A stereotypic idea often expressed about older individuals' conversations is that the persons they talk the most about are family members and the things they talk most about are health problems. Research findings (Stuart, Vanderhoof-Bilyeu, & Beukelman, 1994) reflect differences that appear to be related to gender, as well as to the aging process, in somewhat surprising ways. Men from ages 62 through 85+ years made more frequent reference to their friends than to their families. Women ages 62 through 73 years made more frequent reference to family members than friends (although they often referenced friends), whereas women 75 through 85+ years referenced friends more frequently than family.

Women 62 through 73 years referenced games/sports more frequently even than the men in the study. All participants referenced food, household routines, and games/sports more frequently than they referenced stereotypical topics such as health, emotional status, and finances. Because the subjects in this study lived at home with their spouses, the preparation of food, management of their homes, and recreational games were not unexpected topics of conversation, supporting the idea that considering the context and routine of the individual's daily life-style is vital to determining important topics.

The AAC system designer must find meaningful ways for older clients to talk to friends. These communications reflect a bond of common experience that is often referred to as "age cohort membership." People from the same age cohort have the same associations when certain topics, words, and time periods are mentioned. Word choice and speech register used in AAC must be consistent with cohort membership.

Language Choices: Vocabulary and Register

Each of us incorporates acrolect (formal language), mesolect (informational or ordinary language), and basolect (slang, argot, dialect) into our everyday communication. Every conversation has a "lexicon pitch." Speakers alter their language in response to situation variables. There is an identified expressive value in the use of different speech registers, which must be understood and considered when one is selecting vocabulary for use in an AAC system. For older adults, slang use most frequently includes two elements: at least some of the words that were popular during their young adulthood and slang words that reflect their membership in particular work and/or interest areas. For example, a man in his late 60s who was in the navy and also enjoyed driving fast, might refer to a "zoot suit" in describing a fancy outfit; to a "90-day wonder" in describing an officer or someone who seems to have rapidly assumed authority; and to "step on it" when describing the need for speed.

Colloquialisms and proverbs are also frequently used by older individuals as a standard means of summarizing or providing verbal guidance in life situations. Phrases such as "independent as a hog on ice," "don't buy a pig in a poke," "read them the riot act," and "bury the hatchet" are examples recently overheard in conversations between older adults. From an AAC perspective, in addition to relevant topics, vocabulary items must reflect these age cohort and individual differences. If a client has always used a particular phrase to express humor or to admonish others, that phrase must have priority for inclusion in an AAC system.

Story Telling: Purposes and Forms

Another stereotypic characterization of an older conversationalist is the image of a person who is constantly telling stories about the past (Coleman, 1986). Added to that is the perception that the stories are repeatedly told in exactly the same way. Were this the simple truth, the lives of AAC system designers would be infinitely easier. We could just target a few favorite stories and make them available in a "canned" format. However, considering the perspective that older individuals have become uniquely suited for the task of "telling" in a particularly effective way, it is not surprising to find that their repeated story telling is not simple, nor told exactly the same, nor always about the past (Kemper, Rash, Kynette, & Norman, 1990; Stuart et al., 1994). In comparing stories produced in everyday conversations, Stuart and DuBois (1995) found that the repeated stories of older adults have basic segments that tell the core story. However, these are often told with different vocabulary (e.g., "My Mother passed away," or "My Mom died."). Repeated stories also include expansions that may be used at some tellings and not at others.

Analyses of spontaneous everyday conversations (Boden & Bielby, 1983; Stuart et al., 1994; Stuart & Dubois, 1995) suggest that when, where, and how older adults use stories and select, introduce, expand, and elaborate past experience and events into conversations is a very sophisticated process. Older adults use stories to provide a view of the world, living, and life itself. The summation of this knowledge most often is not articulated directly but instead is woven into a story. This information is the "gist" of the story and represents the purpose for telling the story. Mr. M., an 85-year-old gentleman, commented on this idea one afternoon during one of our visits, "You know, I don't just tell these stories for the fun of it. Sure it's fun, but I want you to have the benefit of all that stuff I learned and I don't wanna get preachy about it—so, I tell a story and you get the idea."

Patterns of three specific identifiable purposes for telling stories have been found: (a) usefulness—sharing information that would assist in performing a task; (b) connectedness—sharing information from another time and place that would expand and enrich understanding of the present; and (c) philosophy—sharing knowledge and wisdom about living that would provide insight and direction for the future (Stuart & DuBois, 1995). The following story of looking into the well is an example of the usefulness category.

During lunch at a senior citizen center, Mr. P. (age 68 years) mentioned that he and his son were going "out to the ranch" later on that day to check on a well. Mr. S. (age 87 years) looked up and said,

> Years ago, I run onto a guy, up there by my place, he had a well . . . he couldn't figure out what was goin' on. I went by there and he was just having a terrible time figuring out how to see down in there. Doin' all kinds of gyrations. I told him, "Go to the house and get your wife's lookin' glass.'" He scratched his head and then decided might as well try it. Did the job. You get yourself a piece of that lookin' glass, you know, a hunk of some you mighta broke 'er somethin', then you hold it just like this [gestures] up against the edge and if you angle it just right you can see down in there. I promise ya."

The story-telling purposes identified here encompass several of the agendas that Light (1988) has defined as being served in communicative exchanges. Her four main agendas are communication of needs and wants, information transfer, social closeness, and social etiquette. Both information transfer and social closeness may well be achieved by the story-telling activities of older adults. As such, they should be considered for AAC interventions.

The purpose of providing story-telling capabilities within an AAC system is to enable an AAC user to participate in a type of communication that is both enjoyable and empowering. Obviously, selection of personally meaningful stories will require input from persons who know the AAC system user well. These persons can compose stories appropriate for the target functions. Ideally, these would be stories the older adult with acquired communication disorders had previously shared many times over a period of years. Interestingly enough, this is the point at which the clinician will often need to counsel family members regarding the communicative function and value of the older age adult's repeated story telling. It is not unusual to encounter a family member who will request, "Please don't put that story he used to tell about trapping muskrats in there; I've listened to that a thousand times." The clinician should attempt to explain the participatory, competence, and membership aspects of this type of communication, facilitating the family's choice of at least one familiar story that fits each of the general purpose categories of usefulness, connectedness, and philosophy. Obviously, if family resistance remains strong, inclusion of selected stories may need to be reconsidered.

Support of enjoyable and empowering participation through story telling means making decisions that accommodate specific aspects of telling and multiple purposes or functions for stories. Once a story is targeted to be included in an AAC system, it will need to be transcribed and the basic segments and expansions identified. Stories should be written to include, when appropriate, reference to past and present, and repeated phrases for emphasis. Variations for the basic segments (e.g., formal vs. informal) will then need to be determined, and mechanisms for ready access to variations must be developed. For example, a basic requirement for any AAC system design is that physical and cognitive demands be minimized so the user is free to focus on interaction with the listener(s). Several different voice output communication aids have software that can be configured to accommodate the unique aspects of basic and expansion selection. In different ways, each of them employs a type of "macro" concept that allows AAC system users to go into a story and step through the various segments, choosing only those they wish to speak at that time. In any case, identifying some key cross-reference codes is be important to allow easy access to particular stories for interactive telling and to allow for use of certain key segments from a story within group discussions and other special contexts.

Customizing for Success

The preceding discussion has focused on unique strengths and communication strategies in normal older adults, as they might be applied to enhancing the success of AAC interventions with some older clients with a communication disorder. Story-telling abilities may be beyond the capability or interest level of some clients because of the specific nature of their communication impairment. In addition, age-associated changes may represent potential barriers to successful utilization of AAC. Clinicians must be sensitive to such variations and make every effort to modify AAC interventions to eliminate or reduce age interference.

Rather than focusing exclusively on deterrents to communicative success, the intent of this chapter has been to challenge clinicians to find positive aspects of aging that can be used to promote AAC communicative adequacy. In addition to the information presented concerning conversational content and story telling, practitioners should search the gerontological literature for skills and attributes that are well preserved into late adulthood, hoping to exploit such skills in AAC design. For example, Howard (1988) isolated semantic activation as one component of long-term memory that remains as consistently accurate for older adults as for younger adults. Semantic activation refers to the fact that the ideas we consider to be somehow related to one another are truly stored together; when one memory node is activated (by a word, picture, or even sensory response) and becomes accessible, this activation spreads along the node's associations, thereby activating nearby semantically related nodes. Storing new information and recalling can be made much easier using semantic association and priming. Obviously a key element is determination of appropriate semantic associations for an individual.

Unfortunately, we do not have research that provides us with a listing of specific associations and semantic priming information for cohorts of older adults. However, we do perhaps have a hint from the intricate topical matrixes used by older adults in discussing past and present. Many older adults use places or historical events as their initial organizer (Boden & Bielby, 1986; Stuart & DuBois, 1995). Examples of this can be seen in the introductions used in stories such as, "Years ago, I run onto a guy up there by my place"; and, "I had a chance to come home at Christmas time, 1944." Using places and times as the overall organizing element, access could be designed specifically for the association and recall of stories and/or phrases. Much of this personalized information might initially be garnered from records and interviews with friends and relatives, then actually placed within the AAC system with the assistance of the system user. This would allow the system user to make personal modifications that would expand the overall meaningfulness of the organization.

Finally, although much of this discussion has been directed toward making voice output communication aids viable for older age adults, a low-technology approach could also be employed in many instances. A favorite theme scrapbook could be designed using photos, newspaper clippings, and actual memorabilia (e.g., ticket stubs, dried flowers, etc.). A relative or friend could write a short synopsis attempting to capture an appropriate story-telling style incorporating vocabulary and phrases often used by the individual. The "write-up" could be pasted within the collage of items. When the AAC system user opened the page of the scrapbook, a communication partner could read the synopsis aloud, allowing the user to make as many verbal or intonational comments as possible. Costs and technology fears would be reduced, but communication empowerment would still be achieved.

Summary

The specific communication disorders seen in elderly clients, and the influences of other aspects of aging, can present formidable challenges to clinicians seeking to implement quality AAC interventions with older persons. Rather than focusing discussion on these challenges, this chapter has chosen instead to highlight the major communicative strategies and strengths of normal older adults. It is suggested that incorporation of appropriate topics, vocabulary, lexical pitch variations, and story-telling options in any augmentative communication intervention should increase the likelihood of successful use of the AAC system for users possessing the necessary skills.

Communication enhancement through AAC, in as natural and functional a way as possible, must be the goal of our interventions. The key to this communication enhancement is the clinician's success in constantly integrating a knowledge of aging with an understanding of augmentative communication service delivery systems and specific communication disorders. As clinicians taking on this task, you join the ranks of those who are constantly challenged and frequently feel inadequate and overwhelmed. Please—persevere, not only with scientific knowledge and creativity, but with a spirit of commitment to enabling not only needs fulfillment in older adults but also the richness of experiential sharing through story telling.

References

Beukelman, D., & Garrett, K. (1988). Augmentative and alternative communication for adults with acquired severe communication disorders. *Augmentative and Alternative Communication, 4,* 104–121.

Beukelman, D., & Mirenda, P. (1992). *Augmentative and alternative communication: Management of severe communication disorders in children and adults.* Baltimore: Brookes.

Blackstone, S. (1988). Amyotrophic lateral sclerosis. *Augmentative Communication News, 1,* 1–8.

Blackstone, S. (1991). For consumers: Intervention with the partners of AAC consumers: Part I: Interaction. *Augmentative Communication News, 4,* 1–8.

Boden, D., & Bielby, D. (1986). The way it was: Topical organization in elderly conversation. *Language and Communication, 6,* 73–89.

Campbell, J., & Lancaster, J. (1988). Communicating effectively with older adults. *Family and Community Health, 11,* 74–85.

Church, G., & Glennen, S. (1992). *The handbook of assistive technology.* San Diego: Singular.

Coleman, P. (1986). *Aging and reminiscence processes.* New York: Wiley.

Denney, N. (1982). Aging and cognitive changes. In B. B. Wolman (Ed.), *Handbook of developmental psychology* (pp. 102–115). Englewood Cliffs, NJ: Prentice-Hall.

Garrett, K. (1992). Adults with severe aphasia. In D. Beukelman & P. Mirenda (Eds.), *Augmentative and alternative communication: Management of severe communication disorders in children and adults* (pp. 331–343). Baltimore: Brookes.

Garrett, K., & Beukelman, D. R. (1992). Augmentative communication approaches for persons with severe aphasia. In K. Yorkston (Ed.), *Augmentative communication in the medical setting* (pp. 245-348). Tucson, AZ: Communication Skill Builders.

Hasher, L., & Zacks, R. (1979). Automatic processing of fundamental information: The case of frequency of occurrence. *American Psychologist, 39,* 444–451.

Howard, D. (1988). Aging and memory activation: The priming of semantic and episodic memories. In L. L. Light & D. M. Burke (Eds.), *Language, memory and aging* (pp. 33–45). Melbourne, Australia: Cambridge University Press.

Kemp, B. (1993). Motivation issues in the use of technology by older persons: A model and recommendations. *Technology and Disability, 2,* 65–70.

Kemper, S., Rash, S., Kynette, D., & Norman, S. (1990). Telling stories: The structure of adults' narratives. *European Journal of Cognitive Psychology, 2,* 205–228.

Light, J. (1988). Interaction involving individuals using augmentative and alternative communication systems: State of the art of future directions. *Augmentative and Alternative Communication, 4,* 66–82.

Lubinski, R., & Higginbotham, D. J. (in press). *Communication technologies for the elderly: Hearing, vision, and speech.* San Diego: Singular.

Salthouse, T. (1985). *A theory of cognitive aging.* Amsterdam: Elsevier/North-Holland.

Straker, J. (1992). Communications technology and older adults: A review of the issues in technology dissemination. *Topics in Geriatric Rehabilitation, 17,* 22–35.

Stuart, S., & DuBois, D. (1995). *Storytelling in everyday conversations of older adults.* Unpublished manuscript.

Stuart, S., Vanderhoof-Bilyeu, D., & Beukelman, D. (1994). Differences in topic reference in elderly men and women. *Journal of Medical Speech-Language Pathology, 2,* 89–104.

Yorkston, K. (Ed.). (1992). *Augmentative communication in the medical setting.* Tucson, AZ: Communication Skill Builders.

Chapter 15

The Breakfast Club and Related Programs

Mary Jo Santo Pietro
Faerella Boczko

Chapters 15 and 16 address issues of communication maintenance programs from two perspectives. In Chapter 15, Santo Pietro and Boczko describe some of the more common approaches to direct communication intervention with Alzheimer's patients, highlighting management recommendations provided by Bourgeois and by Clark. The remainder of the chapter is devoted to discussion of one innovative program, the Breakfast Club, that has been successful in improving communicative and social adequacy in long-term care residents with dementia.

1. *List the types of approaches to direct communication intervention for Alzheimer's patients currently being practiced. Regardless of approach, what practical suggestions does Bourgeois offer for the clinician attempting to develop a successful communication intervention?*

2. *Define the basic elements of the Breakfast Club program. How does the Breakfast Club treatment approach attempt to incorporate Clark's principles of group treatment and Bourgeois' clinical recommendations in one program? Describe social and communicative outcomes of Breakfast Club participation for persons with Alzheimer's disease.*

3. *Think of at least one other setting or activity in which the principles and approaches used in the Breakfast Club could be used to maintain or enhance communication in individuals with dementia.*

※   ※   ※

When we talk about nursing homes, we are talking about Alzheimer's disease. According to the U.S. National Center for Health Statistics (1985), as many as half of nursing home residents across the country have Alzheimer's or a related dementia. That percentage is far higher in many facilities. Typically, Alzheimer's patients are admitted to the nursing home well into mid-stage of the disease, when family members can no longer manage them at home. The communication problems of these advanced dementia patients affect the care not only of the Alzheimer's residents themselves, but also of all other nursing home residents. The quality of life of the staff and administration of every nursing home is influenced as well.

The specific communication problems of Alzheimer's patients have been well documented in recent literature (e.g., Bayles & Kaszniak, 1987; Lubinski, 1991). Typical descriptions of declining communication skills in these patients include the loss of normal pragmatics, loss of auditory comprehension skills, loss of short-term memory, withdrawal from communication encounters, excessive ego-orientation, lack of responsiveness, lack of relevance, lack of cohesion and coherence, inattention, repetitiveness, paranoia, and anxiety. Although one cannot dispute that dementia is a direct cause of deterioration of communication skills, some communication breakdowns in Alzheimer's patients are due to other causes such as depression, concomitant illnesses or disabilities, medication, institutionalization, or even "learned helplessness." The nature of the institutional environment also contributes to communication breakdowns for Alzheimer's patients (Lubinski, 1991). In response to the unique and disturbing nature of this degenerative terminal disease, both family and professional caregivers tend to react in ways that worsen the communication problems (Santo Pietro, 1994).

Deficits in interpersonal communication have been repeatedly ranked as the most difficult of the problems encountered by caregivers in nursing homes (Richter, Bottenberg, & Roberto, 1993; Ripich, Wykle, & Niles, 1995). There are obvious reasons for this. Good communication is important in the institutional setting. Good communication is what nursing home professionals rely on to enlist the cooperation of residents and colleagues. They use it to calm patients, defuse power struggles, prevent catastrophic behaviors, promote personal bonding between patients and themselves, and cut down on both resident and worker stress. Poor communication in the nursing home costs overworked staff precious time and leads to mistakes that are likely to require more work later on. Poor communication leads to caregiver burnout and costs the facility money. In short, the large numbers of Alzheimer's residents in today's nursing homes have created a call for communication crisis management.

Despite the pervasiveness of the problem, only a few treatments aimed at enhancing the communication abilities of Alzheimer's patients have been reported; and even fewer have been scientifically evaluated. Bourgeois (1991) reviewed the literature on communication treatment for elderly adults with Alzheimer's and related disorders and noted, "One conspicuous void in the treatment literature concerns investigations of ways to maintain communicative functioning in aging adults with chronic diffuse and degenerative neurologic disease" (p. 831). She noted that before 1991, the journals of the American Speech-Language-Hearing Association had "not published a single treatment study in this area" (p. 832). "Researchers," Bourgeois declared, "need to identify specific communication deficits in a well-defined patient population, develop a reasonable measurement procedure for tracking the communication deficit before and throughout treatment and plan a replicable and reliably implemented treatment to address the problem" (p. 833).

This chapter first discusses the value of various direct intervention approaches and goals currently being used with Alzheimer's patients. It then describes the development of the Breakfast Club, an innovative attempt to incorporate approaches previously shown to be effective into a single treatment. Ongoing study of the Breakfast Club is also an attempt to carry out Bourgeois' mandate for tracking treatment effectiveness.

Approaches to Direct Communication Intervention for Alzheimer's Patients

Types of Approaches

In her 1991 literature review, Bourgeois reported that four basic approaches to direct treatment of Alzheimer's patients brought about improvements in overall communication effectiveness.

Environmental Approaches. Several specific environmental adaptations were reported to increase and/or improve the communication of Alzheimer's patients. They included making the environment more home-like (Gottesman, 1965), providing conversational partners (e.g., Corson & Corson, 1978), providing group activities (e.g., Blackman, Howe, & Pinkston, 1976), and providing food. Quattrochi-Tubin and Jason (1980) showed increases in the frequency of social interactions (defined as verbally conversing or nonverbal game playing) when 56 cognitively impaired elderly nursing home residents had access to coffee and cookies during activity times. Cartensen and Erickson (1986) reported positive changes as a function of the presence of refreshments. Some more recent studies have suggested a possible direct therapeutic value in traditional dining (Boczko, 1994; Durnbaugh, Haley, & Roberts, 1993; Hallberg, Norberg, & Johnsson, 1993; Sandman, Norberg & Adolfsson, 1988).

Approaches that Control Stimulus Conditions. Although "reality orientation" was generally shown to be ineffective as a protocol for improving communication skills in Alzheimer's patients, the use of external memory aids, such as printed materials and verbal prompts, was reported to have a positive effect on communication success. Bourgeois (1991) was careful to note, however, that "treatment programs utilizing enhanced stimuli need to include training and maintenance procedures to ensure that environmental cues become functional for patients" (p. 834). She cited her own memory wallet protocol, which requires extensive training of caregivers.

Approaches that Provide Ample Reinforcement. Several clinical researchers have reported that providing reinforcements (candy, tokens, etc.) for appropriate behaviors improved the performance of Alzheimer's patients on a variety of verbal tasks. Mueller and Atlas (1972) reported increased conversational interaction in group therapy when positive reinforcers were provided.

Group Therapy Interventions. Lubinski (1978), in words reflecting the sentiments of many geriatric clinicians, called group therapy "a means to establish an interpersonal situation in which meaningful, motivating, and reinforcing communication can occur" (p. 242). Few who cited the importance of group therapy, however, provided clear empirical evidence supporting its efficacy. Bourgeois (1991) noted the need for "group therapy programs that provide descriptions of replicable treatment procedures for operationally defined target behaviors, and that monitor individuals' performance using reliable measurement systems . . . to determine the effectiveness of treatment in groups" (p. 837).

Creating Successful Treatments

Bourgeois (1991) offered three suggestions for clinicians attempting to create successful treatments within the above four approaches to direct communication therapy for Alzheimer's patients.

1. *Choose functional communication skills that directly and significantly alter daily life and that recruit naturally occurring reinforcers in the environment.* Our experience in the nursing home setting tells us that the functional communication skills that most alter daily life and recruit reinforcement in the nursing home setting are the ability to communicate wants and needs, to engage in social rituals, and to engage in two-way conversation.

2. *Choose procedures that exploit a patient's remaining abilities.* The communication-related abilities best preserved in Alzheimer's disease include (a) the use of "procedural memories" (those ingrained, habituated, "know-how" neuromuscular patterns that range from playing the piano and dancing to washing hands and brushing teeth to dealing cards and pouring coffee; (b) the ability to access early life memories (those stored more diffusely and redundantly over the cortex); (c) the ability to sing, recite, pray, and read aloud with preserved pronunciation and grammar; (d) the ability to engage in everyday social ritual; (e) the desire for and capacity to enjoy interpersonal communication; and (f) the desire for interpersonal respect and control over one's environment. In addition, although the Alzheimer's patient's senses of touch, taste, and smell, like the senses of vision and hearing, have begun to diminish, they continue to provide familiar and satisfying input. Stimulation of these senses fosters meaningful activity in the brain.

3. *Select goals to match the constraints and the advantages of the environment.* In the institutional environment, goals must be selected that help patients adapt to constraints like limited freedom and mobility, personnel turnover, rigid schedules, and the clatter and

hubbub of the institutional setting. On the other hand, nursing homes provide many advantages, such as availability of resources, professional understanding and assistance, and large numbers of other individuals with similar needs.

Goals of Direct Communication Intervention with Alzheimer's Patients in Nursing Homes

Considering the strengths and limitations of Alzheimer's patients, the nursing home environment, and the nursing home staff, we have compiled the following five goals for communication intervention in the nursing home setting:

1. Maintain as many of the Alzheimer's patient's residual functional communication strengths as possible.

2. Prevent overresponse to disability, which can lead to "learned helplessness." "Learned helplessness arises when persons learn through repeated experiences that their actions have little effect on the outcome of the situation—especially in the 'restricted' environment of the nursing home" (Foy & Mitchell, 1990, p. 1).

3. Relieve the burden of caregiving; maintain the health and integrity of the caregiver.

4. Improve the quality of life and maintain human dignity of patient and caregiver.

5. Establish harmonious functioning within the nursing home setting.

Protocols for Direct Communication Intervention

Currently the two most common direct treatment protocols reported by speech–language pathologists working with mid-stage Alzheimer's patients in the nursing home are individualized programs, using memory books and/or wallets to maintain function and conversation (Bourgeois, 1991, 1992), and conversation groups (Clark & Witte, 1991; Shoham & Neuschatz, 1985).

Although the effectiveness of Bourgeois' (1990, 1992) individual methodology has been well documented, to our knowledge there are no empirical studies documenting the effectiveness of conversational group therapy. Nonetheless, texts continue to suggest that conversation/communication groups are the most widely used type of intervention in short-staffed nursing homes. The types of group communication therapy for Alzheimer's patients reported in the literature include remotivation therapy, resocialization/conversation therapy, and reminiscence and life review therapy, with resocialization/conversation therapy or the "discourse group" being the most frequently discussed. Nearly all reports of group therapy in the literature cite three common goals: (a) stimulate verbalization, (b) increase interactions among group members, and (c) help group members renew independence and maintain self-esteem.

In her 1995 article on interventions for persons with Alzheimer's disease, Clark talked about the use of discourse group interventions with patients in the more advanced stages of dementia to "enhance group members' feelings of self-esteem, emotional security, and comfort in an atmosphere that fosters adult-to-adult conversational exchanges at persons' functional communication levels" (p. 55). On the basis of anecdotal literature and their own experience, Clark and Witte (1991) and Clark (1995) have made specific recommendations for group therapy with Alzheimer's patients. These recommendations are summarized in Table 15.1.

The Breakfast Club

The Breakfast Club is a multimodal group treatment protocol that seeks to incorporate all that has been written about discourse groups and effective direct communication intervention for Alzheimer's patients in the nursing home setting. The Breakfast Club involves joint action of a small group of Alzheimer's patients in preparing, serving, and eating breakfast, and cleaning up afterward under the direction of a speech–language pathologist.

Goals and Participants

The Breakfast Club seeks to provide the following benefits for its members:

- maintenance of organizational, decision-making, and social skills; conversational skills and early life memories; and interest and involvement;

Table 15.1

Group Principles: Recommendations for Group
Therapy with Alzheimer's Patients

Group Preparation and Scheduling

- Be consistent by conducting the group at the same time and place.
- Schedule the group when members are most alert.
- Prior to implementing group sessions, obtain personal history information on group members for reaffirming values of their previous life experiences and self-worth during sessions.
- Prepare activities ahead of time, but allow members' responses to dictate the thematic flow.
- Ask family members to donate/lend memorabilia.

Physical Environment of the Group

- Hold group sessions in a quiet, distraction-free area with good lighting.
- Seat members in a semicircle.
- Center a table in the middle of the circle. (A table serves as a communication–social barrier in most situations, but it serves as a focal point for persons with Alzheimer's disease.)
- Use a large blackboard or erase board for printing conversational topics and other items.

Communication Principles During Group Sessions

- Provide members with a bridge from their daily routines to the group by introducing, and providing a simple explanation of, the group's purpose while conveying a sense of belonging and specialness to group members.
- Provide models and ways to initially cue members by asking higher functioning members to respond first.
- Present information in a parallel presentation format by separately introducing information to each member in turn.
- Use name tags and emphasize persons' names during group activities, while deemphasizing that members learn persons' names.
- Avoid phrasing questions that require a precise answer, e.g., "What color is this?"
- Ask questions that seek an opinion or comment. Do not directly correct members' inappropriate responses; rather, provide reinforcement and positive feedback by restating and summarizing members' responses for topic cohesion.

(Continues)

Table 15.1 *(Continued)*

- Personalize topics, e.g., "What do you think about _____? Why do you think _____? How do you feel about _____?"
- Use superlatives and intense, emotionally charged phraseology and intonation patterns.
- Relate topics to general life experiences, past experiences, and the generalized present.
- Use familiar multisensory, concrete physical cues and memorabilia associated with the group's theme for triggering intact sensory association and long-term episodic memories.

Management of Emotional and Behavioral Disruptions
- Briefly remove persons from the group who display disruptive behavior and later analyze the circumstances surrounding such behavior.
- Avoid confrontation by distracting attention and changing topics/activities.
- Include only one wanderer per group.

Note. From "Interventions for Persons with Alzheimer's Disease: Strategies for Maintaining and Enhancing Communicative Success," by L. Clark, 1995, *Topics in Language Disorders, 15*, p. 53. Copyright 1995 by Aspen. Reprinted with permission.

- facilitation of retained procedural memories and linguistic abilities in all modalities, and retained reading skills;

- stimulation of auditory, visual, olfactory, gustatory, and tactile senses, and of positive emotions; and

- prevention of isolation and learned helplessness, and prevention of premature deterioration of communication skills.

Over a 2-year period, several groups of 5 mid-stage Alzheimer's patients at the Jewish Home and Hospital for Aged in Bronx, New York, have participated in the Breakfast Club for periods of 6 to 24 weeks each. The 20 residents who participated for at least 12 weeks ranged in age from 75 to 91 years ($M = 84.6$; $SD = 4.15$), scored between 8 and 21 ($M = 15.6$; $SD = 4.01$) out of a maximum of 30 points on the *Mini-Mental State* (Folstein, Folstein, & McHugh, 1975), and scored between 6 and 14 ($M = 10.6$; $SD = 2.28$) on the 25-point *Arizona Battery for Communication Disorders of Dementia* (Bayles & Tomoeda, 1993).

For each Breakfast Club, 1-hour meetings were held five mornings a week in a home-like kitchen setting that was visually and acoustically insulated from the rest of the nursing home. Breakfast Club members, who were not served breakfast trays in their rooms, were seated around a rectangular table with the facilitator at one end. Structure was maintained from beginning to end; a 10-step general protocol was followed each day:

1. Facilitator greets Breakfast Club members and distributes name tags by giving each member a choice of two, one of which is the member's own.

2. Facilitator introduces juices, giving choices and eliciting descriptions and opinions. Visual cues, semantic cues, and carrier phrases are used.

    Examples:

    "Can you read the name of this juice?" (visual cue)

    "This one has lots of vitamin C." (semantic cue)

    "You want a cold glass of _____." (carrier phrase).

3. Facilitator introduces the topic of coffee, again eliciting language through a variety of cues:

    Examples:

    Facilitator shows coffee pot and ground coffee. (visual cue)

    Facilitator passes coffee around for members to smell. (olfactory cue)

    "What's something hot to drink in the morning?" (semantic cue)

    "Do you want your coffee black or with milk?" (paired choice)

    "What are other hot drinks besides coffee?" (semantic associations)

    "How about a chocolate-y hot drink?"

    "Or a drink you need a tea bag for?"

4. Facilitator directs conversation to discussion of various types of breakfast foods and helps group settle on choice for the day. Choices include cereal, eggs, pancakes, and French toast. Facilitator encourages cross conversation by asking one of the members to find out if everyone agrees on the choice of the day.

5. Facilitator prompts members to name the items needed for food preparation.

   Examples:

   "What can we use to break our eggs?"

   "What should we use to cook the eggs? Pancakes? French toast? The fry pan or the plate?" (paired choice)

   "What can we put on the pan so it doesn't stick?" (direct question)

   Facilitator demonstrates mixing the egg or pouring the milk into the cereal and encourages the members to participate (modeling).

6. Facilitator prompts members to correctly sequence their actions while cooking or preparing the selected food.

   Examples:

   "What do we do with the egg first?"

   "How do we know when to add the eggs to the pan?'

7. When the food is deemed ready to eat by group members, it is portioned out equally to all Breakfast Club members. Members generally assist in the serving. The facilitator uses linguistic prompts to encourage members to choose another food to complement the one on their plates.

   Examples:

   "What would taste good with these pancakes? (direct question)

   "Can you read us what kind of jam is in that jar?" (visual cue)

   "What's something warm and brown that you spread butter on?" (semantic cue)

   "Would you like a piece of toast with _____." (carrier phrase)

8. Facilitator offers members another drink option (coffee, tea) to complement the food they are eating and uses direct questioning and paired choice to determine how to prepare the drink as each member prefers.

9. While members are eating and enjoying coffee, the facilitator engages members in conversation. Topics vary and are chosen

in advance. A list of pertinent questions for each topic is used to provide prompts. These questions are open-ended to encourage longer responses and the sharing of opinions; however, choices are also given and questions "narrowed" as necessary.

> *Examples:*
>
> "I wonder what kind of a house you grew up in." (open-ended question)
>
> "What do you remember most about World War II?"
>
> "Did you live in an apartment or in a house?" (forced choice)

10. Breakfast Club is officially concluded. Members are asked to help in the clean-up process. Name tags are returned and individual good-byes are said.

To avoid sensory overload and confusion, the program's food choices are limited, including only those items the participants are capable of preparing. As time goes on, tasks progress from simple (choosing butter or jam for toast) to more complex (actually making French toast or pancakes).

Efficacy of the Breakfast Club

Preliminary results from an ongoing research study at the Jewish Home and Hospital indicate that the Breakfast Club produces positive results and meets its goals in several areas. Over a 12-week period, Breakfast Club participants demonstrated improvement not only in the use of language and communication skills, but also in renewed procedural memories for preparing, sharing, and eating a meal. Their social ritual abilities resurfaced, and they began to show genuine social concern for one another.

The *Resident's Functional and Communicative Independence Scale*, developed and standardized at the Jewish Home and Hospital, was administered by nonbiased certified nursing assistants to the 20 mid-stage patients described above, both the week before the Breakfast Club and after 12 weeks of attendance. The 20-point independence scale measures functional levels of psychosocial interaction, communication/conversation, mealtime independence, and cognitive function. All participants in the Breakfast Club improved on this scale over the 12-week period, with the greatest improvements noted in the psychosocial interaction and communication conversation areas. A *t* test for paired comparisons indicated a significant increase in independence scores for members of the Breakfast Club, t (19) = 8.73, p <.0001. Twenty matched residents who participated only in small discourse/conversation groups showed little or no improvement on the scale. More than half of the matched subjects showed a decline in independence scores.

Speech–language pathologists at the Jewish Home and Hospital also administered the *Arizona Battery for Communication Disorders of Dementia* (ABCD) to Breakfast Club members before and after 12 weeks of participation. ABCD scores of two thirds of the participants increased, one went down, and the rest remained the same. In contrast, ABCD scores of two thirds of the residents in the control group went down.

Additional behavioral changes, less easy to quantify and score, were noted in Breakfast Club participants. Many of these appeared to reflect changes in levels of attention and listening. Breakfast Club members began calling one another by name as early as Week 3. Conversation group subjects never did. By the 12th week of one Breakfast Club, a patient was able to pass out all the name tags to the correct members without prompting.

Videotapes of Breakfast Club sessions revealed a marked increase in eye contact between facilitator and members and among members as the weeks progressed. Members frequently responded to the nonverbal cues and facial expressions of other group members, indicating increased visual attention. Breakfast Club members tended to sit forward in their chairs while they were not involved in breakfast preparation as well as when they were. The incidence of distractibility went down, and Breakfast Club members who frequently stood up and wandered remained seated by Week 5. In contrast, members of the conversation group did not sit forward or orient their bodies to the speaker. Distractibility and the desire to wander appeared to remain constant in conversation group members.

Breakfast Club members appeared to have fewer off-topic utterances and less egocentric speech than did conversation group members. Conversation group members appeared to have more "rambling" speeches and inappropriate interruptions in their interactions than Breakfast Club members did.

Members of the Breakfast Club showed an unexpected ability to participate in hands-on meal preparation, demonstrating use of both the procedural motor memories necessary for making and serving the food and the social rituals required for sharing it. Beyond the

preparation and consumption of the meal, four things happened significantly more often in the Breakfast Club than in the conversation
group: (a) members offered spontaneous humorous remarks and
laughed frequently, (b) members made empathetic statements to one
another, (c) members commented on ongoing activities of the group,
and (d) members broke into spontaneous singing. (On one videotape,
members of the Breakfast Club self-initiated the song "Silvery Moon,"
and all five sang two full choruses with harmony and vocal accompa-
niment.)

Anecdotal comments by direct care staff and families have indicated increased levels of patient involvement in activities of daily living and reduced levels of agitation and anxiety in patients who participated in the Breakfast Club. A nursing assistant observing a
Breakfast Club session said, "I can't believe the patients do what they
do in the club. Mrs. J. used to just sit in the dining room and say, 'Help
me. Help me.' Now she not only eats independently, she helps other
residents." A member of the therapeutic recreation staff noted how 1
patient showed an increase in social interaction. "She now sits in the
core area and engages in conversation with other residents.
Previously, she sat in her own room and isolated herself." Another
patient, who had never left her room, began taking her meals in the
dining room and often sat near the main entry way, pleasantly greet-
ing visitors to the home. Contrary to what the staff had reported about
resident R. at the inception of a Breakfast Club group—"You will have
a lot of problems with her. She won't cooperate and she'll keep getting
lost"—R. actually took on the role of helper in Breakfast Club sessions
and began wheeling other patients to the elevator. "Look," she said,
"I'm needed."

Said the daughter of one Breakfast Club member, "I visit my
mother after the Breakfast Club because she responds so much better
then, and it's easier to talk to her." A supervising nurse who participated in an ongoing Breakfast Club maintenance group reported that
she now saw residents "more as individuals rather than a group of
people with the same needs. Breakfast Club allows some of their former individuality and personality to shine through."

Suggestions for Running a Successful Breakfast Club

1. Form groups carefully. When a program has 5 patients, it is important that they are chosen carefully. As indicated in Clark's (1995)

Group Principles (see Table 15.1), it is probably a good idea to be cautious about including wanderers, criers, and so on. Yet, we have had good luck with persons who have seemed withdrawn or anxious and with some wanderers. The focused activity appears to encourage participation and discourage distraction. Members should, however, have the potential for congeniality.

2. *Anticipate problems in getting patients ready and into the room on time.* Residents need to be awakened, toileted, dressed, and sometimes medicated before they come to Breakfast Club. There are all kinds of excuses—"they're napping, they don't feel well, we can't find them, they've already eaten." If the patients are not on the same unit as the Breakfast Club, the club becomes one of a number of competing activities. More excuses—"The patient went to the day room, the physical therapy clinic, the medical clinic. Transport hasn't arrived; the elevator hasn't arrived; the elevator operator won't cooperate."

3. *Be organized and security conscious in ordering and storing the food.* Having the right breakfast food is essential for this treatment. Decisions have to be made about who will order the food, how and when it will be delivered, and where it will be stored. We recommend weekly delivery of everything, except milk, so that you can plan meals several days in advance. We also recommend that you have the same person in dietary always in charge of the Breakfast Club food order. If one person is responsible, it is more likely that you will know when something has gone wrong. If she or he is ill, you both know that other arrangements must be made. You also need a secure arrangement for storing the food. Even with a locked refrigerator and storage, other staff members with keys often think a few items will not be missed.

4. *Enlist the cooperation of other direct care staff.* Whether or not you have the cooperation of nurses in your facility can make or break your Breakfast Club program. It is important to show the nursing staff that the effort invested in getting residents to the Breakfast Club can actually make their work easier. Once they are convinced that residents who participate in the Breakfast Club do more for themselves, engage in more of the home's activities, become less agitated and depressed, and actually enjoy mealtime, nurses usually become staunch allies of the speech–language pathologist's efforts.

Speech–language pathologists cannot run enough Breakfast Clubs to serve every eligible resident or effect lasting changes throughout an entire facility. They can, however, train other personnel to conduct "maintenance" Breakfast Clubs once they are up and running. Speech–language pathologists at the Jewish Home and Hospital in the

Bronx designed and conducted four 12-week training programs for certified nursing assistants (CNAs) to take over already-formed Breakfast Clubs. Basic information about the communication deficits of Alzheimer's patients and basic facilitative techniques for cuing were taught. The success of the nursing assistants has been remarkable. CNAs have proven apt and enthusiastic facilitators, aided by their day-in and day-out knowledge of individual residents. The residents have responded well to their work and, after 12 weeks of maintenance, have maintained the gains they made in their first 12 weeks in the Breakfast Club with the speech–language pathologist. Perhaps more importantly, the CNAs have learned valuable skills for interacting with Alzheimer's patients. Said one speech–language pathologist after observing CNAs conducting a Breakfast Club, "You know, I think the hardest thing for CNAs to see is that they should do less. I think that in the Breakfast Club, they finally have learned to help less."

Arranging work schedules of CNAs can present an obstacle if there is little administrative support. If CNAs are not available, occupational and recreational therapists or capable volunteers might also be excellent candidates to run ongoing Breakfast Clubs or discourse groups. Speech–language pathologists who are not full-time staff members of nursing homes might offer to create Breakfast Clubs and train personnel as part of a functional maintenance plan.

If creation of a 5-day-a-week Breakfast Club is not viable in your facility, you might take the general principles learned from the Breakfast Club and employ them in other ways. Spend some of your work time in the dining room and make the lunchroom a classroom. Show aides and volunteers how to facilitate independence and communication. Work to alter the policies of the nursing home so that all meals are not selected and delivered to residents on lukewarm trays to be eaten alone in bed. Demonstrate the gains to be made by allowing able residents to interact with companions at the table, choose which foods they will eat, and manage the process independently.

Summary and Implications for the Future

The Breakfast Club is an effective direct communication intervention for nursing home residents who have mid-stage Alzheimer's disease. It was designed to employ all of the approaches to direct intervention that previously have been shown to be effective. For example, it employs environmental supports, ample sensory stimulation, and positive reinforcement in a group setting. Although designed by speech–language pathologists, initial research indicates that it can be carried out successfully by trained nursing assistants or other personnel. Residents who have participated in the Breakfast Club at the Jewish Home and Hospital for the Aged in the Bronx have demonstrated increased independence and involvement and decreased anxiety and isolation for up to 24 weeks; language and cognitive status have not declined measurably.

Current research is seeking to determine differences in effectiveness between standard conversational groups and Breakfast Clubs for Alzheimer's patients, and to document precisely which patient behaviors change over time in response to which types of stimulation by facilitators. Ultimately, it is hoped that a variety of methodologies can be developed using the basic principles of the Breakfast Club.

References

Bayles, K. A., & Kaszniak, K. (1987). *Communication and cognition in normal aging and dementia*. Boston: College-Hill Press.

Bayles, K. A., & Tomoeda, C. K. (1993). *Arizona Battery for Communication Disorders of Dementia*. Tucson, AZ: Canyonlands.

Blackman, D. K., Howe, M., & Pinkston, E. M. (1976). Increasing participation in social interaction of the institutionalized elderly. *The Gerontologist, 16*, 69–76.

Boczko, F. (1994, July/August). The breakfast club: A multi-modal language stimulation program for nursing home residents with Alzheimer's disease. *The American Journal of Alzheimer's Care and Related Disorders and Research*, pp. 35–38.

Bourgeois, M. S. (1990). Enhancing conversation skills in patients with Alzheimer's disease using a prosthetic memory aid. *Journal of Applied Behavior Analysis, 23*, 31–64.

Bourgeois, M. S. (1991). Communication treatment for adults with dementia. *Journal of Speech and Hearing Research, 34*, 831–844.

Bourgeois, M. S. (1992). Evaluating memory wallets in conversations with persons with dementia. *Journal of Speech and Hearing Research, 35*, 1344–1357.

Cartensen, L. L., & Erickson, R. J. (1986). Enhancing the social environment of elderly nursing home residents: Are high rates of interaction enough? *Journal of Applied Behavior Analysis, 19,* 349–355.

Clark, L. (1995). Interventions for persons with Alzheimer's disease: Strategies for maintaining and enhancing communicative success. *Topics in Language Disorders, 15,* 47–65.

Clark, L., & Witte, K. (1991). Nature and efficacy of communication management in Alzheimer's disease. In R. Lubinski (Ed.), *Dementia and communication* (pp. 238–256). Philadelphia: B. C. Decker.

Corson, S. A., & Corson, E. (1978). Pets as mediators of therapy in custodial institutions and the aged. In J. H. Masserman (Ed.), *Current psychiatric therapies* (Vol. 18, pp. 203–206). New York: Grune & Stratton.

Durnbaugh, T., Haley, B., & Roberts, S. (1993, July/August). Feeding behaviors in mid-stage Alzheimer's disease: A review. *The American Journal of Alzheimer's Care and Related Disorders and Research,* pp. 22–27.

Folstein, M., Folstein, S., & McHugh, P. (1975). Mini-Mental State: A practical method for grading the cognitive state of patients for the clinician. *Journal of Psychiatric Research, 12,* 189–198.

Foy, S., & Mitchell, M. (1990). Factors contributing to learned helplessness in the institutionalized aged: A literature review. *Physical and Occupational Therapy in Geriatrics, 9,* 1–2.

Gottesman, L. E. (1965). Resocialization of the geriatric mental patient. *American Journal of Public Health, 55,* 1964–1970.

Hallberg, I., Norberg, A., & Johnsson, K. (1993, May/June). Verbal interaction during the lunch-meal between caregivers and vocally disruptive demented patients. *The American Journal of Alzheimer's Care and Related Disorders and Research,* pp. 26–32.

Lubinski, R. (1978). Why so little interest in whether or not old people talk: A review of recent research on verbal communication among the elderly. *International Journal of Aging and Human Development, 9,* 237–245.

Lubinski, R. (1991). Environmental considerations for elderly patients. In R. Lubinski (Ed.), *Dementia and communication* (pp. 257–278). Philadelphia: B. C. Decker.

Mueller, D. J., & Atlas, L. (1972). Resocialization of regressed elderly residents: A behavioral management approach. *Journal of Gerontology, 27,* 390–392.

Quattrochi-Tubin, S., & Jason, L. A. (1980). Enhancing social interactions and activity among the elderly through stimulus control. *Journal of Applied Behavior Analysis, 13,* 159–163.

Richter, J. M., Bottenberg, D., & Roberto, K. A. (1993, September/October). Communication between formal caregivers and individuals with Alzheimer's disease. *The American Journal of Alzheimer's Care and Related Disorders and Research,* pp. 20–25.

Ripich, D., Wykle, M., & Niles, S. (1995). Alzheimer's disease caregivers: The FOCUSED program. A communication skills training program helps nursing assistants to give better care to patients with Alzheimer's disease. *Geriatric Nursing, 16,* 15–17.

Sandman, P., Norberg, A., & Adolfsson, R. (1988). Verbal communication and behavior during meals in five institutionalized patients with Alzheimer-type dementia. *Journal of Advance Nursing, 13,* 571–578.

Santo Pietro, M. J. (1994). Assessing the communicative styles of caregivers of patients with Alzheimer's disease. *Seminars in Speech and Language, 15,* 236–254.

Shoham, H., & Neuschatz, S. (1985). Group therapy with senile patients. *Social Work, 30,* 69–72.

U.S. National Center for Health Statistics. (1985). *Preliminary data from the 1985 National Nursing Home Survey.* Washington, DC: Division of Health Care Statistics.

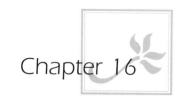

Chapter 16

Functional Maintenance Programs®

Gail K. Neustadt
Joan K. Glickstein

Neustadt and Glickstein broaden the perspective on communication mainte-
nance in this chapter to address functional maintenance programs in gener-
al, particularly as provided in extended care facilities. The authors present the
Tri-Model® philosophy of rehabilitation, which defines rehabilitation as a
restorative process and identifies three naturally progressing phases of recov-
ery. A case example follows one client through all three phases; examples of
reimbursable treatment goals and objectives are also provided.

1. *What are the three phases of recovery identified in the Tri-Model philos-*
   ophy of restorative care? For each stage, identify the setting in which
   services might be delivered and the types of speech–language pathology
   services required.

2. *What are the three primary Functional Maintenance Programs of the*
   Functional Maintenance Therapy® approach as developed by Glickstein
   and Neustadt? How do the programs differ in terms of identified need
   and purpose?

3. *Are communication maintenance programs reimbursable under Medi-*
   care? What populations may be considered for such interventions?
   How must goals be documented to ensure reimbursement?

4. *Why must rehabilitation therapies and restorative nursing operate*
   together to maximize functional potential?

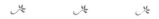

Prior to this decade, little had been written about maintaining function in the geriatric population. In fact, maintenance services were generally not included within the standard practice patterns of physical, occupational, or speech–language therapists. Even the term "maintenance" was avoided in documentation by rehabilitation therapists, as well as nursing staff. For example, nurses might write a resident-focused goal stating that "the resident will not decline in the ability to _____ " instead of "the resident will maintain the ability to_____." This apprehension in using the "m-word" was the result of a long-standing misconception that maintenance always meant custodial, unskilled services not covered by Medicare. Additionally, state and federal surveyors of long-term care facilities often criticize the use of the word "maintenance" as a care plan goal.

The subject of maintenance was not addressed in a comprehensive manner until 1992, when Glickstein and Neustadt wrote *Reimbursable Geriatric Service Delivery: A Functional Maintenance Therapy System.* Today, not only is "maintenance" an acceptable term, but also the proliferation of managed care entities has expanded its meaning into the realm of wellness and prevention. Indeed, the "M" in HMO stands for maintenance (Health Maintenance Organization). This chapter provides a definition of maintenance for rehabilitation professionals, describes the Glickstein and Neustadt (1992) model for service delivery (the Tri-Model), Functional Maintenance Programs (FMP), and discusses supportive Medicare guidelines and documentation. The relationship between rehabilitation and restorative nursing services in provision of FMPs in extended care facilities is also considered. Because the FMP model applies across rehabilitation disciplines, it is presented in general terms, with specific examples highlighting speech–language disorders and services. A case study illustrating the progression of a client with a communication disorder through the phases of restorative care is also presented.

The Tri-Model Philosophy of Rehabilitation

FMPs (Functional Maintenance Programs) are one element of a total service delivery system called the Tri-Model. First proposed in 1992 by Glickstein and Neustadt, the Tri-Model philosophy of rehabilitation provided a new and comprehensive definition of rehabilitation. The

Tri-Model philosophy is put into action via the Tri-Model system, which provides a cost-effective, reimbursable continuum of care that is valid in all provider settings. The Tri-Model philosophy defines rehabilitation as a restorative process, with three phases of recovery requiring skilled services that occur in a natural progression, illustrated by an equilateral triangle of care (see Figure 16.1).

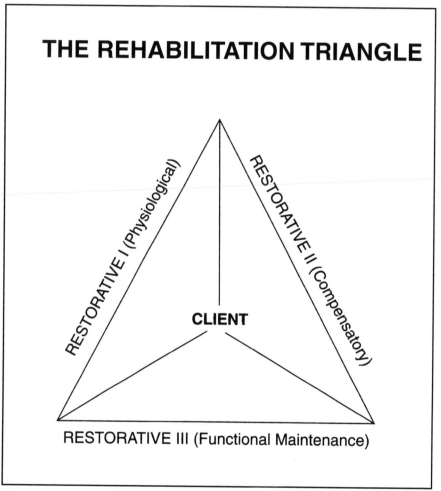

Figure 16.1. Tri-Model system of rehabilitation. *Note.* From *Reimbursable Geriatric Service Delivery: A Functional Maintenance Therapy System*, by J. Glickstein and G. Neustadt, 1992, Gaithersburg, MD: Aspen. Copyright 1994 by GNI. Reprinted with permission of GNI.

Restorative I—Physiological

The Restorative I phase occurs during the acute stage of the disability. During this phase, the individual may experience return of neuro-muscular and cognitive/linguistic functions, enabling varying degrees of recovery. Restorative I programs are designed and imple-mented by rehabilitation professionals immediately following a med-ical diagnosis indicating the need for services. Typically, such pro-grams take advantage of spontaneous recovery, with the nature and extent of recovery being affected by the diagnosis, the severity of the impairment, and the individual's emotional response to his or her impairment. Early intervention stimulates the damaged neurological systems, helping to speed and maximize this stage of recovery. It also assists the individual to recognize and work through a grieving peri-od related to loss of function, in order to promote motivation to achieve greater independence. Restorative I programs traditionally begin in acute care facilities and continue in long-term care settings.

Case Example

A 70-year-old man is admitted to the hospital via ambulance. He is conscious but unable to communicate intelligibly. A neurological evaluation, which includes CT scans of the brain, indicates a left temporoparietal infarct with some involvement of the frontal area (Broca's). Clinical signs include right hemi-paresis, drool on right side of mouth, inability to follow commands. A medical diagnosis of left cerebrovascular accident (CVA) with right hemiparesis and aphasia is made. Medical management includes drug therapy to prevent fur-ther cerebral damage and to dissolve the clot. Rehabilitation is ordered by the physician as soon as the patient is medically stable.

Upon evaluation, the speech pathologist concurs with the physician's diag-nosis of aphasia but refines the diagnosis to a "mixed, expressive/receptive type." Because this is a "fresh stroke," prognosis for recovery is very good and the patient is placed on program five times per week for a period of 6 weeks. At this stage, the speech pathologist's treatment plan might include the fol-lowing statements:

Problem: patient unable to communicate needs due to expressive aphasia.

Goal: patient will be able to verbalize final word in open-ended phrase 65% of the time by _____.

Treatment objective: patient will be able to complete phrases with 75% accuracy by _____.

Note that the treatment objective and goal reflect a measurable degree of progress within a specified amount of time. If the patient does not achieve these goals and objectives within the specified time, he will either be discharged from treatment or the goals and objectives will have to be modified.

Restorative II—Compensatory Phase

The Restorative II phase is an extension of the Restorative I phase, beginning as soon as the rehabilitation professional recognizes that neurological function has started to plateau, no further spontaneous return is expected, and the ability to perform functional tasks without assistance is limited. During this phase, adaptive equipment and compensatory strategies are introduced to assist the individual in independent function.

Case Example:

Our 70-year-old patient has been on program for 4 weeks and is unable to make his needs known orally. A recent CT scan indicates that, although his thrombosis has resolved, there is what appears to be permanent damage. Reevaluation, or ongoing assessment, indicates that he is able to communicate more effectively using a communication notebook. Restorative II documentation reflects these changes.

Problem: patient unable to communicate needs due to expressive aphasia.

Goal: patient will use compensatory strategies to make needs known 65% of the time by _____.

Treatment objective: patient will learn to point to pictures: depicting functional needs by _____.

Note that the problem remains the same but the treatment goals and objectives have been modified to acknowledge the permanence of his loss and to reflect the resident's abilities as well as his needs. Persons seen during the Restorative II stage of recovery are generally on program five times per week as inpatients or three times per week as outpatients.

Restorative III—Functional Maintenance

Although most health care professionals are familiar with professional rehabilitation programs developed during the Restorative I and II phases, there is little recognition and/or understanding of the third phase. In this phase, there will be no "significant" change in the patient's condition. If the patient was in therapy, he or she has reached his or her maximum potential. The objectives of functional maintenance are to

- promote optimum use of identified functional abilities,

- empower caregivers to carry out specialized rehabilitation programs,

- retard deterioration of functional abilities over time,

- improve quality of life,

- assure professional follow-up,

- prevent negative functional outcomes, and

- provide for continuity within a continuum of care.

To achieve these objectives, Glickstein and Neustadt (1992) developed Functional Maintenance Therapy (FMT), which is composed of six elements: screening, evaluation, programming, training, documenting, and quality assessment/improvement. Each of these elements is vital to successfully accomplish the intent of Restorative III. However, the FMP element is the primary focus of this chapter.

FMPs are discharge programs. Within the Restorative III phase, Glickstein and Neustadt (1992) have identified three types of functional maintenance discharge programs (FMPs): (1) FMP II, the Discharge Program, follows traditional therapy at the Restorative I or Restorative II phase. (2) FMP I, the "No-Ongoing Therapy" (NOT) program, is used for persons who received only FMT services. (3) The final program, FMP III, the reassessment and adjustment program, is used when adjustment to an earlier program is necessary.

A major point for the reader to keep in mind as we present these programs is the evolution of focus in our training/teaching. Whereas Restorative I and Restorative II programs require the patient to be the focus of training, Restorative III focuses almost exclusively on training caregivers.

Discharge Program. The purpose of the Discharge FMP is to discharge an individual from a Restorative I or II program in a formalized manner and to deter deterioration of acquired abilities. When an individual receiving ongoing treatment during the Restorative I or II phases reaches his or her maximum potential, continued skilled intervention from a physical, occupational, or speech–language therapist is no longer practical. However, extension of the rehabilitation process is a critical factor in maintaining newly acquired functional abilities. As the individual approaches the Restorative III (maintenance) phase, caregivers as well as the patient/client must be trained to continue the program designed by the rehabilitation professional. A typical scenario would be that of our 70-year-old gentleman, who continues to require the use of a communication notebook. Sometime prior to discharge, the speech–language pathologist designs a program that will help maintain the gains achieved during therapy. This is the FMP. The goal of the FMP is "to maintain the patient's functional communication skills using a communication notebook." The speech–language pathologist continues the patient on program while training the caregiver in the use of the communication notebook. As soon as the training is completed, the caregiver is given written instructions, as part of the discharge plan, and the patient is discharged from treatment.

NOT Programs. Persons with chronic or progressive neurological disorders who require long term care are particularly vulnerable to a decline in functional status. For that reason, it is critical that rehabilitation professionals work in collaboration with caregivers to maintain successful functional outcomes. FMT is often appropriate for individuals who are not candidates for active treatment programs. Since "no ongoing treatment" is warranted, Glickstein and Neustadt (1992) have identified these FMPs as NOT programs. Individuals with dementia frequently fall into this category, as do those persons who have long-standing diagnoses of a progressive nature, such as multiple sclerosis or Parkinson's disease (see Chapters 10, 11, 12, 13, and 15 for sample programs for persons with Alzheimer's disease and related dementias). The NOT program provides a mechanism for accessing untapped functional abilities or preventing the deterioration of functional skills. As environmental and/or behavior modifications are established, functional improvement is often experienced.

For this program, rehabilitation professionals use identified residual functional abilities when providing professional consultation and training to caregivers. The purpose is to assist the individual in utilizing functional abilities in a meaningful capacity. Additionally, NOT programs can be developed with the goal of preventing a decline in functional ability for individuals at risk; thus the FMP may be viewed as a wellness component within the realm of risk management.

Case Example

Three years have passed, and our 70-year-old gentleman is now age 73. He was discharged to home but unable to manage in the community without 24-hour care. His family placed him in a nursing home where he is currently residing. His communication notebook remains in his drawer, unused since his entrance to the facility. Our patient is now called a "resident." The speech–language pathologist discovers our resident and his notebook during a facility screen. Recognizing that he is not living up to his maximum potential and that he is not an appropriate candidate for traditional therapy, she receives a physician order for FMT and places him on program with the goal "resident will communicate functional needs using a communication notebook." She then develops FMP I. The staff and other caregivers are trained and our resident is discharged with the written program. The therapist does not have to train the resident in the use of the communication notebook because he already knows how to use it. She does need to train the staff because they do not. Note here, the entire focus of therapy is on training staff to achieve the positive resident outcome.

Reassessment and Adjustment Programs. An FMP III is appropriate when a change in the effectiveness of the program has occurred. There need not be a change in the patient's/resident's condition. The reassessment and adjustment may be needed whenever there is a change in caregivers or a move to a different room in the same facility. Reassessment and adjustment can be as simple as training a new caregiver in the same program or as complex as a new evaluation with modification to the current program. In either event, the same program is retained.

Case Example

Two months following the establishment of the maintenance program for our 73-year-old gentleman, the speech–language pathologist stops by to see how he is getting along. He has been moved to a new room and there has been a change of caregivers. Once again his communication notebook is in the drawer. Because the program she had designed 2 months ago remains valid, the speech–language pathologist requests a physician order to adjust the program. Her goal is "to prevent deterioration of the resident's current communication abilities."

Medicare Coverage Guidelines
for Functional Maintenance Programs

You will not be reimbursed unless you understand and follow the rules! Most rehabilitation professionals still believe that maintenance programs do not qualify as skilled services, reimbursable under the Medicare Program, the governmental health insurance program established in 1965 as Title XVIII of the Social Security Act for the aged and disabled. Thus, maintenance programs are often not provided or, if provided, are not billed. Confusion exists in distinguishing between "maintenance" as a custodial, unskilled service and "functional maintenance" as a skilled service. In 1992, Glickstein and Neustadt offered the following definitions: "Maintenance is the provision of services intended to maintain the individual at his or her current level in as comfortable a condition as feasible. . . . Functional Maintenance is the provision of services intended to enhance those residual functional abilities identified during an evaluation performed by rehabilitation professionals" (p. 4). The definition of functional maintenance was later amended to include the "provision of rehabilitation services intended to deter decline of functional abilities attained during a professional treatment program and the provision of rehabilitation services intended to prevent negative functional outcomes."

As early as 1981, the Health Care Finance Administration (HCFA) established new guidelines for speech–language pathology services in all provider settings that, for the first time, clearly identified FMPs as covered services. Based on the wording of these guidelines, Glickstein and Neustadt developed the three FMPs.

Although the language in the 1981 guideline clearly establishes the skilled nature of the "NOT" program and the Discharge Program, the language used to substantiate the development of the Reassessment and Adjustment Programs is ambiguous. For example, the statement "and such infrequent reevaluations as may be required," leaves the door open to a variety of interpretations. To some, "infrequent" within the context of the guideline may mean monthly; to others, "infrequent" may mean annually. Later the guideline states, "If a patient has been under a restorative speech pathology program, the speech pathologist should regularly reevaluate the condition and adjust the treatment program." In this instance, the interpretation of the word "infrequent" as monthly would not be acceptable. A quarterly or annual reevaluation might be a more acceptable interpretation of the word "infrequent," depending upon the circumstances. In all cases, appropriate documentation must support that a reevaluation is reasonable, necessary, and infrequent.

In fact, the word "reevaluation" itself is open to interpretation. The question frequently asked is, "What is being reevaluated, the individual or the program?" Again, this depends upon circumstances. When it is determined that the individual has experienced a change in functional status, regardless of the origin, it is reasonable and necessary to provide skilled rehabilitation services. If functional change is due to physiological or cognitive alterations, the individual needs to be reevaluated and the prior FMP adjusted accordingly. However, if it is clear from the outset that there is no physiological basis for the individual's change in functional status, it is only reasonable and necessary to reevaluate and adjust the program, not the individual. In both instances, the physician's order should state, "reevaluation and adjustment of prior FMP," leaving the interpretation up to the therapist. To assure positive coverage outcomes, proper and adequate documentation is imperative.

A question then arises regarding the word "required." Who or what requires the reevaluation—the physician, the family, the patient, or perhaps governmental regulations? The interpretation of the word "required" leads to a host of dilemmas, too numerous to address here. However, fundamental to the question of what is required is the fact that whenever an individual experiences a change in functional status, good clinical judgment dictates that the problem(s) be addressed. For individuals residing in nursing facilities, it took an act of Congress to state that all residents in nursing facilities must function at their highest level feasible. By inserting the word "their" before highest, the federal government forced nursing homes to focus on providing all of the services a resident might require in order to function at his or her optimal level. The Nursing Home Reform Act of 1987, which was contained in the Omnibus Reconciliation Act of 1987, known as OBRA-87, set forth stringent requirements regarding quality-of-life and quality-of-care issues. The very fact that OBRA-87 stated that individuals residing in nursing facilities must function at their highest level feasible creates the need for Reassessment and Adjustment Programs on an ongoing basis.

Functional maintenance has been delineated throughout the years in many Medicare manuals for a variety of disease states and is identified as a skilled service that is covered under both Part A and Part B of Medicare when provided by physical, occupational, and/or speech–language therapists. For example, Functional Maintenance Therapy is discussed as appropriate for Parkinson's disease, old stroke, terminal illness, Alzheimer's disease, multiple sclerosis and amyotrophic lateral sclerosis, and decline in functional status (Health Care Financing Administration, 1987, 1989a, 1989b).

Documenting Functional Maintenance Programs

The second key to reimbursement is documentation. The adage, "if it wasn't written, it wasn't done," remains a truism; however, today's documentation must also focus on meaningful, functional outcomes. "Meaningful," in this context means "purposeful." An individual may be able to function on an imitative level, but if there is no purposeful outcome to his or her utterance, speech is considered functional but not meaningful. Communication implies an exchange of information regardless of how rudimentary or basic the means.

In order to be reimbursable, documented goals must be not only meaningful and functional, but also time based, and measurable. For example, an individual with expressive aphasia achieves the goal of pointing to pictured objects with 90% accuracy within 1 month of therapy. This may be measurable, functional, and time based; but it is not meaningful. On the other hand, if the client is now able to communicate basic functional needs to caregivers using a language board, then a meaningful and functional goal has been established. When this type of goal is communicated via documentation to Medicare claims reviewers, a positive coverage decision is likely to occur.

Communicating positive meaningful outcomes for FMPs provided under the NOT program can be difficult because the programs are short. Not only must documentation be clear, concise, correct, and consistent, but it also must provide reviewers with sufficient documentation to paint a clear picture of the skilled nature of the service. In addition to the evaluation, timely progress notes are required. The intent of the progress note is to document the progression of the individual throughout the duration of the treatment program, as opposed to necessarily documenting improvement. For documentation to be adequate, for the purposes of FMPs, the rehabilitation professional documents a progress note each time a skilled service is provided. Thus, in addition to documenting time spent with the individual for whom the FMP is being completed, it is important to document all caregiver training and teaching activities, professional consultations, and time spent designing the program. The program itself must be reduced to writing in a formal manner and included as part of the individual's medical record, as well as incorporated into the care plan. This is true for any setting—a nursing facility, a rehabilitation hospital, or within the home and/or community.

To convey the skilled nature of the FMP to third-party payers, it is important to include information specific to each type of program (NOT, Discharge, and Reassessment and Adjustment). Three types of FMP report forms developed by Glickstein and Neustadt (1992) are shown in Figures 16.2, 16.3, and 16.4. The front of each form contains identifying information and other information pertinent to the particular program type. For example, the FMP I (NOT program) form contains language found in the 1981 Medicare guideline intended to establish the skilled nature of the program; the FMP II (Discharge Program) form contains space for documenting functional abilities; and the FMP III (Reassessment and Adjustment) form contains space for identifying the change in functional status necessitating skilled rehabilitation services. The back of each form provides space for writing the program instructions. In all cases, the language of the instructions needs to be simple and easily understood by caregivers. Because the FMP is designed to be used by laypeople with no background in speech–language pathology and minimal reading skills, the rehabilitation professional should refrain from using professional jargon.

For services to be reimbursable, a physician referral is required for FMP I (NOT) and FMP III (Reassessment and Adjustment). A separate physician referral for the FMP II (Discharge) is unnecessary because the Discharge FMP is the natural conclusion of any active treatment program that was initially physician ordered.

Skilled FMPs and Restorative Nursing— A Relationship Model

Thus far, this chapter has focused on the Tri-Model philosophy of rehabilitation and functional maintenance programs for provision of skilled rehabilitation programs provided by rehabilitation professionals.

(Continues on page 374)

FUNCTIONAL MAINTENANCE PROGRAM II (FMP II)
Discharge Summary/Program

P.T. ☐   O.T. ☐   SLP. ☐   DYSPHAGIA ☐

Resident _____ B.D. _____

Medical Diagnosis _____ Onset _____

Rehab. Diagnosis _____ Onset _____

Physician _____ Referral Date _____

Facility _____Therapist _____

Initial Evaluation Date: _____ FMP Date _____ Discharge Date_____

Reason for DC _____

Treatments to Date _____

Functional Abilities at beginning of therapy:

Functional Abilities upon discharge:

In order to maintain current Functional Levels, a functional maintenance program (FMP)
has been designed. It will be monitored periodically as required.

Figure 16.2. FMP discharge form. *Note.* From *Reimbursable Geriatric Service Delivery: A Functional Maintenance Therapy System*, by J. Glickstein and G. Neustadt, 1992, Gaithersburg, MD: Aspen. Copyright 1994 by GNI. Reprinted with permission of GNI.

FUNCTIONAL MAINTENANCE PROGRAM I (FMP I)
No Ongoing Treatment (NOT)

P.T. ☐   O.T. ☐   SLP. ☐   DYSPHAGIA ☐

Resident _____ B.D. _____

Medical Diagnosis _____ Onset _____

Rehab. Diagnosis _____ Onset _____

Physician _____ Referral Date _____

Facility_____Therapist _____

Initial Evaluation Date: _____ FMP Completion Date _____

Based on the results of the Initial Evaluation, it has been determined that

_____ is not an appropriate candidate for an ongoing

treatment program. In order to maximize identified functional abilities, Functional Main-

tenance Therapy was provided. The Functional Maintenance Therapy took

_____ hours to develop and institute and includes the initial evaluation, the

designing of an individualized Functional Maintenance Program (FMP), the inservicing

of staff, and the education/training of the individual and/or family caregivers. The FMP

will be monitored if required on an infrequent basis by the rehabilitation professional.

Figure 16.3. FMP "NOT" form. *Note.* From *Reimbursable Geriatric Service Delivery: A Functional Maintenance Therapy System,* by J. Glickstein and G. Neustadt, 1992, Gaithersburg, MD: Aspen. Copyright 1994 by GNI. Reprinted with permission of GNI.

Attention is now directed to Restorative Nursing, another aspect of care that is related to the Tri-Model system of rehabilitation. Whereas skilled nursing services are provided within the framework of the Tri-Model during the Restorative I (Physiologic) and Restorative II (Compensatory) phases, nursing Restorative III (nursing functional maintenance) does not include any skilled nursing services. As defined in the *Resident Assessment Instrument Training Manual and Resource Guide* (Morris et al., 1991), *restorative nursing* refers to "nursing interventions that assist or promote the resident's ability to attain his or her maximum functional potential." Because restorative nursing

---

FUNCTIONAL MAINTENANCE PROGRAM III (FMP III)
Program Adjustment

O.T. ☐   P.T. ☐   SLP. ☐   DYSPHAGIA ☐

Resident _____ B.D. _____

Medical Diagnosis _____ Onset _____

Rehab. Diagnosis _____ Onset _____

Physician _____ Referral Date _____

Therapist _____ Reeval Date. _____

Prior Date of Service: From: _____ To _____

Last Evaluated on _____ FMP Adj. Completed On _____

Because the previous FMP designed for _____
was no longer effective, a reevaluation and adjustment has been provided. It took ____
hours to develop this FMP and includes the reevaluation, the time spent in revising the
individual Functional Maintenance Program, the inservicing of staff, and the education/
training of the individual and/or family caregivers. The FMP will be monitored if required
on an infrequent basis by the therapist.

---

reason for revision:

_____

functional abilities at time of last FMP:

_____

functional abilities at time of monitor:

_____

functional abilities after FMP adjustment:

Figure 16.4. FMP reassessment and adjustment form. *Note.* From *Reimbursable Geriatric Service Delivery: A Functional Maintenance Therapy System*, by J. Glickstein and G. Neustadt, 1992, Gaithersburg, MD: Aspen. Copyright 1994 by GNI. Reprinted with permission of GNI.

interventions are generally carried out by nonskilled personnel, these services do not meet Medicare guidelines for coverage purposes.

In order for individuals, and particularly residents of nursing facilities, to attain and maintain their highest feasible functional levels, the two aspects of care (rehabilitation therapy and restorative nursing) must operate at a collaborative level. When conflict, competition, and separation exist between these two vital departments, the ability to achieve positive functional outcomes for residents is undermined. Only through open communication, team building, staff stability, and adequate cross-training can collaboration be achieved. The point at which skilled rehabilitation services are discontinued and restorative nursing services commence is a juncture requiring great balance.

Prior to the discontinuation of any skilled service, it is the responsibility of the rehabilitation professional to provide inservice training to caregivers. Training needs to be sufficient to assure the safety of the individual and the effectiveness of the FMP as designed by the rehabilitation professional. It is the responsibility of the caregiver to carry out the program and communicate any changes noted to the rehabilitation professional. Figure 16.5 shows the relationship between the therapy Tri-Model and the nursing Tri-Model. The space between the two aspects of care represents that domain where cross-training from the rehabilitation professionals to caregivers occurs as well as the domain where communication from caregivers back to rehabilitation professionals occurs. Ideally there is a convergence within the domain of functional maintenance. The result of successful convergence is a transdisciplinary team that is involved in cotreatment.

As our current health care system continues to evolve, FMPs will play an increasingly significant role in providing a vehicle for service delivery and achieving positive treatment outcomes in a cost-effective manner. FMP is the bridge between the professional and the layperson. Under current Medicare regulations, FMPs are reimbursed through Part A and Part B. They are physician driven and, under Medicare law, a skilled service. But perhaps the most important aspects of FMPs, when placed in the context of a total rehabilitation system such as the Tri-Model, are the opportunity and challenge they offer the therapist; the opportunity to develop new and innovative programs for persons who would otherwise do without treatment, and the challenge to work as equals with professionals from other disciplines as well as with laypersons.

References

Glickstein, J., & Neustadt, G. (1992). *Reimbursable geriatric service delivery: A functional maintenance therapy system.* Gaithersburg, MD: Aspen.

(Continues on page 378)

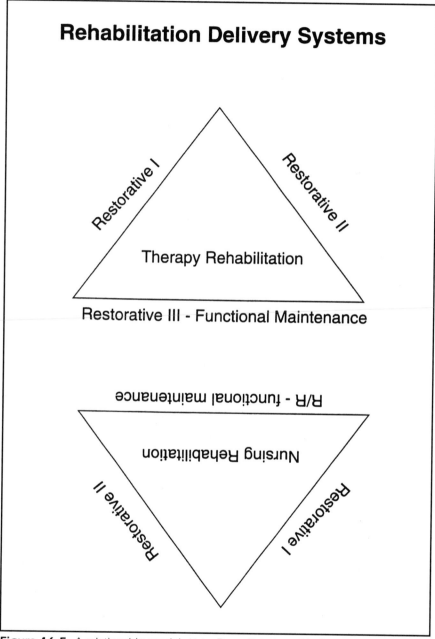

Figure 16.5. A relationship model. *Note.* From *Reimbursable Geriatric Service Delivery: A Functional Maintenance Therapy System,* by J. Glickstein and G. Neustadt, 1992, Gaithersburg, MD: Aspen. Copyright 1994 by GNI. Reprinted with permission of GNI.

Health Care Finance Administration. (1981). *Medical outpatient physical therapy and comprehensive outpatient rehabilitation facilities manual* (Publication 9, Transmittal 46). Washington, DC: Author.

Health Care Financing Administration. (1987). *Medicare skilled nursing facility manual* (Publication 12, Transmittal 262). Washington, DC: Author.

Health Care Financing Administration. (1989a). *Medical review* (Transmittal 3905). Washington, DC: Author.

Health Care Financing Administration. (1989b). *Medicare skilled nursing facility manual* (Publication 12, Transmittal 281). Washington, DC: Author.

Morris, J., Hawes, C., Murphy, K., Nonemaker, S., Phillips, C., Fries, B., & Mor, V. (1991). *Resident assessment instrument training manual and resource guide.* Natick, MA: Eliot Press.

Omnibus Budget Reconciliation Act of 1987. Public Law 100-203.

Social Security Act of 1965. Public Law 89-97.

Chapter 17

Targeting Dysphagia in the Elderly: Prevention, Assessment, and Intervention

Mary Ann Toner

Toner describes the effects of primary, secondary, and tertiary aging on swallowing and eating functions in older adults. A case example is used to illustrate the potential contributions of all of these aspects of aging to swallowing dysfunction in a single client. A variety of assessment approaches are identified, and management considerations are addressed from the particular perspective of the aging population. The need for appropriate inservice and education of caregivers and older adults for home-based and long-term care is discussed.

1. *List the primary, secondary, and tertiary aspects of aging that may affect eating and swallowing behaviors in older adults. For the case example provided in the chapter, identify aspects of the client's situation that fit under each of these categories.*

2. *Identify the different approaches to dysphagia assessment described in the chapter. How is one's choice of assessment approach influenced by aging realities?*

3. *What types of preventive approaches might be appropriate in dealing with eating and swallowing problems related to primary and secondary aging?*

4. *What are some of the practical elements of a successful intervention program for older persons with dysphagia? What types of training may be required to assist family caregivers and health professionals to identify and manage swallowing disorders in the elderly?*

Eating is part of our socialization and reflects our culture. People don't eat only to stay alive or when they are hungry; they eat to celebrate, to mourn, to socialize, and to occupy their time. As a result, swallowing disorders affect not only physical status, but also psychological, social, and cultural status. This may be particularly true for older persons who are trying to maintain their roles and identities while facing the inevitable effects of aging. Unfortunately, it is this age group that is at particular risk for developing dysphagia. Although it would be valuable to know the incidence of feeding and swallowing disorders in the elderly in all settings, estimates are obtained most easily in institutional settings. Reports of the incidence of dysphagia in the elderly indicate that 35% to 59% of nursing home residents experience swallowing difficulty, and 74% exhibit feeding problems (Donner, 1985; Trupe, Siebens, & Siebens, 1984). Cooper and Cobb (1988) reported that 12% to 70% of older adults in institutions demonstrate evidence of malnutrition. Although these statistics suggest that many elderly will experience difficulty swallowing, it should not be concluded that aging is the cause or best indicator of a swallowing problem. In fact, most elderly persons continue to eat without significant difficulty throughout their life span.

To provide appropriate care for the geriatric population, it is important that health care professionals be knowledgeable about the effects of the aging process on swallowing. Because the elderly are more likely to demonstrate a clinically significant swallowing disorder, professionals should be aware of the factors that may influence the effectiveness of standard assessment and remediation procedures. No attempt will be made in this chapter to provide detailed descriptions of assessment and intervention strategies; excellent descriptions are available in numerous other sources (e.g., Cherney, 1994; Groher, 1992; Logemann, 1983). In this chapter, effects of aging on swallowing and nutrition will be reviewed. Potential influences of these factors on assessment and remediation will be discussed, and examples of programs designed to enhance the success of intervention will be provided. A case study describing an older dysphagic patient's progression through the health care system will be presented at the end of each section.

Effects of Aging

Normal aging does have an effect on the swallowing process. A useful framework for considering the effects of aging was suggested by

Granieri (1990), who placed factors that affect the elderly into three categories: primary aging, secondary aging, and tertiary aging. Primary aging factors include those that result from the normal aging process. Secondary aging factors are those that result from a pathological condition. Tertiary aging includes effects of social, psychological, and environmental factors.

Primary Aging

The effects of primary aging on feeding and swallowing behaviors include changes in motor functioning, sensory perceptions, and nutritional requirements. Some of these effects are discussed briefly in other chapters in this text (see Chapter 3 and Chapter 6).

As a result of the aging process, there is a decrease in the strength and tension of the muscles of the lips, tongue, craniomandibular area, and pharynx. These changes may result in slower oral manipulation and transit, extra tongue effort and motion, reduced biting force, and reduced tongue force (Sonies, 1991). Additionally, the elderly are more likely to demonstrate a delayed onset of the pharyngeal swallow, filling the valleculae prior to the onset of laryngeal elevation (Tracy et al., 1989). They also demonstrate stasis in the valleculae and pyriform sinuses after the swallow, without subsequent aspiration or awareness of pharyngeal pooling (Cook et al., 1994; Dejaeger, Pelemans, Bibau, & Ponette, 1994).

Cook et al. (1994) hypothesized that the reduced efficiency of the oropharyngeal swallow may be due to age-related changes in the function of the upper esophageal segment (UES). Dejaeger et al. (1994), using manofluorography, confirmed this hypothesis. They found no significant difference in oral and pharyngeal transit times when UES relaxation was complete; however, incomplete relaxation of the UES was identified in 18% of their elderly subjects (0% in young subjects). That older group also demonstrated reductions in tongue driving force, oral–pharyngeal propulsion, pharyngeal transit time, hypopharyngeal transit time, and velocity of bolus movement. No correlation between the observed increased stasis and presence of incomplete UES relaxation was found. If elderly subjects exhibited stasis in the valleculae and pyriform sinuses, however, they were also more likely to exhibit lower tongue driving force and lower amplitude of pharyngeal contraction. Thus, it appears that oropharyngeal efficiency is affected in some older persons by reduced ability to create both the positive pressure of the oropharyngeal pump using the tongue and the negative pressure of the hypopharyngeal suction pump by opening the UES.

The esophageal stage of the swallow is also affected by muscular changes. Consequently, esophageal peristalsis may be weakened and reflux may be more common. Such changes can result in the elderly person experiencing more frequent "heartburn," but no significant interference with swallowing should be evident.

Sensory changes must also be considered in examining feeding and swallowing in the elderly. As part of the aging process, taste detection and recognition thresholds increase. Older persons are also more likely to have food complaints and experience a "background" taste in the oral cavity; however, these changes may actually be related to unidentified secondary or tertiary aging factors. Because taste perception is a complex process, the exact physiological bases of the age-related changes are not easy to identify. Decreases in the number of taste buds and changes in other senses, particularly olfaction, appear to be major influences on the taste perception changes experienced (Schiffman, 1983).

The elderly demonstrate elevated detection and recognition thresholds for olfactory stimuli. Thus, an odor must be more concentrated before they become aware of it; and they will be less likely to be able to identify the odor. Elevation of olfactory thresholds correlates with changes in the olfactory membranes, changes in the endocrine system, and neurological changes affecting the olfactory nerve and brain (Schiffman, 1983; Sonies, 1991).

Although taste and smell may be the sensory functions most commonly associated with swallowing and nutrition, other sensory perceptions also play an important role. The visual appeal, temperature, consistency, weight, volume, and "sound" of the food can affect overall perception of and preference for the food. In fact, as taste and olfactory functions decline, these additional perceptions may become even more important contributors to the elderly person's enjoyment of food (Toner & Helmer, 1992).

Oropharyngeal sensorimotor changes are not the only factors that should be considered in determining if the patterns an older adult is demonstrating are consistent with primary aging. General physical changes, such as decreased muscle mass, increased total body fat, and decreased basal metabolic rate, affect nutritional requirements (Granieri, 1990). This results in lower caloric requirements for the elderly. A gradual decrease in the amount of food consumed, therefore, may not be an indication of disorder.

It would be convenient if all older persons demonstrated the same changes at predictable times, allowing us to give an exact description of the normal swallowing behaviors of the geriatric population. Unfortunately, this is not the case. Even when researchers find no significant difference in the swallowing patterns shown by young and elderly adults, greater variability within the elderly population is often reported (e.g., Dejaeger et al., 1994). Thus, it is very difficult to predict which patterns will be demonstrated by an individual client. In general, what can be concluded safely about the primary effects of aging on swallowing is that we can expect to see a wider range of normal functioning in the older population than will be seen in the young adult population. Additionally, it appears that, if an elderly person demonstrates one swallowing change, he or she is more likely to demonstrate additional changes. The healthy older adult is able to make appropriate adjustments to changes in functioning. For example, older people often eat more slowly, take smaller bites, use more chewing "strokes," and avoid foods that are hard to manipulate orally (e.g., tough, dry, or sticky foods), hard to digest, or irritating to the esophagus. They may show preferences for foods with stronger tastes or smells, adding more salt or sugar to foods. They may also develop taste/food aversions. All of these changes may occur in the absence of a pathological condition.

Secondary Aging

The elderly are prone to many pathological conditions that cause dysphagia. Etiologies commonly associated with dysphagia in older persons include cerebrovascular accidents (CVA), arthritis, diverticula, hernias, progressive neuromuscular disorders, and dementia. The elderly also experience dysphagia secondary to etiologies that are not linked as strongly with aging, such as head injury, carcinoma, and head and neck surgery. These pathologies may be characterized by numerous motor and sensory difficulties. Older persons who have already experienced some changes in motor and sensory swallowing behaviors and implemented natural adaptations may have more difficulty compensating for any new difficulties. As a result, they often develop problems earlier and demonstrate more severe symptoms than would a younger person.

Swallowing symptoms associated with these common etiologies are well described in several texts (Cherney, 1994; Groher, 1992; Logemann, 1983). Motor impairments often include weakness of the lips, tongue, velum, pharyngeal musculature, and laryngeal musculature. Such motor deficiencies can result in the patient having difficulty removing food from a utensil or cup, keeping liquids in the mouth, chewing adequately or in a coordinated manner, avoiding scattering of the bolus, shaping an adequate bolus, and preventing all or part of the bolus from escaping into the pharynx before the pharyngeal stage of the swallow can be initiated. If the velum is weak, food/liquid may escape into the nose. Weak pharyngeal muscles can result in slow, inadequate clearing of the pharynx. If the laryngeal muscles are weak, airway protection is compromised and aspiration, particularly of liquids, is likely to occur. Fatigue and discomfort during the swallow are also common symptoms associated with poor muscular function.

Sensory impairments can result in many of the same symptoms and often co-occur with motor difficulties. Even if motor functions are intact, patients with tactile deficits can "lose" the bolus in their mouth, making it difficult to perform appropriate oral preparation and transit. Additionally, the bolus may enter the pharynx without pharyngeal or laryngeal response, and perhaps a lack of reaction/cough when the bolus is aspirated. Significant deficits in taste and smell can also occur as a result of several pathologies, reducing the person's appetite and willingness to eat.

Etiologies that affect cognition, such as Alzheimer's disease or traumatic brain injury, may also impair eating and swallowing abilities. Cognitively impaired patients often demonstrate misperception or lack of awareness of food, primitive motor patterns, and distractibility while eating. Their swallow may be characterized by poor bolus preparation, "forgetting" to swallow, and/or loss of the bolus from the oral cavity.

Some elderly people experience difficulty eating, swallowing, and maintaining nutrition in the absence of significant disease or trauma. This group is composed of older people who experience several "minor" health problems that, in combination, decrease resources to a level that makes it difficult to maintain normal functioning. As a result, they are more likely to demonstrate problems related to strength, endurance, and sensitivity. Even relatively minor health problems may significantly reduce the swallowing efficiency and safety of these older people, causing problems that they are unable to adapt to without assistance.

Obviously, these disorders are not exclusive to the elderly; however, some conditions occur so frequently in older adults that they are often thought of as "normal." Two such areas, loss of dentition and reduction of saliva, were introduced in Chapter 6. Although the incidence of tooth loss and other oral–dental conditions is high in the geriatric population, improvements in dental care and treatment techniques allow healthy elderly people to retain their teeth throughout their lives. Lack of dental care, poor diet, illness, and many medications contribute to dental disease and tooth loss. These conditions may be accompanied by oral pain, bad breath, xerostomia (dry mouth), mucositis, temperature sensitivity, and/or altered taste perceptions (Martin & Martin, 1992). As a result, affected older persons may restrict their diet inappropriately, be unable to prepare the bolus adequately, or be reluctant to eat at all.

Similarly, many elderly complain of a dry mouth. Occasionally, this lack of oral moisture is due to the person restricting fluids for reasons unrelated to swallowing ability, for example, those who decrease intake of fluids to avoid urinary frequency. Salivary flow can also be affected by over 300 medications (Winkler, 1989), and the average elderly person takes 13 prescription drugs per year (Nix, 1989). Reduction of saliva can have both motor and sensory implications for the elderly. Food must be mixed with an adequate amount of saliva to allow "spreading" across the taste buds and formation of a cohesive bolus. If the mouth is dry, efficiency of bolus movement through the oral cavity is reduced, and it is more difficult to clear debris. Elderly people who experience xerostomia are at higher risk for developing oral lesions; as a result, they may experience significant pain when eating.

The line between primary and secondary aging effects is not always clear. Sensory changes similar to those experienced in normal aging may be due to chronic disease or the effects of medication (Olsen-Noll & Bosworth, 1989). Declines in the senses of taste and smell have also been identified as a major factor in anorexia in the elderly (Schiffman & Warwick, 1988). The older person who becomes anorexic may experience significant weight loss before he or she is aware of any difficulty. This can also happen as a result of other etiologies, such as degenerative neuromuscular problems, making any rapid or unexpected weight loss a potential indicator of disorder. Thus, discrimination between normal and disordered is often a question of degree; it is essential that the clinician consider a wide variety of etiologies, normal changes, and potential interactions to ensure accurate identification of clinically significant swallowing problems.

Tertiary Aging

Social, psychological, and environmental factors can affect health, appetite, nutrition, and swallowing in any age group. The elderly are no exception. In fact, it has been suggested that older people may eat for social reasons more than physiological need (Olson-Noll & Bosworth, 1989; Weinberg, 1972). Factors that diminish an elderly person's motivation to eat or ability to enjoy socialization during mealtime increase the potential for malnutrition. Conversely, positive mealtime experiences can be used to facilitate other areas of functioning; for example, such activities have even been used to enhance cognitive functioning in the elderly (see Chapter 15 for a discussion of the Breakfast Club). Consequently, tertiary aging factors affecting nutrition and/or swallowing should be considered when one is examining an elderly client and when planning intervention.

The social network of older people is often altered by retirement, death of friends, or loss of mobility. Additionally, death of a spouse or children moving away reduces access to family supports. Financial problems and deteriorating health may force some elderly to move from their homes. It is not surprising, therefore, that some older individuals experience depression. Problems commonly associated with depression that affect eating and swallowing include loss of appetite, rejection of foods, reduction in activity level, agitation, and lack of motivation. Depressed patients may also report that it is difficult to swallow because their throat is tense, swallowing is uncomfortable, or eating makes them tired.

Some elderly cannot afford the kinds of foods needed to maintain adequate nutrition, or they may be physically unable to prepare meals. The environment older persons live in can have a significant effect on eating and swallowing. Dining rooms in retirement communities and long-term care settings may provide a tense, noisy, distracting environment in which the older person feels rushed to eat, making it difficult to enjoy meals and difficult to use adaptations for a safe swallow. Even if the elderly are living in their own home, changes in family structure can leave them alone. If they have no one to eat with or "cook for," they may be unwilling to prepare adequate meals or may not "feel hungry."

It has been theorized that malnutrition can result in dysphagia, increasing risk of aspiration by altering muscle and nerve function (Veldee & Peth, 1992). If left unidentified and untreated, these problems can compound each other—lack of appetite leads to malnutrition, which causes dysphagia, which in turn results in less motivation to eat.

Case Example

Approximately 1 year after retiring from her position as an executive secretary, Mrs. J, a 66-year-old woman, reported feeling unusually tired following her usual daily activities (shopping, housekeeping, golf). She stated that she "felt fine" on some days, but on others, she was "too tired to even eat." She also stated that her hands seemed weak. She was examined by her family doctor, who diagnosed arthritis and anemia. He also suggested the she might still be adjusting to retirement. He prescribed iron supplements and multivitamins. Mrs. J. reported feeling better for approximately 2 months, but then experienced more severe episodes, with particular difficulty chewing. A friend told her about someone who had similar problems that were relieved by getting dentures. Mrs. J. had experienced dental problems for several years, so she consulted her dentist. Although her dentist did not feel it was truly necessary, she had her upper teeth extracted and was fitted with a full upper denture.

This case demonstrates several of the difficulties encountered in attempts to discriminate between primary, secondary, and tertiary aging factors. It would not be unexpected for someone Mrs. J.'s age to tire more easily because of a normal decline in physical endurance. The secondary aging factors (i.e., arthritis, anemia, and dental disease) also appeared to be contributors to her problem. Tertiary factors that may have influenced her condition included the potential social and psychological effects of retirement. It is interesting that, when medical avenues did not relieve her symptoms, she relied on the experience of a friend to determine a course of treatment. Unfortunately, the identified factors were not the actual basis for her difficulties.

Implications for Assessment

Primary, secondary, and tertiary aging factors should be considered when one is assessing an elderly patient's swallowing and nutritional status. Typically, a swallowing evaluation is performed after a patient complains of difficulty swallowing or a health care professional identifies risk factors. Unfortunately, age biases can diminish the effectiveness of this referral system. Older people are at increased risk for many health problems, often experiencing more than one condition at a time. Symptoms of a co-occurring health problem are frequently more prominent than those of the dysphagia; consequently, swallowing problems may be overlooked by health care professionals (Zimmerman & Oder, 1981). Another aspect of the effect of age bias was reported by Chappell-Potter, Poole, and Stephenson (1991), who found that nurses in skilled care facilities were less likely to refer a 90-year-old patient than a 70-year-old patient, although they expected significant improvement in swallowing function following intervention, even if prognostic factors were poor. Additionally, older people themselves may contribute to the problem. For example, they may fail to report dysphagia symptoms if they have adapted to the new difficulties or they may attribute the problems to "just getting old."

Simple screening devices/questionnaires can be used to reduce the potential of such biases interfering with early identification of swallowing or nutritional problems. These information-gathering procedures serve two functions. First, they provide a means of identifying the at-risk elderly. Second, they increase public and professional awareness of the significance of swallowing, eating, and nutritional changes. Fishman (1994) suggested use of a nutritional screening instrument that can be self-administered by the elderly person. In addition to examining dietary habits, that protocol obtains information about general health, physical disabilities, dental problems, and social and financial issues that might affect eating (Greer, Margolis, Mitchell, Grunwald, & Associates, Inc., 1993). Other screening tools address swallowing behaviors more directly. A sample protocol is shown in Table 17.1. This questionnaire was administered as part of a larger speech-language-hearing screening program (Scheib, LeMay, & Toner, 1990). Referrals for medical evaluation and additional swallowing assessment were made if the person reported significant eating/swallowing difficulties, a sudden onset of a problem, or unexpected weight loss.

An essential part of any swallowing evaluation is a thorough case history. In addition to information provided by the elderly patient, it may be not only beneficial but also necessary to obtain input from additional informants. If an older person is suffering from a dementia-causing disorder, the primary caregiver must be relied upon to provide eating, swallowing, and nutritional information. Even when the elderly patient is not cognitively impaired, spouses, family members, and caregivers may be aware of subtle or gradual changes not observed by the patient. In a nursing home setting, several caregivers

Table 17.1

Eating/Swallowing Questionnaire

Y	N	Do you experience any difficulty eating or swallowing?
Y	N	Have you experienced significant weight loss recently?
Y	N	Do you have trouble with food "going the wrong way?"
Y	N	Do you need to clear your throat frequently?
Y	N	Does food enter your nose frequently while you are eating?
Y	N	Do you have difficulty keeping some foods or liquids in your mouth?
Y	N	Does food stick in your mouth even after several swallows?
Y	N	Do you experience any pain, soreness, or numbness in your mouth?
Y	N	Do you have difficulty chewing?
Y	N	Do you have dentures?
Y	N	Do you experience frequent heartburn?
Y	N	Do you experience pain or discomfort in the neck, chest, or stomach after eating?
Y	N	Does your mouth feel dry often?
Y	N	Does your saliva feel thick?
Y	N	Have you noticed a change in the way foods taste?

Circle any foods that you have difficulty chewing or swallowing or that you avoid eating.

Thin liquids (water, coffee)	Stringy foods (celery)	Meats
Soft, thick foods (puddings)	Sticky foods (peanut butter)	Pills
Dry, crumbly foods (toast, cookies)	Others _____	

Are there any medical conditions for which you are receiving treatment? If so, what?

_____

What medications are you taking currently?—_____

_____

_____

_____

can provide valuable information. For example, nurses are often able to report medical and nutritional status changes, while aides may be in a better position to report changes in eating patterns and difficulties experienced during actual meals.

The ideal method for assessing swallowing in the elderly would be one that allows visualization of all portions of the swallow using unaltered foods, with no limit on time or number of swallows examined. It could be performed in any environment any number of times, would not affect the patient's typical swallowing pattern, and would be cost-effective. No single assessment technique meets all of those requirements; therefore, two or more different strategies may be required to obtain a complete and accurate description of the person's swallowing problem.

Most evaluations begin with a clinical assessment. The results of this examination are often used as a basis for determining candidacy for other forms of assessment. It may include brief assessments of cognitive status and language abilities to determine the patient's ability to cooperate and follow instructions. Before foods are presented, motor and sensory functions are assessed. Usually, the person is observed while swallowing a variety of foods. The oral and pharyngeal stages of the swallow are observed by feeling and watching oral and laryngeal movements during the swallow and visual inspection of the oral cavity after the swallow. Effects of different food consistencies, temperatures, and weights, as well as bolus size, can be assessed in this way. Because several "swallows" can be assessed, indications of "warm-up" and/or fatigue may be observed. Although this assessment can be performed in any setting using unaltered foods, it still constitutes an artificial situation that may cause patients to alter their typical swallowing patterns. Additionally, if the patient does not cough after the swallow or demonstrate other obvious signs of aspiration, the clinician's conclusions regarding presence/absence of aspiration are necessarily limited. This is a primary reason why a clinical examination is not considered sufficient in most cases.

Videofluorography allows the clinician to view all stages of swallowing. Although it is often referred to as the "gold standard" for assessment techniques, it does have some disadvantages for use with the geriatric population. Obviously, this procedure cannot be performed in all settings, continued indefinitely, or repeated any number of times.

An assessment technique that allows more frequent observation and assessment in a wider variety of settings is fiberoptic endoscopic evaluation of swallowing (FEES). FEES allows visualization of the pharyngeal portion of the swallow and provides a video recording that allows comparisons for long-term monitoring. The introduction of the endoscope may affect the "naturalness" of the patient's swallow, and it may be difficult to perform FEES with a confused or agitated patient. Advantages and disadvantages of FEES are still being examined (Kidder, Langmore, & Martin, 1994), but it appears to hold great promise as a dysphagia assessment tool.

A procedure that is often not included as part of a formal assessment is observation of a meal. This provides assessment in the most natural eating setting and allows observation of adaptations the patient has made (good or bad), food preferences, reactions to the environment, and changes across time (e.g., breakfast vs. dinner; beginning of meal vs. end of meal). Clinicians often obtain information about mealtime behaviors during the interview; however, actual observation may reveal details that either were not addressed by the clinician's questions or that the patient did not identify during the interview.

Because the elderly often have complex swallowing problems, a combination of these strategies would be optimal. Zenner, Losinski, and Mills (1995) reported that the performance of their elderly, confused patients was often affected by the structure and environment of a videofluoroscopic swallowing study, with some performing more poorly than usual and some showing better than usual swallowing. As a result, assessment relied on clinical examination alone. They recommended that in such cases, accuracy of the clinical examination can be enhanced if it is supplemented with cervical auscultation, suggesting that this combination provides a means of assessing clients in more natural settings and allows frequent monitoring of status.

Choice of assessment strategies is often dictated by setting. Obviously, the patient must be in a health care facility to perform videofluoroscopy. FEES may be performed in a wider range of settings; however, for many nursing home residents and home care patients, clinical examination, cervical auscultation, and observation of meals are the only strategies available or feasible.

Case Example

Mrs. J. continued to experience fatigue and difficulty eating. She also experienced significant weight loss. She attended a health fair and obtained information about nutritional needs of the elderly and warning signs of nutritional and swallowing problems. Mrs. J. took this information to her family physician, who referred her to a neurologist. Seven months after her concerns were initially reported to her physician, Mrs. J. was diagnosed with amyotrophic lateral sclerosis (ALS). (Interestingly, at a later date, she needed medication for an infection when her usual physician was gone. She contacted another local physician and advised him of her health status. Without ever seeing her, he informed her that she was "too old to have ALS.")

Mrs. J. was referred to a speech–language pathologist (SLP) for a swallowing evaluation. She was accompanied by her husband. Mrs. J. reported difficulty chewing meats but identified no other specific food or swallowing problems. She attributed much of her fatigue while eating to the energy required to cut the food into bite-sized pieces and sit up throughout the meal. Although she admitted losing weight, she associated this more with her medical condition than with her difficulty eating. Her husband identified several additional problems. Mr. J. reported that his wife had reduced her fluid intake. He also felt that she ate more rapidly and took bigger bites, perhaps trying to finish her meal before she fatigued. Finally, he observed that she "choked" or coughed frequently while eating the evening meal.

During clinical examination and videofluoroscopy, Mrs. J. demonstrated no apparent difficulty with any substances, but was judged to swallow very deliberately. Her husband identified this pattern as typical for early meals, but not for later meals. Following this, the clinician went to Mrs. J.'s home to observe her at lunch and dinner. During dinner, Mrs. J. demonstrated slow oral preparation. As the meal progressed, swallows began to appear more effortful and she coughed after several bites. A severe coughing episode was observed when she sipped water.

Intervention

In designing a program of intervention, the clinician must balance physical/medical needs with quality-of-life issues. Strategies recommended must not only be acceptable to the patient or caregiver, but must also be feasible for long-term implementation. For example, if patients initially agree to make broad changes in their eating/swallowing habits, but later find that many areas of their life have been affected, they may decide that continued strict adherence to the initial recommendations "just isn't worth it." Clinicians should try to avoid this problem when planning intervention, but the possibility should be discussed with patients and family members. If the problem arises, the clinician should be prepared to make adjustments in the intervention plan.

Prevention may be the ideal goal of any intervention program. Diminishing the risk for development of the targeted problem is obviously a basic preventative measure; however, current research has not provided a way to stop the effects of aging on the swallowing mechanism. Thus, prevention of dysphagia in the geriatric population may be limited to minimizing the severity of symptoms and preventing unnecessary medical complications through early identification and intervention. To accomplish these objectives, public and professional awareness needs to be enhanced, and early intervention services must become more widespread. For example, health care professionals would need to assess the swallowing and nutritional status of all elderly patients, with periodic monitoring for changes. If older people became more aware of swallowing and nutritional risk factors, they might be more cautious when they experienced any illness, perhaps choosing their foods carefully and being sure to maintain adequate nutrition. Unfortunately, these are still ambitious goals. At the present time, most of our efforts in dysphagia intervention continue to be more reactive than proactive.

The effects of some of the secondary aspects of aging may be addressed with relatively simple strategies that inhibit development of further problems. For example, Martin and Martin (1992) described several strategies that reduce the negative impact of poor oral conditions on chewing and swallowing. Obviously, regular dental care can help a patient who experiences difficulty chewing resulting from loose or painful teeth. For some older people, pain is eliminated by avoiding extreme temperatures and sweets. To reduce problems related to xerostomia, Martin and Martin suggested that elderly people drink sugar-free carbonated beverages and avoid caffeine, tobacco, alcohol, and spicy foods.

Quality of life can be affected unnecessarily if clinicians are "too safe" in their recommendations or do not reevaluate long-term patients periodically to determine if all recommendations are still appropriate. For example, clinicians may make recommendations to alter diet unnecessarily or be slow to change unnecessary recommendations based on inappropriate assumptions regarding an older person's abilities or conclusions that an older person will not improve. Groher and McKaig (1995) found that a mechanically altered diet was recommended for 31% of a group of older patients (mean age 72.9 years). In that group, 91% of the patients were assigned a diet below the level they could tolerate, 4% were above the level they could tolerate, and only 5% were at the appropriate level.

When a swallowing disorder is identified, successful intervention starts during the assessment process. Allowing family/caregivers to observe as much of the evaluation as possible and including them in the discussion of the results promotes their understanding of the problem and their acceptance of the dysphagia team's recommendations. Family members may also provide valuable input that will help the swallowing team modify recommendations to fit the individual patient's needs and preferences. When recommendations for intervention are made, several areas must be considered to facilitate successful implementation, including food preparation, menu planning, preparation of the patient for eating, swallowing strategies, and after-meal care. The social/psychological effects of each recommendation must be considered. In fact, the emotional response of the patient and family may be the most important determiner of success. The need for alternate feeding methods must also be addressed in many cases. Finally, long-term success of any intervention plan is largely dependent on the ability of the patient and primary caregiver to carry out appropriate recommendations. This requires effective training and inservicing techniques.

Although dysphagia intervention strategies do not differ significantly for young versus elderly adults, it may be necessary to make appropriate accommodations for the effects of aging. As previously stated, the following discussion will not provide an in-depth presentation of remediation techniques. Instead, those areas that are likely to be affected by the distinctive aspects of aging will be discussed. Much of the following discussion is oriented toward settings in which clinicians are likely to provide services to the geriatric population (e.g., hospitals and long-term care facilities). With slight modifications, however, the recommendations presented can apply to any setting.

Meal Planning and Preparation

Often an elderly dysphagic patient cannot maintain adequate nutrition and swallowing efficiency in the standard three meals a day. Several small meals and snacks may be required, making meal planning and preparation more time and energy consuming. Daily menus must include the necessary nutrients as well as the necessary number of calories. Foods selected must have the characteristics that will facilitate a safe swallow, plus account for the patient's preferences. Clinicians must be careful not to avoid this complex issue by simply telling patients/caregivers what the patient should not eat. Instead, they should provide lists of foods that can be eaten, with specific instructions regarding how foods can be prepared to be safe yet appealing. It is in this area that the dietitian is invaluable.

During preparation of the foods, the patient's taste perceptions and preferences must be considered. In addition to age-related declines in taste and smell, the elderly patient often experiences additional changes caused by the swallowing disorder. Flavor enhancement is recommended to counteract these declines, but it is important that enhancements do not exacerbate existing health conditions. For example, the patient may prefer higher concentrations of sweet or salt, but addition of these elements would not be appropriate for diabetic patients or patients who require a low-sodium diet. Method of preparation can also affect the flavor of foods. Hotaling (1992) recommended preparation of pureed foods using a food processor instead of a blender, eliminating the need to "water down" the food, thereby preserving flavor and nutrient density. Older patients may also react negatively to recommended changes in liquid consistency. Even the normal elderly have been found to report a significant decrease in preference for thickened liquids and often perceive thickened liquids as "bitter" (Toner & Helmer, 1992). The temperature at which food is served is also an important consideration. Frequently, it is recommended that foods be served at certain temperatures to facilitate swallowing responses or to allow for a patient's temperature intolerance. Such factors may prohibit serving some foods at the temperature the patient preferred prior to becoming dysphagic; but every attempt should be made to provide the patient with foods at a temperature that enhances flavor and that the patient finds acceptable. Because so many elements affect perception of the taste of the recommended foods, enhancement of "other sensations," such as the smell and visual appearance, may be essential to its acceptability.

Hotaling (1992) suggested that foods may be more acceptable if menus are planned that can be served to all, with the texture or consistency varying appropriately for different patient needs. Although this recommendation was directed toward long-term care facilities, it also has valuable implications for home care patients. Primary caregivers often feel that they have to prepare special meals for the dysphagic patient. This doubles (at least) the time and energy required for this activity. Family members may also feel uncomfortable eating together when one member is unable to eat the same foods. If caregivers are provided with menu and preparation ideas that allow them to serve the same basic foods to everyone, the patient and the family are more likely to enjoy meals.

Patient Preparation

Before the patients are served a meal, it is important that they "have all of their senses." The older patient may wear a hearing aid, glasses, and dentures. Each of these should be functioning well and in place before mealtime. If xerostomia is a factor, artificial saliva may be required. Dry mouth and "background taste" may also be reduced by oral cleaning prior to eating.

For some elderly patients, time must be allotted to allow them to "wake up" and become alert before eating. Caregivers often find that meals are interrupted because eating stimulates a bowel movement in the patient. For some, this may be solved by planning a regular bathroom trip a sufficient period of time before serving the meal. Other patients seem to need the stimulation of the food and respond better if a time is set aside for a small snack followed by a scheduled bathroom time.

Mealtime/Eating Strategies

The environment in which the person eats may determine the success of all other strategies. If patients cannot tolerate visual and auditory distractions, it may be necessary for them to eat in a quiet room, with one other person or alone if they do not require assistance or monitoring. In contrast, some elderly persons are not motivated to eat meals without the social aspects of eating; and some cognitively impaired patients may need the situational cues of other people eating to demonstrate appropriate eating/swallowing behaviors. For example, one elderly nursing home patient responded to food only when his wife was present and encouraging him to eat or when he was placed in the dining room with other patients. In those cases, he required monitoring to control impulsivity but swallowed foods safely.

When patients are in the appropriate environment, it may be necessary to position them for eating. This may require supporting them in an upright position or slanting their upper bodies in an appropriate direction. For some elderly, limited mobility, arthritis, and lack of endurance can make body positioning and maintenance of a position difficult. Positioning of the patient's head during the swallow must also be considered, with some positions being difficult or uncomfortable for an older person with limited flexibility.

Many patients require some level of assistance in feeding. Patients with cognitive impairments may need reminders before and during each swallow. Some patients require assistance putting the food in their mouth plus reminders to chew and swallow, whereas others need only visual reminders of necessary swallowing strategies, such as feeding cards that contain simple pictures or instructions. In long-term care facilities, providing assistance at meals can be complex and frustrating. Aides often feed several patients at one time. If the patients differ in the degree or type of assistance required, it is difficult for aides to provide appropriate assistance to each. Additionally, the patients may be distracted by each other or disrupt the meal with inappropriate behaviors. Some of these problems can be controlled by reducing the number of patients in each feeding group, grouping patients with similar needs, and keeping the room as calm as possible. It is also helpful if the aide is provided with a clearly visible feeding card for each patient. Reminder cards also facilitate a smooth transition when aides assume feeding responsibilities for a new patient or when new aides are hired. In a home setting, reminder cards can be used to facilitate a the transfer from hospital to home and can assist a patient in habituating a new swallowing pattern.

After-Meal Care

Following a meal, older patients' teeth (or dental appliance) and tongue should be thoroughly cleaned. If their mobility is limited, they might also appreciate assistance in washing their face and hands and being helped to the bathroom. To reduce the risk of reflux, many elderly must maintain an upright position following a meal. For individuals in wheelchairs, this may result in sleeping in uncomfortable, awkward positions following a meal. If eating fatigues them, they may return to bed if the head of the bed can be elevated adequately and they can be supported in that position.

Tube Feeding

When a patient cannot maintain adequate nutrition through oral feeding or demonstrates significant aspiration that cannot be controlled through facilitation strategies or diet recommendations, it may be necessary to implement an alternative feeding method. Ciocon (1990) stated that a nasogastric tube may be the preferred option if a feeding tube is needed to maintain nutrition for only a short period, such as when a patient is acutely ill or when a malnourished patient is being prepared for surgery. If a feeding tube will be required for 4 weeks or longer, Ciocon found that gastric tubes or jejunostomy tubes are preferred. In addition to severe dysphagia, Ciocon listed protein-calorie malnutrition with inadequate oral intake for 5 days or normal nutritional status with less than 50% of required nutritional intake for 7 to 10 days as indications for tube feeding.

Although the need for and potential benefits of alternative feeding methods often seem apparent to the professional, many older people are reluctant to agree to this recommendation. This recommendation is often made at a time when the patient and the family are under significant stress, resulting in difficulty thinking clearly and understanding information they are given. In some cases, the patient may be cognitively unable to make a competent decision. Under the best of circumstances, older patients and their families may have many misconceptions about feeding tubes and their implications. It should be established that feeding tubes are not recommended only to extend life; in fact, some studies indicate that they do not have this effect for many patients (Krynski, Tymchuk, & Ouslander, 1994). However, feeding tubes can help relieve many of the discomforts and complications caused by disease. Krynski et al. found that long-term care residents and community-dwelling elderly people seem to have little information about tube feeding. After they participated in an educational program that provided them with simple, pictured explanations of tube feeding, including advantages and complications, their knowledge was found to increase significantly. These authors stated that such education encourages elderly couples to discuss their feelings about feeding tubes before one is needed. This helps a spouse determine what the patient would want if he or she is ever forced to make that decision.

If the patient rejects a feeding tube recommendation, the dysphagia team must decide whether or not to provide further intervention.

A similar decision must be made when it is recommended that the patient receive nothing by mouth (npo status). The patient may agree to a feeding tube but refuse to stop eating orally. In these cases, the health care professionals must decide whether or not further intervention should be provided to help the person swallow as safely and comfortably as possible for the rest of his or her life. There is no clear standard in determining the answer to this ethical question. Regardless of the clinician's decision, it is essential for the clinician to document recommendations and the patient's wishes. Krynski et al. (1994) indicated that such decisions may become even more important as larger portions of the population survive into old age and suffer cognitive and functional disabilities.

Training and Inservice Models

Caregivers are an essential component of a dysphagia intervention program and, as such, they need to receive adequate instruction and support for successful performance of their role. Training needs differ depending on the type of setting, the prior experience/training of the caregiver, and the patient care responsibilities. Very different challenges are presented by patients who remain in their home with an elderly spouse as the primary caregiver versus those who are placed in a long-term care facility with multiple caregivers. Following is a discussion of two models of caregiver training, one designed primarily for home care patients and the other for long-term care settings. Many of the components of these models were based on caregivers' responses to questionnaires regarding their perception of obstacles to providing long-term care for a dysphagic patient (Toner, 1992). A summary of the problems identified by each group of caregivers is presented in Table 17.2.

Home-Based Care. Chapter 10 presents a discussion of many of the issues that confront caregivers in the home and describes model training programs designed to meet caregiver needs. In the area of dysphagia, caregiver training often begins during the assessment phase. In this training model, the family caregivers are included in the diagnostic procedures and the intervention planning. While the patient is in acute care, the caregiver can observe intervention strategies and discuss menu planning. Gradually, the caregiver assumes some of the

Table 17.2

Obstacles to Long-Term Dysphagia Intervention:
Perceptions of Professionals and Caregivers

Obstacles Identified by Family Caregivers:

- Time and energy required for all care requirements
- Food restrictions without provision of adequate recommendations for appropriate foods
- Patient rejection of recommended foods/liquids
- Loss of social aspects and enjoyment of mealtime
- Change in relationship with patient
- Lack of personal and professional support

Obstacles Identified by Nursing Home Personnel:

- Lack of consistency of care due to inadequate training personnel turnover
- Large number of patients resulting in difficulty implementing individual plans
- Scheduling difficulties
- Nature of patients (lack of cooperation and appreciation)
- Nature of feeding area
- Lack of professional support, lack of availability of experts for consultation
- Interference from patients' families

Obstacles Identified by Home Health Professionals:

- Lack of family/patient consistency in following recommendations
- Inappropriate patient/family response to improvement
- Patient self-medication
- Family reactions of anger, fear, helplessness

---

responsibilities of care under the observation of a team member. If the patient is moved to the hospital's extended care unit, which provides a more home-like environment, the caregiver can practice assisting the patient while trying to maintain a relatively normal mealtime interaction. During the time the patient is in the hospital, the caregiver is provided with menu suggestions and preparation instructions and is helped in planning schedules and checklists for patient care. The caregiver is also provided with information about local resources, such as home health providers, support groups, and medical supply stores. Before the patient is discharged, a member of the team visits the home to help identify potential problem areas or needs, such as a bed that allows elevation of the head, a chair that allows positioning, or a supply of tube-feeding formula. On the day of discharge, a team member may make another home visit to help the caregiver and patient make a smooth transition. If a home health agency will be providing assistance, one of the agency's caregivers is invited to visit the patient and caregiver in the hospital and review the intervention plan. If possible, the home health professional makes the home visit on the day of discharge.

Following discharge, the status of the patient is monitored on a regular basis, and problems are discussed with the patient and caregiver. One problem that arises frequently when an elderly spouse is the primary caregiver is a decline in the spouse's health and nutritional status. The spouse's energies are directed so much toward the patient that he or she neglects his or her own needs. Occasionally, the solution to the problem is as simple as ordering "meals-on-wheels" to provide the spouse with a meal that he or she doesn't need to prepare. If possible, "fast food" or restaurant foods that a patient can eat should be suggested. Spouses are also encouraged to seek help from family and friends, who could cook extra quantities when they fix meals and bring leftovers for the patient and spouse. Spouses may also be helped to find respite care so that they can have some time for themselves each week.

Long-Term Care Inservice Training. Results of a survey of caregiver knowledge of dysphagia identification and intervention suggest that traditional inservice training has not been effective in the long-term care setting (Bessler & Toner, 1990). As a follow-up to that research, nursing home personnel, including nurses, aides and dietitians, and speech–language pathologists who had provided dysphagia inservice training in nursing homes, were asked to identify factors that influence effectiveness of inservice training. On the basis of those responses, it was determined that effective inservice presentation should include provisions for variations in employees' academic training, patient contact responsibilities, and experience. A need for accommodation to time limitations and frequent turnover in personnel was also identified. Finally, the caregivers felt a need for information oriented toward treating large numbers of patients instead of individual patient needs. These concerns were addressed with a four-component training model (Toner & Bessler, 1991).

The first component of the model is needs assessment. Prior to training sessions, all caregivers complete a questionnaire that identifies their previous training/experience and their patient care responsibilities. Using this information, employees are grouped according to the types of information that will best supplement their prior training and will be most relevant to their present responsibilities.

The second component is information presentation. Using the groups identified in the needs assessment, participants are asked to attend 1-hour inservice sessions that are relevant to their needs. Each session addresses a major content area, such as patient preparation, feeding strategies, group feeding, meal preparation, or monitoring patient status. Information presentation is coordinated with techniques to enhance audience involvement. These procedures include simulating swallowing dysfunctions (swallowing while lying down or holding something under the tongue), hands-on training with current patients, presentation of case studies, videotapes, and use of feeding/diet reminder cards. Written information summaries are provided as well as checklists for patient identification, referral, and follow-up. As part of this component, special sessions are conducted for family members to help them understand the rationale for the procedures used by the caregivers and to provide suggestions for ways family members might facilitate care.

A third component of the program involves techniques to provide continuing training. Videotapes of specific swallowing problems and patients or patient groups are used to provide ongoing training. Self-study and reference materials are also furnished. Initially, these materials were also intended to serve as a means of training new employees.

The final component involves assessment of training effectiveness. Various forms of knowledge evaluation have been attempted, with participant examination of case histories and observation of skill application being identified as the most beneficial. Both participants and presenters judged an objective, knowledge-based assessment instrument to be the least effective means of evaluating training effectiveness.

When asked to evaluate the training model, participants reported that differential grouping encouraged interaction and participation.

Information presented was judged to be appropriate to group needs, with particular benefit attributed to participant involvement techniques, family training sessions, and reminder cards. Although the videotapes provided for continuing training were considered helpful, they were not considered adequate for training new personnel. It was felt that contact with training personnel and group interaction facilitated understanding and carryover of the information.

This model was designed to address the specific needs of long-term care facilities, but its components can also be adapted for use in other settings. Subacute and acute care settings often require similar staff training. The training and reference materials can be used to assist home-based patients and their families. Presentation of similar information to various support groups might be particularly beneficial in promoting understanding of swallowing problems and acceptance of the recommended remediation procedures.

Case Example

After evaluation, it was recommended that Mrs. J. be given a feeding tube to allow her to maintain nutrition and hydration. She was concerned that this would limit her mobility, until it was explained that a feeding tube did not require being "hooked up" to a machine. It was also explained that, if she did not maintain adequate nutrition, her physical abilities would actually deteriorate more rapidly and she would lose her independence sooner. Mrs. J. was informed that a feeding tube would not prohibit eating orally, but dietary and swallowing strategies would be needed to help her swallow more easily and safely.

Mr. J. and the couple's adult daughter were shown how to perform tube feedings and care for the feeding tube. They were also shown how to perform the Heimlich maneuver. They were provided with information regarding types of tube feeding formulae and stores at which it was available. Before Mrs. J. left the hospital, her family had assumed responsibility for her tube feedings. Mrs. J. did not require assistance with oral feeding at that time, but was provided with reminder cards that illustrated recommended swallowing strategies. The family was provided with a list of symptoms that would indicate advancement of her condition and a need for further alteration of her diet/swallowing plan.

Mrs. J. reported difficulty adhering to a recommendation to avoid thin liquids, stating that thickened liquids tasted bitter. The clinician presented several common fluids at thickened consistencies, adding sweetener to some. Mrs. J. identified the fluids she found acceptable, primarily sweet or salty samples. She used those fluids to keep her mouth moist and relied on the feeding tube for hydration. Mrs. J.'s physical status remained fairly constant for several months, and she followed swallowing and diet recommendations with no complications. When her condition progressed, she began to aspirate her secretions and experience difficulty with all foods. She was advised that continuing to eat orally would affect her health status. Mrs. J. chose to continue to eat orally. Her family was shown how to suction, and additional dietary and swallowing recommendations were made. Mrs. J. did not adhere closely to the diet recommendations. She began to eat only one meal each day, usually requesting something from a fast food franchise that provided high olfactory and visual stimulation (e.g., mashed potatoes and gravy from Kentucky Fried Chicken). At that point, Mr. J. began to demonstrate weight loss, so the daughter began to bring meals that he could eat alone or that could easily be modified to feed his wife and himself. The daughter also stayed with her parents on most weekends to relieve Mr. J. of his caregiver responsibilities. A hospice organization was contacted, and an aide was assigned to help with daily care of Mrs. J. Mrs. J. contracted pneumonia but refused to be hospitalized. She recovered, but experienced another episode within a month. She suffered respiratory failure and died in her home.

Conclusions

Mrs. J. illustrates many of the issues encountered when one is dealing with the dysphagic elderly. First, health care professionals must be careful not to assume that changes in eating and swallowing are age related. Healthy older people may experience subtle changes but rarely report significant swallowing difficulty. An increase in public awareness programs would help older persons realize when they are experiencing a problem. If an elderly person expresses concern, a careful examination should be done to identify the basis of that complaint to ensure that symptoms of a disorder are not overlooked. To identify swallowing problems in the elderly, a combination of available procedures may be necessary. The cognitive and physical status of the geriatric patient should be considered in selecting assessment methods, and the family's input should be solicited. The special needs and desires of the older patient and older caregiver must also be considered in planning intervention. The effects of dysphagia are not limited to the changes in the patient's eating behaviors. Changes in the patient's (and family caregiver's) life-style, social interaction, psychological adjustment, and self-esteem are also common. Appropriate preparation and training of caregivers can relieve some of the problems that patients and caregivers will encounter.

In the end, health care professionals can only make recommendations. The final decisions must be made by patients and their families.

Throughout the process, the health care professional should try to ensure that patients and families have all of the information they need to make informed decisions. If the patient rejects one or all of the recommendations made by the dysphagia team, health care professionals may either remove themselves from the case or support the patient's choices by providing any help the patient will accept. Hopefully, before making that decision, each professional will weigh quantity-of-life issues against quality-of-life issues. For many elderly people, quality will be more important.

References

Bessler, C. D., & Toner, M.A. (1990). Nursing home personnel's awareness of dysphagia issues. *Rocky Mountain Journal of Communication Disorders, 7,* 29–32.

Chappell-Potter, R., Poole, M., & Stephenson, G. K. (1991, November). *Dysphagia management of the elderly: How nurses view our role and why it's important.* Paper presented at the annual meeting of the American Speech-Language-Hearing Association, Atlanta.

Cherney, L. R. (Ed.). (1994). *Clinical management of dysphagia in adults and children* (2nd ed.). Gaithersburg, MD: Aspen.

Ciocon, J. O. (1990). Indications for tube feedings in elderly patients. *Dysphagia, 5,* 1–5.

Cook, I. J., Weltman, M. D., Wallace, K., Shaw, D. W., McKay, E., Smart, R. C., & Butler, S. P. (1994). Influence of aging on oral–pharyngeal bolus transit and clearance during swallowing: Scintigraphic study. *American Journal of Physiology, 266,* 972–977.

Cooper, J. W., & Cobb, H. H. (1988). Patient nutritional correlates and changes in a geriatric nursing home. *Nutritional Support Services, 8,* 5–7.

Dejaeger, F., Pelemans, W., Bibau, G., & Ponette, F. (1994). Manufluorographic analysis of swallowing in the elderly. *Dysphagia, 9,* 156–161.

Donner, M. (1985). Editorial. *Gastrointestinal Radiology, 10,* 194–195.

Fishman, P. (1994). Detecting malnutrition's warning signs with simple screening tools. *Geriatrics, 49,* 39–45.

Granieri, E. (1990). Nutrition and the older adult. *Dysphagia, 4,* 196–201.

Greer, Margolis, Mitchell, Grunwald, & Associates, Inc. (1993). *Nutrition screening initiative: Nutrition interventions manual for professionals caring for older Americans.* Washington, DC: Author.

Groher, M. E. (1992). *Dysphagia: Diagnosis and management* (2nd ed.). Stoneham, MA: Butterworths.

Groher, M. E., & McKaig, T. N. (1995). Dysphagia and dietary levels in skilled nursing facilities (Abstract). *Dysphagia, 10,* 62.

Hotaling, D. L. (1992). Nutritional considerations for the pureed diet texture in dysphagic elderly. *Dysphagia, 7,* 81–85.

Kidder, T. M., Langmore, S. E., & Martin, B. J. W. (1994). Indications and techniques of endoscopy in evaluation of cervical dysphagia: Comparison with radiographic techniques. *Dysphagia, 9,* 256–261.

Krynski, M. D., Tymchuk, A. J., & Ouslander, J. G. (1994). How informed can consent be? New light on comprehension among elderly people making decisions about enteral tube feeding. *The Gerontologist, 34,* 36–43.

Logemann, J. L. (1983). *Evaluation and treatment of swallowing disorders.* San Diego: College-Hill Press.

Martin, K. U., & Martin, J. O. (1992). Meeting the oral health needs of institutionalized elderly. *Dysphagia, 7,* 73–80.

Nix, R. J. (1989, February). Polypharmacy: Drug-induced illness in the elderly. *Focus on Geriatric Care and Rehabilitation, 2,* 1–2.

Olsen-Noll, C., & Bosworth, M. (1989). Anorexia and weight loss in the elderly. *Postgraduate Medicine, 85,* 140–144.

Scheib, R., LeMay, A., & Toner, M. A. (1990, November). *Screening communication abilities of the elderly.* Paper presented at the annual meeting of the American Speech-Language-Hearing Association, Seattle.

Schiffmann, S. S. (1983). Taste and smell in disease. *The New England Journal of Medicine, 308,* 1275–1343.

Schiffman, S. S., & Warwick, Z. S. (1988). Flavor enhancement of foods for the elderly can reverse anorexia. *Neurobiology of Aging, 9,* 24–26.

Sonies, B. C. (1991). The aging oropharyngeal system. In D. N. Ripich (Ed.), *Handbook of geriatric communication disorders* (pp. 187–203). Austin, TX: PRO-ED.

Toner, M. A. (1992). *Swallowing disorders in the elderly.* Paper presented at the Nutrition and Aging III: Rehabilitation, Little Rock.

Toner, M. A., & Bessler, C. D. (1991, November). *Dysphagia inservice model for nursing home personnel.* Paper presented at the annual meeting of the American Speech-Language-Hearing Association, Atlanta.

Toner, M. A., & Helmer, D. (1992, November). *Effect of fluid consistency on taste perception and preference.* Paper presented at the annual meeting of the American Speech-Language-Hearing Association, San Antonio, TX.

Tracy, J. F., Logemann, J. A., Kahrilas, P. J., Jacob, P., Kobara, M., & Krugler, C. (1989). Preliminary observations on the effects of age on oropharyngeal deglutition. *Dysphagia, 4,* 90–94.

Trupe, E. H., Siebens, H., & Siebens, A. (1984). *Prevalence of feeding and swallowing disorders in a nursing home.* Paper presented at the Third National Leadership Conference on Long Term Case Issues: Future World of Long Term Care, Washington, DC.

Veldee, M. S., & Peth, L. D. (1992). Can protein-calorie malnutrition cause dysphagia? *Dysphagia, 7,* 86–101.

Weinberg, J. (1972). Psychologic implications of the nutritional needs of the elderly. *Journal of the American Dietetic Association, 60,* 293–296.

Winkler, S. (1989, October). Dental aspects of aging and dental health guide for those who care for and about elderly persons. *Focus on Geriatric Care and Rehabilitation, 3,* 1–8.

Zenner, P. M., Losinski, D. S., & Mills, R. H. (1995). Using cervical auscultation in the clinical dysphagia examination in long-term care. *Dysphagia, 10,* 27–31.

Zimmerman, J. E., & Oder, L. A. (1981). Swallowing dysfunction in acutely ill patients. *Physical Therapy, 61,* 1755–1763.

Chapter 18

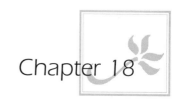

Managing Hearing Loss in Aging: Seniors as Adaptation Experts

Laurel E. Glass
Holly H. Elliott

Glass and Elliott examine management of hearing loss in older adults through consideration of the adaptive attitudes and behaviors that facilitate coping with hearing impairment. Most of the chapter focuses on developing a better understanding of the experience of adult onset hearing loss, so that professionals can provide effective, broad-based services. Findings from the authors' Adult Onset Hearing Loss Project are used to isolate four focal points for clinicians, including recognition that (a) dealing with hearing deficits means dealing with loss, (b) acknowledgment of hearing loss is prerequisite to effective adaptation, (c) many reasons exist for denial of hearing difficulties, and (d) the single most important need after acknowledgment is information.

1. *What are some differences between the experience of being Deaf (defined as born deaf or becoming deaf before speech has developed) and acquiring hearing loss in late adulthood? How do the differences between these experiences affect management and coping strategies?*

2. *What kinds of losses are experienced by adults with gradual onset hearing loss? Why is acknowledgment of hearing loss considered critical to successful intervention? What reasons are offered for the commonly observed denial of hearing impairment by older adults?*

3. *What types of information are needed by adults attempting to deal with adult onset hearing loss?*

4. *According to these authors, what are the advantages of self-help consumer organizations oriented toward individuals with hearing impairment?*

Not too many years ago, a debate occurred at the annual meeting of a large, prestigious association of highly trained professionals skilled in the assessment and delivery of care to persons with hearing loss. The issue was whether the definition of *normal hearing* and of *hearing impairment* should be changed for persons 65 years of age or older. The outcome would determine the degree of hearing loss at which it was appropriate professionally to recommend hearing aids for a client. If passed, the proposal would mean that older people would be described as normal hearing even if their hearing was the same or worse than that of a younger person with similar audiological findings suggesting hearing loss.

The debate ended when a former member of the association's executive committee went to the microphone. Pointing to his ears, he said, "Last year I was not wearing hearing aids; this year I have aids in both ears. I hear more with them. I hear more accurately with them. I am 63. Are you telling me that if I go for a hearing assessment 2 years from now, when I am 65, I should be informed that—although hearing aids help me—I have normal hearing and do not need them? What nonsense!" The debate was finished. The descriptors of hearing status were not changed. Not that time.

Can seniors really get by with hearing less? What nonsense! It is only in a statistical sense that hearing less is "normal" for seniors; a higher proportion of seniors do have more serious hearing dysfunction than do middle aged and younger persons in the same sized population. So? It could only be middle aged and younger persons who interpret that to mean that seniors have fewer (less important) problems than younger people in coping with the communication difficulties created by hearing loss.

The emphasis in this chapter will be on the attitudinal and behavioral adaptations that help an older person with hearing impairment cope successfully with hearing loss. The technologies of intervention—hearing aids at several levels of technological sophistication, cochlear implants, and the variety of "assistive listening devices" available—are detailed in other sources (e.g., Palmer, 1995; Stach & Stoner, 1991). Helpful programs for aural rehabilitation, stress reduction, speechreading, and other learnable skills about "how-to-hear-when-you-don't-hear" also are described well in other publications (e.g., Kaplan, in press; Lesner & Kricos, 1991; Trychin, 1993), as well as in Chapter 12 of this text. It is hoped that the research-based information presented here may enlarge the context within which current technologies and rehabilitation programs are utilized.

The Population of Adventitiously Hearing Impaired Persons—And What It Is Not

There is no firm estimate of the number of persons who have become hard-of-hearing or deafened as adults; all figures are estimates and based on a variety of more or less objective criteria of hearing loss. There seems to be some agreement that roughly 28 million adult citizens in the United States have some degree of hearing loss (National Institute of Deafness and Other Communication Disorders [NIDCD], 1989), although this estimate keeps changing upward. This is between 8.6% and 9.1% of the population. Of that number, only about 2% are deaf (Holt & Hotto, 1994). It is relevant to note that most persons with hearing impairment in this country have been raised as hearing, and have experienced a gradual, often unrecognized, decrease in the accurate processing of sound. Both demographic and a variety of audiological data clearly indicate that the prevalence and the severity of hearing loss tends to increase as a population ages; more than one third of the U.S. population has a significant hearing impairment by age 65.

Recognition that deaf ≠ Deaf has been relatively recent. Individuals born deaf or who became deaf before speech was established were raised in the context of a visually based communication system, with its multiple implications for life-style, interpersonal relationships, learning mode, and so on. These individuals are now acknowledged as "culturally Deaf," with a unique, complex language based on visual signs. In contrast, persons who became deaf or became hard of hearing as adults were raised in an environment in which auditory cues were available from unseen as well as from visible sources. Sound has a radically different meaning to such "culturally hearing" persons than it does to Deaf individuals; sound has been a primary purveyor of significant information and is depended on for that function. The loss of sound-based information, with its subtlety and flexibility in conveying emotional as well as object-based meaning, is an enormous loss to someone raised with a sound-based communication style. The loss may be likened to the loss of vision for a Deaf person raised to be dependent on visual communication modes (Glass & Elliott, 1994c).

Differentiation between the therapeutic needs of these two (grossly defined) populations should have a substantial effect on the focus of therapy and on the modalities used in assistive therapies with such clients. This reality has yet to affect significantly the allocation of funds to public and private agencies, and the current political climate suggests that it will not soon have such an effect. However, recognition of the major differences between these groups must affect the ways clinicians work with individuals who come to them. Though the audiological deficit may be similar, these persons come from substantively different cultural traditions relative to sound, and the kinds of assistance needed are enormously different.

Psychosocial Aspects of Hearing Loss in Adulthood

From 1990 through 1993, the authors were funded by the National Institute on Disability and Rehabilitation Research for a research project on adult onset hearing loss (formally titled "Psychosocial Aspects of Hearing Loss in Adulthood"). In the following chapter sections, we share some of our research data and insights, seasoned with clinical experience and supplemented by the work of others. A brief description of the Adult Onset Hearing Loss Project will provide necessary background (Glass, 1994; Glass & Elliott, 1994a, 1994b, 1995).

Initially, 70 adventitiously hearing impaired persons participated in a series of small face-to-face focus groups. In addition, a one-page questionnaire was sent to approximately 14,000 members of Self-Help for Hard of Hearing Persons, Inc. (SHHH) and approximately 500 members of the Association of Late Deafened Adults (ALDA). In addition to demographic questions, the survey requested information about hearing loss, its onset, how it was perceived, and why the respondent joined a self-help consumer group. More than 7,000 responses were received, with return rates of over 50% for each organization.

Information from focus groups and questionnaires was used to construct an interview instrument for face-to-face, 2- to 3-hour interviews with 131 individuals across the country who were nominated by themselves or others as having "coped successfully with hearing loss." The interview probed descriptions of the onset of hearing loss, as well as its effects on relationships, feelings about oneself, and various daily activities. Interviewees also completed pencil-and-paper personal information questionnaires and the short form of the *16 Personality Factor Questionnaire* (16PF), a well-standardized inventory of independent personality factors (Institute for Personality and Ability Testing, 1986). A copy of a recent audiogram was obtained from most interviewees.

Finally, all data sources were used to construct a 13-page questionnaire requesting information about the demographic, auditory, and general health attributes of participants and including questions about the effects of hearing loss on interpersonal relationships, work, recreational and volunteer civic activities, prior and present adaptations to the hearing loss, coping styles and strategies, and feelings about the experience of losing hearing. Forty-two hundred participants, equally divided between men and women, were selected randomly from the respondents to the one-page survey. Persons interviewed previously were excluded. A total of 2,731 questionnaires (65.4%) were completed, many with marginal notes or accompanying letters.

Of those completing the survey, 64.9% had become hard-of-hearing or deafened between the ages of 18 and 65. Because mean age at the time of the survey was 67 years, information is retrospective. Roughly the same number of men and women responded, with the majority being White, married, and from a suburban or urban community (two thirds). About four fifths had 1 or more years of college and more than a fourth had done graduate work; about 15% had professional or academic doctorates. Four fifths said their income was adequate or comfortable. Three fourths had experienced a progressive hearing loss; four fifths reported that their loss was at least moderately severe at the time of completing the questionnaire. Almost half of the respondents were working when they "began to recognize hearing loss was a problem."

Focal Points Derived from Research

Findings of the Adult Onset Hearing Loss Project, plus clinical experience, suggest at least four focal points that can be useful in guiding clinicians working seniors with hearing impairment:

1. Hearing loss is *loss*.

2. Acknowledgment of hearing loss is resisted by clients; without acknowledgment, successful adaptation to the loss is difficult and may be impossible.

3. Failure to acknowledge hearing loss ("denial"?) happens often; its reasons are poorly understood, and helping clients overcome resistance to acknowledgment is very difficult.

4. Early on, accurate information about hearing loss helps clients more than emotional support.

The implications of each focus will be expanded in the following sections.

First Focus: Loss. Hearing loss is *loss.* It is rarely benign in its effects on anything in the life of the person experiencing it. Hearing loss affects the perception of self; it affects relationships; it affects work and play. Not only is it all of the above, but it is also thoroughly inconvenient! Things that were easy become difficult.

Our clinical impression is that older people may have an edge over younger ones in coping with hearing loss and its implications. No one reaches seniority without experiencing multiple losses, many trivial but some of intense challenge. The old know intimately that some pain does not ease, but that most gradually subsides. They have no doubt that one way or another they will find a way to cope. This does not mean that they escape the frustration, anger, anxiety, stress, and all the other unpleasant accompaniments to the *loss* of hearing; it only means that older people may adapt more quickly to the realities of their situation. In a sense, life experience has made the old experts at adaptation.

To lose hearing—and to begin however hesitantly to acknowledge it—is more threatening to self and function, more frightening, more anger creating, more challenging, and more unpleasant than others can recognize (see, e.g., Weinstein & Ventry, 1982). From an interviewee:

> I remember the fear, the terror with not being able to cope with the hearing loss. And not being able to sustain my own earning ability and keep a job. So I tried to hide it. Futile. Everybody probably knew it. I would misinterpret something over the telephone and then I would have to figure out how to cover up. I would misinterpret things at meetings so I would get to the point where I wouldn't say anything, which, of course, gave the impression that I was stupid. This went on for about five years—the enjoyable parts of the job were overshadowed by the increasing stress at the hearing loss. (Woman, middle management, aged 48 at onset of hearing loss)

Her experience is not unique. The effects of adult onset hearing loss on life quality were explored in a study at the University of California, San Francisco, Audiology Clinic (Glass, Nguyen, Carman, & Flower, 1989). Sixty-five persons coming to the Audiology Clinic for their first audiological examination agreed to fill out a Likert format, pencil-and-paper questionnaire about the effects of hearing loss on their life-style. Audiograms showed that about half (49%) had only a mild hearing loss, and slightly more than a third (37%) had a moderate loss. Nearly half (46%) had tinnitus.

Despite what is generally described as a minor loss by the professional field, more than half (54%) of the patients reported that the hearing loss "affected my activities":

94% said, "I miss out on lots of conversations."

86% said, "I feel tension in many listening situations."

83% said, "I feel left out of things."

69% said, "My family and friends want something done about my hearing."

51% said, "I avoid situations I used to enjoy."

Respondents reported that they had stopped or had difficulty in several areas: wanting TV or radio louder than others do (86%); conversing with two or three people at the same time (62%); going to the movies (62%); attending large parties (60%); attending church (60%); going to lectures (57%); and attending meetings (54%). Hearing loss, even mild, is not benign.

The only activity seemingly "protected" from the effects of hearing loss may be contacts with family members. Sixty percent of the participants reported continued, but eroded, family contacts. An additional 34% noted that family interactions were carried out "with difficulty." As an 80-year-old interviewee, a mother, said, "I don't stay long at my children's homes anymore. They're busy, involved in their lives, people are always dropping in. The TV usually is on. Family dinners with a lot of people are a nightmare. I know they love me and they try hard but it is just too tiring to stay there and not know what is going on."

Clinicians were sometimes, but not always, helpful. Respondents to the 13-page questionnaire gave quite different assessments of the quality of help received from differently trained professionals

(Table 18.1). Fortunately, audiologists and ear-nose-throat physicians were experienced by clients as the professionals who did the best job of understanding their problem, helping them understand the loss, and giving good advice about how to deal with it. Unfortunately, the family doctor, from whom a person with a hearing impairment is most likely to seek initial help, seemed less likely to provide it well. Of the 600 or so respondents answering this question, only a third thought their family doctor really understood; fewer than a third thought the doctor had really helped them understand, and only a quarter thought the family doctor had given first-rate advice.

The problem can be thought of as bidirectional. The intense fear and denial of persons learning to deal directly with their dysfunctional hearing often makes them difficult to treat. Helping professionals prefer to help, not have their help rejected. While family doctors are in the business of helping people stay well, the traditional model of physician-delivered health care is that of helping acutely ill people become well again. Busy, tired physicians do not recognize hearing loss as a critical loss; certainly it is not life threatening. The person who is struggling with diminished hearing may get little attention.

Second Focus: Acknowledgment. Acknowledgment of hearing loss is necessary if one is to adapt successfully to it. Without acknowledgment, adaptation is difficult and may be impossible. This may be the single most important reality about coping well.

The more we look at persons who have adapted well to their hearing loss, the more it seems true that there are few ways adaptation can occur without conscious acknowledgment of the uncomfortable new "given"—the fact that auditory information can no longer be processed with ease. One of the benefits of self-help consumer organizations like SHHH and ALDA may be that the groups are filled with role models who have acknowledged their hearing deficiency and are embarked on the devious, demanding road of adapting life-style to the reality of hearing loss—in relationships, in the use of technology, in the tolerance of anxiety, and in the expectation of outcome (see Appendix 18A for helpful addresses).

Acknowledgment that one is hearing impaired allows the helpful recognition that recurrent difficulty in comprehending auditory information is not anyone's fault—neither one's own nor that of other people. With acknowledgment that the problem is biologically based (not a character defect), one can begin to deal directly with feelings of guilt

Table 18.1
Assistance Received by Hard-of-Hearing and
Deafened Adults from Professionals

Audiologists

Understanding?
- Not very — 12.0%
- Yes, OK — 26.7%
- Very — 59.2%
- (*N* = 1,178)

Helped me understand
- Not much — 15.2%
- Yes, OK — 29.0%
- Yes!! — 55.2%
- (*N* = 1,162)

Gave good advice
- Not really — 15.3%
- Yes, OK — 28.0%
- Yes!! — 54.8%
- (*N* = 1,241)

Ear, Nose, and Throat Physicians

Understanding?
- Not very — 23.0%
- Yes, OK — 21.6%
- Very — 53.8%
- (*N* = 435)

Helped me understand
- Not much — 24.8%
- Yes, OK — 21.8%
- Yes!! — 52.1%
- (*N* = 427)

Gave good advice
- Not really — 23.4%
- Yes, OK — 23.2%
- Yes!! — 53.1%
- (*N* = 457)

Family Doctors

Understanding?
- Not very — 35.6%
- Yes, OK — 25.3%
- Very — 35.6%
- (*N* = 567)

Helped me understand
- Not much — 48.0%
- Yes, OK — 22.8%
- Yes!! — 27.8%
- (*N* = 485)

Gave good advice
- Not really — 31.2%
- Yes, OK — 31.9%
- Yes!! — 25.5%
- (*N* = 609)

(e.g., for being a bother to other people, for messing up others' plans or activities, for misunderstanding others' requests or comments). Self-denigration, guilt, and self-doubt often accompany the loss of auditory understanding; not infrequently, there is an initial loss of felt competence, self-assurance, and self-acceptance. Associated with these, the "perception-of-self-as-still-adequate" is protected by a spectrum of defensive behaviors, some of which are unpleasant to others. For example, some hard-of-hearing persons talk nonstop, thereby preventing others from saying something they would not hear clearly enough to respond to sensibly. Acknowledgment can allow the client and the clinician to begin to work directly on such erosions of self-esteem.

Acknowledgment also allows persons with hearing impairment to adopt intentional strategies to control the effects of their dysfunctional hearing. Hearing loss is fatiguing; it is tiring to strain to interpret words and meanings that are heard only partially or in distorted form. Hearing loss causes stress, especially on the job or in significant personal relationships, when the outcome of important transactions may depend on the accurate comprehension of auditory cues. Acknowledgment can give the person the courage, for example, to control the configuration of a room, change the placement of participants in a conversation, insist on a quiet environment, or mandate appropriate nonglare lighting.

Acknowledgment, therefore, is linked to successful coping. This conclusion is supported by three statistically significant findings that emerged from analysis of the 16PF inventories completed by interviewees who were selected as persons who had "coped successfully with hearing loss." The 16 pairs of independent personality factors assessed by the inventory are cool/warm; concrete-thinking/abstract-thinking; affected by feelings/emotionally stable; submissive/dominant; sober/enthusiastic; expedient/conscientious; shy/bold; tough-minded/tender-minded; trusting/suspicious; practical/imaginative; forthright/shrewd; self-assured/apprehensive; conservative/experimenting; group-oriented/self-sufficient; undisciplined self-conflict/following self-image; relaxed/tense. The scores of successful copers tended to be quite balanced between the extremes of the 16PF pairs; that is, the distribution of their scores resembled that of the normal population. However, three pairs of personality factors were associated by 16PF with "successful copers": *Forthrightness* in contrast to deviousness or shrewdness, *dominance or assertiveness* in contrast to submissiveness, and *expediency* in disregard of the rules in contrast to rule-bound staidness were all associated with successful coping. We suggest that, in combination, these can be freely interpreted as behaviors that "make the situation work." In coping with hearing loss, we think this means an insistence on adaptations that make comprehension possible despite the hearing deficit.

Two final comments about acknowledgment are relevant. When one acknowledges dysfunctional hearing, it often is possible to move to an acknowledgment that *not everything said is worth hearing*. This can allow the development of a conscious or partly conscious hierarchy of importance within which the "effort to hear" is allocated differentially.

Perhaps more important, acknowledgment of hearing impairment can allow the associated acknowledgment that *not all relationships are of equal value*. To hear what the butcher says is pleasant, but not usually imperative. To hear what one's boss says is absolutely necessary if one wants to continue working. To hear what one's lover or close friend says allows movement into deeper commitment, understanding, and sharing. Such acknowledgments allow the person with hearing impairment to choose to put the greatest amount of energy-dependent effort at hearing where it is personally most important.

Third Focus: Denial. Failure to acknowledge hearing loss ("denial"?) occurs very often; its reasons are poorly understood, and overcoming resistance to acknowledgment is very difficult. Clinically, the term *denial* is applied to patients who consciously or unconsciously try to relieve their anxiety by pretending that the serious situation described to them by their clinician is either exaggerated or nonexistent. In relation to hearing loss, both clients and clinicians have suggested a number of reasons why the reality of intrusive hearing loss is denied. None are well supported by data, but most make intuitive sense:

- To acknowledge a disability harms one's self-image.

- Hearing loss is associated by the public with aging. To many, getting old implies decreased competence, diminished resources, less freedom, and lowered attractiveness. "Aging" is frightening.

- In these contexts, people with hearing impairment might deny hearing loss for fear of denigration by others and because others might misinterpret failure to hear as loss of mental alertness.

- Denial may be related to a pragmatic fear of losing one's job if one's capacity to understand others and communicate with them is impaired.

- Denial may also relate to the strong feeling that "I want to go on doing what I'm doing; if I acknowledge hearing impairment, I may not be able to!"

None of these can be excluded. Probably all are true to a greater or lesser degree.

From the standpoint of the person beginning to work through difficulties communicating, the issues are not simple "denial" or "acknowledgment." More than half of our respondents had their hearing tested as soon as they suspected they had a hearing loss. However, of the 44% who delayed, about half waited between 1 and 5 years; more than 40% of those who postponed testing waited more than 5 years before getting their hearing checked (Table 18.2). When asked why they had delayed in obtaining a hearing test, about a third reported blaming other people; "I was sure I could hear; other people were mumbling." Half felt their loss was so mild that they could deal with it without help, and about a third didn't want to wear a hearing aid or didn't want others to know they needed a hearing aid.

Whether a hearing test was obtained immediately or was delayed, the reasons given by respondents for getting their hearing tested were substantial: communication was stressful; their jobs were affected; tinnitus was troublesome; they were withdrawing; their family thought they needed their hearing checked. Although almost 70% felt relief after hearing loss was diagnosed, other emotions were frequent: fear, depression, anger, disbelief (Table 18.2). In addition to these elements, which characterize most who resist the acknowledgment of hearing loss, our impression is that there may be an even stronger, hidden impulse supporting denial. In a sense, "denial" may be an appropriate defense; that is, denial may be necessary for self-preservation (Cousins, 1984; Glass, 1987). This can be illustrated by two unpleasant anecdotes.

> "You're deaf. It's only going to get worse. A hearing aid won't help." (Said by an otolaryngologist to a 19-year-old undergraduate woman majoring in music at a distinguished west coast university.)

> "You're going deaf. You won't be able to continue running your own shop. You'll have to expect sharply reduced income and will probably end up working for someone else." (Said by a vocational rehabilitation counselor to a 42-year-old-male, owner of a small business in the automotive industry.)

Table 18.2

Respondents' Reactions to Getting Their Hearing Tested

Respondents' Reactions	Percentage Responding
A. After I suspected I had a hearing loss, I	
☐ immediately had my hearing tested	55.3%
☐ put off getting my hearing tested	44.3%
For how long? ☐ < 1 year	11.1%
☐ 1 to 5 years	47.0%
☐ > 5 years	41.6%
	(N = 1,903)
B. I delayed in getting my hearing tested because: (Check all that apply)	
☐ I could hear; I thought other people were mumbling	32.8%
☐ I didn't want to wear a hearing aid	18.3%
☐ It was only a mild loss; I could deal with that	53.9%
☐ I didn't want others to know I needed a hearing aid	14.5%
☐ I felt afraid to find out what was wrong	7.2%
	(N = 1,110)
C. I made an appointment to have my hearing tested because:	
☐ my hearing loss was affecting my job	25.6%
☐ my family suggested that I needed a hearing aid	11.8%
☐ I was withdrawing from group activities	12.0%
☐ communication was becoming stressful	47.9%
☐ I wanted relief from the tinnitus	25.3%
	(N = 1,903)
D. When you heard the diagnosis, did you feel:	
☐ disbelief	12.8%
☐ relief that I knew what the problem was	30.3%
☐ relief that there was help out there	38.2%
☐ anger because this was disrupting my life	9.6%
☐ depression	11.8%
☐ fear—"what did this mean for my life?"	26.8%
☐ it confirmed my suspicion	11.1%
	(N = 1,819)

Therapeutic? No way. Helpful? Hardly! Both clients were furious (and frightened). Both withdrew from "therapy." Both *denied* what their clinician told them. Both went their own way. Both made it. Both made it with difficulty.

The first incident occurred more than 40 years ago; the second happened recently—only 4 years ago. We suggest that the reaction of both "deniers" illustrates very clearly a positive effect of denial. In each instance, the denial fueled anger, and the anger gave each the energy *not* to submit passively to the negative, frighteningly disastrous prognosis given them. The denial and noncompliance with recommended behaviors led to intense—and beneficial—efforts to explore other options.

It is clear that persons who have lost hearing, that is, those who have become hard of hearing or become deafened as adults, have lived with a complex matrix of discomfort, composed partly of denial and partly of acknowledgment. Finally, they reach the stage of seeking professional help to understand and cope with their impairment. We suspect that the clinicians most successful in working with such clients are those most sensitive to these complexities.

Fourth Focus: Information. After hearing loss is acknowledged, the single most important need is for information about it. This is more important than the need for supportive people. Unexpectedly, and contrary to the "everyone knows" perception, our research revealed that information is the strongest felt need of persons who acknowledge their lost hearing. For example, when SHHH members were asked to rank a group of 10 reasons for joining SHHH, needs for information were listed as the top four (Table 18.3). SHHH confirmed this in a subsequent study.

We suggest that there are several types of information needed. One type is objective, fact-based straight talk about the biological/medical realities of hearing loss. Adults with hearing impairment also need to know explicit "things-to-do-that-help," for example, the strategies of where to sit in a room, what to say when someone asks an unexpected question, how to remain part of a conversation without becoming obnoxious (e.g., Boone, 1988; Elliott, 1985). Information about available technologies and therapy techniques is also required. Another piece of information that persons with hearing impairment need to know is that, until now, no technology (not even the most sophisticated cochlear implants or the most carefully programmed

Table 18.3
Reasons for Joining SHHH
(ranked from most to least important)

1. Technical information
2. Coping strategies
3. Information about services
4. Medical information
5. Emotional support
6. Socialization
7. Advocacy
8. Information about legal rights
9. Professional interest

digital aids) can restore hearing as satisfactorily as well-fitted glasses can restore visual acuity. Although clinicians still do not understand completely what causes hearing loss, some explanation of current thought about contributing factors and of the progressive nature of hearing loss across the life span is needed by the client whose hearing has been impaired (see Chapter 5 of this volume).

Persons who have difficulty hearing also need to know that their hearing will fluctuate from time to time; they are neither "making it up" nor faking hearing loss. (Early on, at least, their associates may be full of blame; "John can hear when he wants to.") Hard-of-hearing and deafened persons need to have their family informed, too, and clinicians can usually do this more accurately and forcefully than can John. Persons with hearing impairment also need to be informed that they do hear less well when they are ill, when they are distracted, when they are taking certain medications, when they are in a noisy environment, when the light is poor, when they cannot see the speaker, or when communication is coming from a distance or over a poor amplifying system.

Although amplification often helps, people with hearing impairment need to know that loudness does not necessarily mean better hearing; it may exacerbate the distortion that accompanies some hearing loss. If they experience this distortion, persons with hearing impairment need to know that some hearing losses are accompanied by an acute, often painful, sensitivity to particular pitches. If they suffer from "head noises" (tinnitus), it sometimes helps to learn that at least 15% of the U.S. population is affected by tinnitus and that persons over the age of 50 are twice as likely to have this problem (NIDCD, 1989).

Probably most important, people learning to cope with hearing loss need to be reassured that others have experienced what they are experiencing. After those others adapted in all the ways available to them, most survived with lives more successful and satisfying than they had dared hope in the midst of their struggles to cope. One helpful example is shown in Table 18.4. People who were employed when they experienced the onset of hearing loss were asked to compare whether they felt less, the same, or more successful, competent, or appreciated at work *after* making adjustments to help manage their hearing loss as they had *before* their hearing loss occurred (Glass & Elliott, 1993a). More than half reported that they felt as successful, competent, and appreciated at work and that their earnings had not been affected adversely.

Conclusions

Adaptation to hearing loss is not easy; questionnaire and interview data plus clinical experience show that repeatedly. However, adaptation does happen. Adventitiously hard-of-hearing and deafened people learn by persistence, grace, and intelligence to continue or regain productive, fulfilled, and satisfying lives. Respondents to the 13-page questionnaire, engaged in the retrospective assessment of experiences that had caused deep pain and anxiety for them, affirm that to a large degree. The outcome of those reassessments can be reassuring both to clinicians and to persons still actively engaged in the struggle. Few clients have access to such reassurance; it helps when the clinicians with whom they work can provide it.

Both research and clinical experience cause us to emphasize the reality that hearing loss is *loss*; it is not benign. More than a third of people over the age of 65 in the United States are hearing impaired, and their hearing loss is associated with increased stress, anxiety, anger, fatigue, and isolation. All these are secondary to impaired communication caused by the diminished hearing. Acknowledgment of hearing impairment is necessary if appropriate and successful adapta-

Table 18.4

Perception of Work Achievement After Hearing Loss

Gender	N	% Successful	% Competent	% Appreciated	% Earning
Women	538	47.8	50.9	52.8	54.3
Men	771	56.2	55.5	57.2	55.5
Total	1,309	52.7	53.6	55.4	55.0

Note. Percentage of respondents who felt the same or more *successful, competent,* or *appreciated* at work or who felt their *earning power* was unaffected or increased after their hearing loss. From "Work Place Success for Persons with Adult-Onset Hearing Impairment," by L. E. Glass and H. H. Elliott, 1993, *Volta Review, 95,* 403–415.

tion to the hearing loss is to occur. Nonetheless, denial of hearing loss is common, and this makes acknowledgment and successful adaptation more difficult. Denial may also protect the hearing impaired person from despair and passive submission to negative prognoses. Early in the adaptation process, the need for accurate information about hearing loss is more important even than the need for supportive people. Access to current technical interventions, whether through use of hearing aids, cochlear implants, and/or the multitude of assistive listening devices presently available, helps adaptation. Additionally, participation in good aural rehabilitation programs and training in speechreading, stress management, and other coping skills does help achieve successful adaptation. The more aware clinicians are of the kinds of situational evaluations made by hard-of-hearing and deafened clients, as presented here, the more quickly appropriate adaptations by clients can occur—in attitude, coping skills, and technologies.

Authors' Note

This work was supported in part by Research Grant No. H133A90003 from the National Institute on Disability and Rehabilitation Research, U.S. Department of Education. Persons assisting in the Adult Onset Hearing Loss Project include Helen Luey, Nancy Grant, Marcus Krafft, Susan Hager, Sylvia Acquino, Marjorie Crossman, Robert Scholtz, and Linda Mitteness.

References

Boone, M. (1988, November/December). On-the-job hearing problems: Making a personal check list. *SHHH Journal*, pp. 7–10.

Cousins, N. (1984). *The healing heart* (pp. 139–144). New York: Avon.

Elliott, H. H. (1985, November/December). Acquired hearing loss: Shifting gears. *SHHH Journal*, p. 23.

Glass, L. E. (1987). Adventitious hearing loss: Some aspects of denial. In G. Lesnoff-Caravaglia (Ed.), *Aging in a technological society* (pp. 91–94). New York: Human Sciences Press.

Glass, L. E. (1994). The challenge to independence. In S. E. Boone, D. Watson, & M. Bagley (Eds.), *The challenge to independence: Vision and hearing loss among older adults* (pp. 15–24). Little Rock: University of Arkansas Rehabilitation Research and Training Center for Persons who are Deaf or Hard of Hearing.

Glass, L. E., & Elliott, H. H. (1993a, March). *Evaluation and rehabilitation of individuals deafened as adults.* Workshop for Rehabilitation Counselors for the Deaf, California State Department of Rehabilitation Annual In-Service Training Meeting, Ventura, CA.

Glass, L. E., & Elliott, H. H. (1993b). Work place success for persons with adult-onset hearing impairment. *Volta Review, 96,* 403–415.

Glass, L. E., & Elliott, H. H. (1994a, November). *Coping with adult onset hearing loss: Implications for aural rehabilitation.* Paper presented at the annual convention of the American Speech-Language-Hearing Association, New Orleans.

Glass, L. E., & Elliott, H. H. (1994b, March). *Coping with adult onset hearing loss: Seniors as adaptation experts.* Paper presented at the annual meeting of the American Society on Aging, San Francisco.

Glass, L. E., & Elliott, H. H. (1994c). On signing with a hearing accent. In M. D. Garretson (Ed.), *Deafness: Life and Culture, Deaf American Monograph 44* (pp. 59–64). Silver Spring, MD: National Association of the Deaf.

Glass, L. E., & Elliott, H. H. (1995, November). *Research update on adult onset hearing loss.* Workshop for Graduate Course on *Psychosocial Implications of Deafness and Hearing Loss,* San Francisco State University, San Francisco.

Glass, L., Nguyen, M., Carman, C., & Flower, R. (1989). *Some effects of hearing loss on social behavior.* Unpublished manuscript.

Holt, J. A., & Hotto, S. A. (1994). *Demographic aspects of hearing impairment: Questions and answers* (3rd ed.). Washington, DC: Gallaudet University Center for Assessment and Demographic Studies.

Institute for Personality and Ability Testing, Inc. (1986). *The 16 personality factor questionnaire.* Champaign, IL: Institute for Personality and Ability Testing.

Kaplan, H. (in press). Adjustment and informational counseling. In M. J. Moseley & S. J. Bally (Eds.), *Communication therapy for deaf and hard-of-hearing adults.* Washington, DC: Gallaudet University Press.

Lesner, S. A., & Kricos, P. B. (1991). Audiologic rehabilitation: Candidacy, assessment, and management. In D. N. Ripich (Ed.), *Handbook of geriatric communication disorders* (pp. 439–461). Austin, TX: PRO-ED.

National Institute of Deafness and Other Communication Disorders. (1989, April). *National strategic research plan.* Washington, DC: U.S. Government Printing Office.

Palmer, C. V. (1995). Improvement of hearing function. In R. A. Huntley & K. S. Helfer (Eds.), *Communication in later life,* (pp. 181–223). Boston: Butterworth-Heinemann.

Stach, B. A., & Stoner, W. R. (1991). Sensory aids for the hearing-impaired elderly. In D. N. Ripich (Ed.), *Handbook of geriatric communication disorders* (pp. 421–438). Austin, TX: PRO-ED.

Trychin, S. (1991). *Manual for mental health professionals, Part II. Psycho-social challenges faced by hard of hearing people.* Washington, DC: Gallaudet University.

Weinstein, B. E., & Ventry, I. M. (1982). Hearing impairment and social isolation in the elderly. *Journal of Speech and Hearing Research 25,* 253–259.

Appendix 18A
Other Resources Helpful to the Clinician

The Journals of SHHH and the Newsletters from ALDA are filled with specific, consumer-useable information. Some helpful addresses are as follows:

SHHH (Self-Help for Hard of Hearing People, Inc.)
7910 Woodmont Avenue, Suite 1200
Bethesda, MD 10814
Phone: (301) 913-9413 (Voice); (301) 657-2249 (TTY)

ALDA (Association of Late Deafened Adults)
10310 Main Street, Box 274
Fairfax, VA 22030
Phone: (815) 899-3049 (TTY)

Additional helpful information may be obtained from

National Information Center on Deafness
Gallaudet University
800 Florida Avenue NE
Washington, DC 20002
Phone: (202) 651-5051 (Voice and TTY)

An excellent booklet to give to clients newly diagnosed as hearing impaired and their families is

Luey, H. S., & Per-Lee, M. (1983). *What should I do now? Problems and adaptations of the deafened adult.* Washington, DC: Gallaudet University.

(This booklet is out-of-print but Gallaudet plans to publish a new edition; requests might spur them to move more quickly.)

Also available is

Luey, H. S. (1980). Between two worlds: The problems of deafened adults. *Social Work in Health Care 5,* 253–263.

One of the first books published on psychosocial aspects of adult onset hearing loss, and still among the most useful, is

Orlans, H. E. (Ed.). (1985). *Adjustment to adult hearing loss.* San Diego: College-Hill Press.

Selected references to literature before 1988 are listed in

Glass, L. E. (1988). Hearing. In M. Abramson & P. M. Lovas (Eds.), *Aging and sensory change: An annotated bibliography* (pp. 17–23). Washington, DC: The Gerontological Society of America.

Chapter 19

Collaborative Services: Working Together in the Aging Network

John A. Krout
Susan E. Durnford
Carol S. Crichley

Krout, Durnford, and Crichley provide an interdisciplinary perspective on the aging services network. The reader is provided with a description of the network itself, as well as the relevant mandates and programs of the Older Americans Act (1965). Barriers to collaborative interaction between communication disorders professionals and the aging services network are identified, and tentative solutions and model programs for collaboration are described.

1. *What is meant by the term "aging services network?" How does this term relate to the Older Americans Act (OAA)? Which "title" of the OAA is of greatest importance to communication disorders professionals, and what services and programs are served by this title?*

2. *How well do speech–language pathologists and audiologists interact with the aging services network? What are some of the primary barriers to better interaction and communication disorders service delivery to older community-dwelling adults? How might these barriers be overcome in the future?*

3. *Develop a plan for improving communication disorders professionals interactions with the aging services network in your community.*

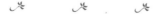

Hearing loss is one of the four most common chronic conditions experienced by older adults (U.S. Senate, 1986). Speech–language–cognitive–communication disorders have a significant impact on one third of the 65+ population (Sayles & Adams, 1979). These problems become more common with increasing age, and their prevalence will increase dramatically as the "baby boom" cohort ages. Thus, audiologists and speech–language pathologists are finding increasing numbers of older persons in their client base, a trend that will only accelerate in the future. Currently, many community-dwelling older individuals with speech–language and hearing problems are not being identified, nor are they receiving evaluative or therapeutic services. To improve service delivery to these older adults, communication disorders professionals need to become more knowledgeable of and increase their interaction with the aging services network.

The term *aging services network* refers to the collection of public agencies (federal, state, and local) and private agencies (usually not-for-profit) that provide a broad array of nonacute health and social services designed to assist older adults live independently in the community. The term does not refer to hospital-based or nursing home care. Many of the agencies in this network have developed under the administrative and funding umbrella of the Older Americans Act (OAA, 1965).

There are numerous benefits to improved interaction between communication disorders professionals and the aging services network. For example, although there is a clear need for audiology and speech–language pathology services among community-dwelling adults, traditional points of contact, such as hospitals and long-term care facilities, do not promote access. In fact, more older adults are served by the aging services network than by nursing homes each year (Krout, 1989). The aging services network can provide contact points with both older adults and agencies that can act as information and referral sources for speech, language, and hearing services. These points of contact will become even more important in the future as changes in health care policies and reimbursement practices designed to increase service coordination and decrease costs will move more forms of service delivery into home and other noninstitutional settings. Community-based services will become the source of job opportunities for many health care professionals.

Increased speech–language pathology and audiology involvement with the aging services network will also promote increased understanding of communication disorders and available services on the part of network professionals. In turn, these aging services network professionals will become more effective in serving their communicatively disordered older clientele, while making more efficient and appropriate referrals for communication disorders services. Finally, improved access to the aging services network would promote collaborative, multidisciplinary research efforts that would increase the understanding of both normal and disordered communication processes and interactions involving older adults (Shadden & Barr, 1988).

It is fitting that this last chapter in a text written "For Clinicians by Clinicians" should remind the reader that service delivery to any age group or disorder type does not occur in a vacuum. This chapter provides an overview of the aging services network with an emphasis upon aspects of the Older Americans Act of particular relevance to speech–language pathologists and audiologists. Barriers that may impede interaction between the aging services network and communication disorders professionals are discussed, and strategies for overcoming these barriers are described. Examples of innovative programs involving collaboration between the aging services network and speech–language–hearing specialists are provided. The chapter closes with a brief review of the research, resource, and policy issues that need to be addressed to increase the involvement of communication disorders professionals with the aging services network.

Aging Services Network

The Older Americans Act

Legislative Components. Several federal programs significantly affect the availability of the aging services network, as defined here, including the social services block grant of the Social Security Amendments of 1965 (formerly Title XX), provisions of both Medicaid and Medicare, and state programs. Perhaps the most significant piece of federal legislation for the purposes of this chapter is the Older Americans Act (OAA). Initially passed by Congress in 1965, the OAA recognized the need to develop a coordinated system of services to meet the diverse and unique needs of all persons aged 60 or over and to acknowledge the ability of most older adults to make significant contributions to their communities. The focus was on social services that would assist older persons to live independently in the community, even as their health and resources might decline. Acute health care or long-term care for seriously ill persons was not to be a priority. The OAA has been reauthorized 11 times, most recently in 1992, and was scheduled for reauthorization in 1995.

The original legislation was significantly affected by the 1961 White House Conference on Aging. Over the years, the specific programs and priorities of the OAA have evolved and changed in some significant ways. One trend has involved targeting of OAA dollars increasingly toward elders with greatest social and economic need (low-income in general and low-income minorities, specifically), along with a growing emphasis on cost sharing by participants in OAA program funding. Future reauthorizations may bring even more change if funding is reduced and the "block grant" approach to allocating federal monies becomes a reality.

Title I of the 1965 OAA legislation included 10 rather sweeping objectives, which remain governing principles for this legislation (Gelfand, 1993, p. 12):

1. an adequate income

2. the best possible physical and mental health

3. suitable housing

4. full restorative services

5. opportunity for employment without age discrimination

6. retirement in health, honor, and dignity

7. pursuit of meaningful dignity

8. efficient community services when needed

9. immediate benefit from proven research knowledge

10. freedom, independence, and the free exercise of individual initiative

The vast majority of these objectives relate directly or indirectly to adequacy of communication behavior and services to the older individual with a communication disorder. Issues of physical and mental health, full restorative services, independent functioning, and benefit from research knowledge are, or should be, fundamental objectives of speech–language and hearing professionals as they seek to improve communicative functioning in older adults.

Not all provisions of the OAA, as defined in its seven "titles," are of direct interest to speech–language pathologists or audiologists. A brief description of each of these sections of the OAA is provided in Table 19.1, followed by a more extensive discussion of those policy and funding priorities that provide opportunities for improved service delivery to older persons with communication disorders.

Programs of Interest and/or Benefit to Communication Disorders Professionals. The Administration on Aging (AoA) is charged with carrying out the provisions of the OAA and administering the funds authorized by Congress for its various titles. Other responsibilities include providing information on aging issues and the needs of older persons, developing policies and programs to meet these needs, collecting statistics on the programs funded under the OAA, advocating for older persons throughout the federal government, and coordinating federal, state, and local efforts in aging services, including those involving public and private organizations. The AoA can provide communication disorders professionals with information on issues facing older adults and on the activities of the aging services network. Thus, audiologists and speech–language pathologists should consider contacting the AoA to explore partnerships in service to older adults.

The title likely to be of greatest interest and importance to communication disorders professionals is Title III—Grants for State and Community Projects and Programs. This title identifies the services that should be provided at the local level and the monies authorized for specific programs. The term *supportive services* under Title III is used to refer to a broad range of initiatives, including various types of health-related care, transportation, recreation and education, nutrition, legal assistance, housing assistance and repair, job counseling, crime prevention and personal safety, and the ombudsman program intended to protect the rights and investigate the complaints of long-term care facility residents. Newer services include translation services for non-English-speaking elders, insurance counseling, guardianship representation, additional types of therapies (e.g., dance, music, and art therapy), disease prevention and health promotion activities, and counseling for persons providing informal care for older adults (Gelfand, 1993). Nutrition services, both congregate and in-home, have historically received the largest allocations and

Table 19.1

Main Titles and Provisions of the Older
Americans Act (1965) and Subsequent Amendments

Title I. Objectives

Title II. Administration on Aging (housed in Department of Health and Human Services [DHHS])

Purpose: To establish the Administration on Aging (AoA) charged with carrying out the provisions of the OAA, administering authorized funds, providing information on aging issues and the needs of older persons and developing appropriate policies and programs to meet needs, advocating for older persons throughout the federal government, and coordinating aging services efforts at all levels and across the public and private sectors.

Title III. Grants for State and Community Programs

Purpose: To identify and fund the provision of supportive and nutrition services at the local level, via a network of state units on aging (SUAs) that fund and oversee local area agencies on aging (AAAs) that in turn provide direct services and contract with other community agencies to provide services to older adults in geographically defined planning and service areas (PSAs).

Title IV. Training, Research, and Discretionary Projects and Programs

Purpose: To provide direction and funding for the training of gerontological practitioners, for gerontological education in general, and for the conduct of applied research and demonstration projects. Recent priorities have included the funding of institutes to address specific issues such as needs of minority elderly, rural aging, transportation, and long-term care.

Title V. Community Service Employment for Older Americans

Purpose: To fund and coordinate a number of contractors that provide job training and placement for lower income persons aged 55 and over who are unemployed or who have difficulty finding employment. Funding is provided by the U.S. Department of Labor through contractural arrangement with 10 national organizations.

Title VI. Grants for Native American Tribes

Purpose: To fund tribal development of social and nutritional services not already provided by Title III.

Title VII. Allotments for Vulnerable Elder Rights Protection Activities (authorized in 1992)

Purpose: Support state long-term care ombudsman programs; prevent elder abuse, neglect, and exploitation; support state elder rights and legal assistance development; and promote state outreach, counseling, and assistance programs for insurance and public benefit.

---

serviced the largest numbers of elders under Title III of the OAA. Congregate meal programs are often located in senior centers, an important part of the aging service network.

Obviously, not all of these services can draw on the expertise of communication disorders professionals, but several certainly appear likely to provide them opportunities for serving older adults. For example, disease prevention and health promotion services, translation services, care provider counseling, and in-home services for the more frail would seem to be appropriate. It is important for speech–language pathologists and audiologists to know that Title III of the OAA also establishes and governs the operation of the aging services network organizational structure. This network consists of state units on aging (SUAs) that fund and oversee the operations of local area agencies on aging (AAAs) that in turn both provide services directly and contract with other community agencies to provide services to older adults in geographically defined planning and service areas (PSAs). These service providers and AAAs can provide communication disorders professionals access to older populations potentially in need of their services in their communities.

Finally, Title IV (training, research, and discretionary projects and programs) has been extremely important for the training of gerontological practitioners, gerontological education in general, and the conduct of applied research and demonstration projects. Although the funding has not been large, it has had far-reaching effects. Over the years, the research and training priorities of Title IV have varied considerably. In recent years, priorities have focused on funding institutes to address specific issues, such as the needs of minorities, rural aging, transportation, and long-term care. This title of the OAA offers opportunities for audiologists and speech–language pathologists to collaborate with other allied health professionals and organizations such as senior centers and area agencies on aging to offer education and, in some cases, programs and services to older adults.

Allocations for the OAA have remained fairly flat since the 1970s, despite the large growth in the number of persons 60 years and older and added service expectations (Hudson, 1995). For example, the total OAA allocation (administration and programs) was approximately $1.4 billion in 1995; anyone age 60 or over is eligible to receive OAA services. The congregate and in-home meal programs were funded for $453 million in 1993 ($470 million in 1995) and provided 135 million congregate meals to 2.5 million older persons and 106 million in-home meals to 825,000 home-bound older persons. Waiting lists for in-home meals are common in many communities (White House Conference on Aging, 1995). Thus, some services are not available at all in some areas, and waiting lists are common for specific programs. In some cases, the service that is available does not necessarily meet the needs of the older person, or the service is not easily accessible because of a lack of transportation. This is not an unanticipated or even unintended consequence of the OAA legislation, given that one of the primary responsibilities of the aging services network is to develop community partnerships to generate nonfederal resources for these programs. This lack of adequate resources can be seen as a challenge for those speech–language pathologists and audiologists who wish to work within the network.

Major Points of Contact: Communication Disorders Professionals and the Aging Services Network

The aging services network administered by the OAA is represented schematically in Figure 19.1 (Torres-Gil, 1991). As you can see, the network includes federal, state, and local agencies as well as a network of service providers. Currently, there are 57 SUAs, 670 AAAs, and some 25,000 providers of services.

Area Agencies on Aging. The key link in this system at the local level is the Area Agency on Aging (AAA). AAAs were first developed as a national demonstration project funded by the Administration on Aging. The main charge of the AAA is to develop a local system of comprehensive and coordinated services for the elderly by determining needs in the local area, evaluating the effectiveness of resources used to meet these needs, and arranging with local service providers for the provision of needed services (U.S. Department of Health, Education, and Welfare, 1977). In addition, federal legislation emphasizes that AAAs play two other roles—program development and advocacy. Program development refers to AAA actions to increase the emphasis on serving the needs of the elderly in non-AoA funded programs. AAAs are also charged with advocating for greater attention to and resources for elderly programs at the local level.

Today, AAAs support over 30 services, including nutrition, access/transportation, legal aid, information/referral, multipurpose

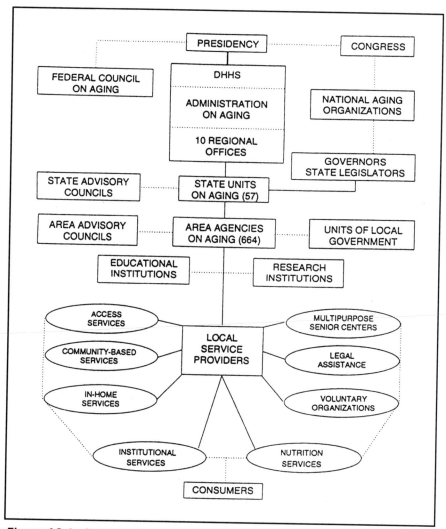

Figure 19.1. Older Americans Act Network. From *The New Aging: Politics and Change in America* (p. 56), by F. M. Torres-Gil, 1991, Westport, CT: Greenwood Publishing Group, Inc. Copyright 1991 by Greenwood Publishing Group, Inc. Reprinted with permission.

senior centers, and employment (Binstock, 1987). AAAs appear to be fairly evenly based in three different organizational contexts: not-for-profit; council of government; and city/county government (public) (Krout, 1994). Almost 4 out of every 10 AAAs serve one county, whereas 30% are responsible for seven or more counties. Whereas 18% of the

AAAs cover less than 500 square miles each, another 20% contain over 6,500 square miles each. The mean number of persons aged 60 and over in the PSAs is 63,000. Finally, it is important to note that OAA funding accounts for slightly less than half of AAA budgets. Thus, it is clear that OAA/Title III funding and priorities do not define in total the activities of AAAs (Krout, 1994).

AAAs can provide information to audiologists and speech–language pathologists and can also serve as an entry point into other components of the aging services network. AAA staff may be able to identify services that can meet the additional needs of an older person receiving treatment for a communication disorder. However, AAA staff typically have little specific knowledge of speech–language and hearing problems. Thus, communication disorders professionals should also consider working with AAAs to educate staff as well as other practitioners in the aging services network about these problems, and to help design service delivery systems to meet them. Some AAA funds may be available for support of information/education and screening programs for speech–language and hearing disorders.

Senior Centers. A senior center is not a service per se, but rather an organization through which many services can be made available to older adults and which provides a physical location for those services and for older adults to gather for social, recreational, educational, and volunteer opportunities. Such centers can provide communication disorders professionals valuable points of contact with older adults.

The number of senior centers has grown to between 10,000 and 15,000, depending on how one defines the term (Krout, 1989). Many, but by no means all, senior centers fit under the umbrella of AAAs. Most are multipurpose in that they provide a range of activities and services and are multifaceted in terms of the functions they fulfill for older participants as well as the roles they play in local social and health service networks. In addition, many centers perform "focal point" functions through information and referral and collocation of services with other organizations, even in the absence of a formal designation as a focal point. Throughout their history, senior centers have responded to the needs of both frail and well older persons.

Krout (1994) has found that a significant number of senior center participants have "aged in place" over the last two decades. This means that the general senior center population has gotten older, more frail, and more prone to experiencing communication disorders. Thus, senior center staff and participants have particular needs for information on communication problems and appropriate referrals for services.

Speech–Language and Audiology Services in the Community

Many older individuals are receiving services for communication disorders, but the services are being provided mainly for residents of extended care facilities, rehabilitation facility patients, or community-dwelling elders. Far fewer older individuals are being served via the aging services network. In limited instances, small research or service provision grants may be utilized to serve those living in the community. In areas where a university speech and hearing clinic is located, older individuals may be offered speech, language, and hearing services free or at a reduced cost. These university clinics may participate in third-party payment, or the individual may need to pay for the service and submit the costs to a third-party payer for whole or partial reimbursement.

Some data are available on the involvement of aging service network agencies with services for older adults with communication impairment. Nationwide, probably between 10% and 15% of the older people participating in senior centers are vision or hearing impaired, frail in health, or cognitively impaired (Krout, 1995). These persons do not necessarily receive any services at the center for their communication problem. On the other hand, the Maryland Association of Senior Centers (1984) found that almost half of the centers surveyed reported services for persons with visual impairment, one third for individuals with hearing impairment, and almost two thirds for those with mobility impairment. Another study of senior center-based programming revealed some focus on education/information on speech and hearing issues (Freedman & Friedmann, 1986). There is a conspicuous absence of information on speech–language disorders.

Several articles have described programs aimed at increasing the involvement of older people with hearing and visual impairment in senior centers. Becker and Nadler (1980) described the integration of older prelingually deaf people into senior center activities. A key factor in this program was the center's hiring of a social worker who was active in the deaf community and could use sign language. As a result of a slow and careful process, deaf older people eventually began to participate in many of the center's activities, after first staying together and then apart from center users who could hear. Hearing staff and users were educated about deafness and signing, and interpreters helped to ensure that the deaf were fully informed about center programs. The center eventually gained 61 deaf members.

One of the unintended consequences of the program was that center staff and participants became visually more aware of their surroundings and were said to have gained an understanding of working with a "subculture." Thus, though existing data are sparse, it would appear that parts of the aging services network, such as senior centers, can offer communication disorders professionals an organizational context that affords them contact with noninstitutionalized older adults who may need their services. However, the data also indicate that screening and other services are much more likely to focus on hearing loss, not speech–language communication issues.

There remains limited information about the interaction between speech–language and hearing professionals and the aging services network. Perhaps communication disorders professionals in many communities have become involved with activities sponsored by aging network agencies. However, the dearth of presentations of these activities at conferences and in professional journals would suggest otherwise. This absence may validate the notion that speech–language and audiology are seen as only an ancillary service (Jakobs-Condit, 1984). It would appear that significant barriers limit the involvement of communication disorders professionals in the aging services network and that these barriers should be identified and eliminated.

Overcoming Barriers to Receiving Communication Disorder Services

We now turn to an identification of those barriers that limit the degree of contact between communication disorders professionals and the aging services network. For each barrier, a discussion of how it can be lessened, if not overcome, is provided.

Lack of Knowledge of the Aging Services Network Among Communication Disorders Professionals

Perhaps the most basic reason for the lack of interaction between speech–language pathologists and audiologists and components of the aging services network is the fact that few communication disorders professionals have a good understanding of what the network is, how it operates, and how it can be accessed. One obvious way to increase this awareness is to contact aging service network organizations, such as your local AAA. A listing of several key national organizations that can provide information on state and local agencies is provided in Appendix 19.A, and a list of questions that can be utilized to survey resources and needs at these agencies can be found in Appendix 19.B (Shadden & Barr, 1988). Invite representatives from the AAA to present inservices to your local speech–pathology and audiology organization regarding the scope of services provided to elders in your community, or visit the AAA personally to acquaint yourself with its personnel and services. Additionally, seek information from the American Speech-Language-Hearing Association (ASHA) about recognized gerontological conferences to provide incentives for professionals in the communication disorders field to become better acquainted with the broad spectrum of professionals and services involved in gerontology.

For communication disorders professionals in academic settings, another strategy for gaining knowledge of and access to older adults in the aging services network is to develop externships for students (and faculty) in sites such as senior centers, adult day programs, and case management offices. These interactions provide students with valuable experiences with older adults and help them learn first-hand about how older persons experience and respond to communication problems. A framework for understanding normal aging is also promoted. Speech–language pathologists and audiologists could also explore the possibility of forming partnerships with aging services network agencies to conduct research and evaluation studies, in addition to community outreach and education efforts.

Another way to increase the understanding of communication disorders professionals is to include information on the Older Americans Act and the aging services network in existing communication disorders core curriculum coursework. Students should be encouraged to take at least one gerontology course *before* the fieldwork experience. Such preservice training should ideally encourage interdisciplinary academic and clinical/fieldwork experiences. Students particularly interested in working with older adults should be encouraged to add a gerontology minor. Models for incorporating content in the communication disorders curriculum have been provided by others (Weinstein, Clark, Shadden, & Peavey, 1993).

Lack of Understanding of Communication Disorders and Related Services Among Aging Services Network Personnel

Few aging service network practitioners understand the nature of communication disorders and the types of services that speech–language pathologists and audiologists can provide to older adults. Communication disorders professionals will need to take the lead in working with components of the aging services network to promote understanding of these problems and services. For example, local area agencies on aging, senior centers, and other community-based services for older adults (including other allied health professionals) can be provided with written materials or staff presentations on communication problems. Videotapes can be used as an effective way to provide information on communication disorders to service practitioners. Such tapes can also be distributed to libraries, doctors' offices, and similar locations. These educational/outreach programs should be offered at little or no cost. Arranging for continuing education units (CEUs) for other professions will also serve as an incentive for aging network practitioners to attend such programs. Additionally, many aging services network agencies offer programs for caregivers that could also be utilized as a format for inservices.

The role of computer technology should also be considered. For example, computerized inservice programs regarding common communication disorders of the elderly could be developed for aging service network agencies. An example of one such approach to training staff was designed at the Seattle Veterans Administration Medical Center to inservice physicians regarding adult neurogenic communication disorders. For agencies that are on-line, e-mailing of information can be very effective and cost-efficient. The Internet can also be utilized to provide information to seniors directly through sources such as Senior Net and America OnLine.

Communication Disorders Terminology

Aging service network practitioners and communication disorders specialists use terminology that is unfamiliar to each other; lack of understanding and inadequate communication between professionals may result. The clinical terminology used by speech–language pathologists and audiologists in the diagnosis and treatment of communication problems is likely confusing and could even be intimidating to aging service network practitioners and older adults. Speech–language pathologists and audiologists should explore ways to communicate their expertise in language that is more easily understood and less intimidating to older persons and those who provide care for them. One strategy includes the provision of inservices or informational literature (e.g., a glossary of terms) explaining commonly misunderstood communication disorders terminology to elders, family, and aging service network professionals.

Interaction and Referral

It is important for aging network practitioners and family caregivers to understand communication problems so that they can make referrals to the appropriate communication disorder professionals. It is also likely that many people do not understand how and where to access speech–language pathology and audiology services. One way to reduce this barrier is for communication disorders professionals to work with agencies and develop an informal or formal referral mechanism. A communication problem hotline that provides information on communication problems associated with aging could be established jointly by a local speech–language pathology/audiology professional organization and an area agency on aging or senior center. Speech–language pathologists and audiologists could volunteer at the hotline or provide the training for other volunteers, including older adults. Of course, direct contact with older adults at program sites could provide information on service access though presentations. Preliminary screenings could also be conducted at such settings.

Funding and Personnel

These strategies to overcome barriers to interaction between communication disorders professionals and the aging service network generally will require communication disorders professionals to volunteer their time and energy. Most of the activities discussed as solutions are not reimbursable under existing public and private payor regulations, and aging service network agencies generally lack the resources to pay for them. Indeed, lack of reimbursement for services provided by audiologists and speech–language pathologists outside acute care and long-term care settings may be one of the main reasons otherwise healthy older persons do not seek treatment for communication problems. Thus, aging service network agencies may not provide communication disorders education, screening, or maintenance services because they are not generally reimbursable through government programs, such as Medicare or Medicaid, or private insurance.

To change this, communication disorders professionals could work with private insurers and federal/state governments to alter existing reimbursement policies. Emphasis should be placed on obtaining funding for services outside traditional health care settings and for less disabled older persons that generally utilize aging services network services. Another strategy is to work with other community agencies to provide services through support groups for older adults with communication problems. As these agencies and the individuals they serve recognize the expertise of speech–language pathologists and audiologists, they may initiate future referrals for reimbursable services. Communication disorders professionals could also provide aging network agencies with information on reimbursement options, as well as identifying other speech–language pathologists and audiologists in the community. Other options include enlisting the help of volunteers (Shadden & Barr, 1988) to develop and implement grant-supported projects and, where appropriate, providing group therapy at a cost savings to agencies and participants.

Model Programs

Examples of model programs initiated to overcome barriers to communication disorders professionals working with and within the aging services network are outlined in the following section. These model programs illustrate the diversity in funding sources, from small internal grants to major private or government-funded grants. Additionally, these grants demonstrate how audiology and/or speech–language pathology professionals can potentially provide grant-funded services in the aging services network.

The Summer Gerontology Internship program, funded by Ithaca College, is a good example of how internal grant funds provide faculty additional experience working with the aging population (Svitko-Crichley, 1991). The project, conducted at three senior centers over a 5-week period, involved presenting informational sessions on hearing loss and hearing aids to the center's users and professionals, hearing screenings, and follow-up counseling. Additionally, a brochure was developed providing information on hearing loss and hearing aids, as well as defining the qualifications and roles of audiologists and otolaryngologists. The grantee also developed a resource list of area professionals and gave the lists and brochures to senior citizen centers for distribution to center users.

The US WEST Rural Speech–Hearing Outreach Program provides a model of how corporate grant funds can be utilized to improve service provision to elderly adults and facilitate collaboration between professionals serving that population through the provision of information and the development of a referral network (Scheib, LeMay, & Toner, 1990; Scheib, Honsvick, & Jelinek, 1991). Informational brochures were developed to provide factual information and to dispel common misperceptions about communication and aging. Brochures were distributed to relevant personnel (e.g., physicians) and at key sites (e.g., health fairs, senior citizen centers, etc.). Inservices and workshops were provided at many of those sites. To develop a referral network, informational letters describing the incidence of communication disorders in the elderly, early signs of these disorders, and the roles of audiologists and speech–language pathologists were sent to professionals serving older adults. These professionals had the option of being included on a referral list that would then be distributed to the elderly and other professionals. Feedback by senior centers regarding the program was positive, as senior center personnel felt this was a viable approach to meeting the needs of the older adult. Professionals benefited not only by receiving referrals but also by networking with other professionals and agencies in the area.

Project KEEP (KEEP ELDERS COMMUNICATING) demonstrates how federal funding can be generated to meet the communication needs of the older adult in rural settings (Glista & Bate, 1995). This project was generated by the Department of Speech–Language Pathology and Audiology at Western Michigan University (WMU) and approved for funding by the Health Resources Services Administration of the U.S. Department of Health and Human Services. The purpose of this grant is to increase the quantity and quality

of audiologists and speech–language pathologists who have specialized competencies for (a) diagnosing, assessing, and treating older
Americans using meaningful and relevant methodologies and technologies to extend their years of high-quality human communication;
(b) enhancing treatment decisions by adopting another's perspective
and collecting data on age, family, and culture; (c) providing care to
older Americans within the framework of interdisciplinary health care
teams; (d) working with older Americans and their families in natural,
functional life environments to facilitate optimal communication,
including those in rural areas; and (e) implementing strategies for preventing communication impairment and disability among older Americans while promoting and accommodating full participation in
social and avocational settings. Specialized coursework and practicum
opportunities have been designed to support preservice audiology
and speech–language pathology graduate students. This grant is
unique in that it was designed to closely interface with the Interdisciplinary Rural Health Grant awarded to WMU's College of Health
and Human Services.

Finally, there is the example of a federally funded grant awarded
by the Administration of Aging under Title IV of the Older Americans
Act to the Helen Keller National Center for Deaf-Blind Youth and
Adults (Brady & Bagley, 1992). The purpose of the grant was to provide training for those older individuals with sensory losses to cope
better with daily living activities. In addition, the grantee hoped that
professionals in the aging services network would become more
aware of the effects of sensory losses during everyday activities. The
grantee, along with a variety of other allied health care professionals,
developed a 6-week educational program focused on coping strategies
for older individuals with hearing and/or vision problems.
Additionally, this educational program was implemented locally by a
contract with an Area Agency on Aging.

Program, Policy, and Research Issues

Currently, there is a dearth of information on the interaction between
speech–language pathologists and audiologists and the aging services
network. The scant data we do have clearly suggest that communication disorders professionals know very little of the components and
operation of the aging services network, and rarely access the network

as a way to increase the knowledge and utilization of speech–language and audiology services among older adults. Likewise, aging services network practitioners know little of the communication disorders that speech–language pathologists and audiologists are trained to address or of the services they provide. More research is needed to determine the relative importance of various barriers in creating this lack of knowledge and interaction as well as on the factors that create these barriers.

Once more data are available on these barriers and their causes, program interventions can be designed, implemented, and evaluated to overcome the barriers. The efficacy of potential strategies to increase the interaction between the aging services network and communication disorders professionals needs to be investigated through carefully designed and executed research projects. Successful models must be developed and disseminated, and replication studies testing both their short-term and long-term impacts should be conducted.

Such research, demonstration, and dissemination efforts will require funding as well as the support of both aging services network and communication disorders professional organizations. Because it is unlikely that these organizations have sufficient monies for these tasks, they should explore working together to obtain public and private (including corporate) funding. This will require a joint effort to educate those in control of program allocations about the benefits of greater collaboration in serving the communication needs of older adults. An example might be taken from the field of music therapy, where a well-planned and executed education and lobbying effort resulted in the inclusion of demonstration project monies for music therapy programs for older adults in the 1992 reauthorization of the Older Americans Act (Krout, 1995).

The music therapy example demonstrates the need for action at the state and federal policy level as an important strategy if resources for greater aging service network/communication disorders professionals interactions are to be forthcoming. Because funding follows policy, attention must be paid to the rules that govern reimbursement for audiology and speech–pathology services and how those rules need to be altered. The advent of managed care as an important component not only of private health insurance but also of Medicare and Medicaid may actually provide opportunities for increased funding for communication disorders services delivered outside of nursing homes and hospitals. Whether as a cause or an effect, managed care has shifted the site of the receipt of some health care from acute care to community settings. Senior centers and other points in the aging services network may be seen increasingly as cost-effective delivery sites, as well as places where health promotion activities (e.g., dysphagia prevention) can reach large numbers of older adults. Speech–language pathologists and audiologists should explore opportunities to work with the aging services network and develop health services that could be reimbursed under managed care.

Conclusions

The aging services network serves a large and diverse population of older adults through scores of community-based programs located in every community in the nation. Many of these programs focus on health education and promotion and ultimately aim to improve the quality of life of older adults by helping them to continue living independently. However, programs relating to hearing, and especially speech–language problems, are often not provided by this network or are provided sporadically and superficially. This is unfortunate given that so many older adults will experience problems in these areas.

This paucity of programs presents an excellent opportunity for audiologists and speech–language pathologists to collaborate with practitioners in the aging services network to increase the knowledge of communication problems among older adults and increase the use of appropriate clinical services. As discussed earlier in this chapter, this collaboration can take many forms and can have many benefits for communication disorders professionals and the aging services network. Fundamentally, it is most important for communication disorders professionals to take the initiative to learn more about the operation and activities of the aging services network and its participants through direct contact with its practitioners and programs. Much of what audiologists and speech–language pathologists do is not well known in the community, and it is often cloaked in terminology that is both confusing and intimidating to even well-educated laypersons. These and other barriers to improved service interactions between communication disorders professionals and the aging services network do exist, but they can be overcome. Doing so will help ensure that older adults become informed about and receive appropriate services for speech–language and hearing problems; quality of life will be enhanced significantly.

References

Becker, G., & Nadler, G. (1980).The aged deaf: Integration of a disabled group into an agency serving elderly people. *The Gerontologist, 20,* 214–221.

Binstock, R. (1987). Title III of the Older Americans Act: An analysis and proposal for the 1987 reauthorization. *The Gerontologist, 27,* 259–265.

Brady, D., & Bagley, E. (1992). *Community based confident living programs for at-risk elderly with sensory losses.* Project funded under Title IV of the Older Americans Act. Washington, DC: Administration on Aging.

Freedman, F., & Friedmann, S. (1986). "Project Stay Well" does well in New York City. *Aging, 353,* 2–3.

Gelfand, D. (1993). *The aging services network* (3rd ed.). New York: Springer.

Glista, S., & Bate, H. (1995). *KEEP ELDERS COMMUNICATING (KEEP).* Project funded by the Health Resources Service Administration of the U. S. Department of Health and Human Services.

Hudson, R. B. (1995). The Older Americans Act and the defederalization of community-based care. In P. K. H. Kim (Ed.), *Services to the aging and aged: Public policies and programs* (pp. 45–75). New York: Garland.

Jakobs-Condit, L. (Ed.). (1984). *Gerontology and communication disorders.* Rockville, MD: American Speech-Language-Hearing Association.

Krout, J. (1989). *Senior centers in America.* Westport, CT: Greenwood Press.

Krout, J. (1994). Changes in senior center participant characteristics: A longitudinal analysis. *Journal of Gerontological Social Work, 22,* 1–21.

Krout, J. (1995). Senior centers and services for the frail elderly. *Journal of Aging and Social Policy, 7,* 59–76.

Maryland Association of Senior Centers. (1984). *Report on MASC survey of senior centers.* Unpublished manuscript.

Older Americans Act of 1965. Public Law 89-73.

Sayles, A. H., & Adams, J. K. (1979). *Communication problems and behaviors of the older American.* Rockville, MD: American Speech-Language-Hearing Association.

Scheib, R., Honsvick, C., & Jelinek, J. (1991, November). *Implementing an elderly screening program: A marketing strategy.* Paper presented at the annual meeting of the American Speech-Language-Hearing Association, Atlanta.

Scheib, R., LeMay, A., & Toner, M. (1990, November). *Communication disorders in the elderly: A screening model.* Paper presented at the annual meeting of the American Speech-Language-Hearing Association, Seattle, WA.

Shadden, B. B., & Barr, J. A. (1988). Networking strategies for enhancing inter-disciplinary service provision. In B. B. Shadden (Ed.), *Communication behavior and aging: A sourcebook for clinicians* (pp. 360–376). Baltimore: Williams & Wilkins.

Social Security Amendments of 1965. Public Law 89-97.

Svitko-Crichley, C. S. (1991). *Hearing screening and hearing loss education programs in senior centers.* Project funding by Ithaca College Gerontology Institute. Ithaca, NY: Ithaca College.

Torres-Gil, F. M. (1991). *The new aging: Politics and change in America.* Westport, CT: Greenwood Press.

U.S. Department of Health, Education, and Welfare. (1977). *Local area agencies on aging help the aging but problems need correcting.* Washington, DC: Administration on Aging.

U.S. Senate, Special Committee on Aging. (1986). *Developments in aging 1985: Part III.* Washington, DC: Government Printing Office.

Weinstein, B. E., Clark, L. W., Shadden, B. B., & Peavey, J. (1993, November). *Doing the impossible: Incorporating coursework on aging into the curriculum.* Miniseminar presented at the annual meeting of the American Speech-Language-Hearing Association, Anaheim, CA.

White House Conference on Aging. (1995). [Official 1995 White House Conference on Aging, Background Materials]. Washington, DC: Author.

Appendix 19A
Aging Network Service
Resources and Information

Administration on Aging (AoA)
Office of Human Development
U.S. Department of Health and Human Services
330 Independence Avenue, SW
William J. Cohen Building
Washington, DC 20201
(202) 619-0641

American Society on Aging (ASA)
833 Market Street, Suite 512
San Francisco, CA 94103
(415) 882-2910

National Council on the Aging, Inc. (NCOA)
409 Third St., SW
Second Floor
Washington, DC 20024
(202) 479-1200

Gerontological Society of America (GSA)
1275 K Street, NW
Washington, DC 20005
(202) 842-1275

**National Association of Area Agencies
on Aging (NCOA)**
1112 16th Street, NW
Washington, DC 20036
(202) 296-8130

**National Association of State
Units on Aging (NASUA)**
2033 K Street, NW
Washington, DC 20006
(202) 785-0707

Directory of Aging Resources
Business Publishers, Inc.
951 Pershing Drive
Silver Spring, MD 20910-4464
(301) 587-6300

National Guide to Funding in Aging
The Foundation Center
79 Fifth Avenue
New York, NY 10003-3076

Appendix 19B:
Questionnaire for Local Area
Agencies on Aging

1. Is there a need for discounted/free speech, language, and hearing screenings?

2. Are collaborative inservice opportunities available?

3. Do opportunities exist to write a column in a local gerontologically oriented publication?

4. What are the specific problems or needs of older persons with communication or cognitive impairments?

Hearing impairment	Swallowing concerns
Speechreading needs	Word-finding problems
Speech unintelligible	Writing impaired
Reading impaired	Unable to initiate a conversation
Decreased problem solving	Impaired memory
Impaired orientation	
Maintain use of assistive listening devices	

5. What informal resources currently address these needs? Note any limitations.

6. What formal resources currently address these needs? Note any limitations.

7. What relationship exists between formal and informal resources? How could these linkages be enhanced?

8. What problems or needs are not currently being met by existing resources?

9. List the current number of adult day-care centers and/or senior citizens' centers in the area. What services does that person provide? How many of these are informally or formally serviced by an audiologist? What services does that person provide? Limitations?

10. Are collaborative grant-writing opportunities available? Which grants were written and funded?

Note. From "Networking Strategies for Enhancing Interdisciplinary Service Provision," by Barbara B. Shadden and Jane A. Barr, 1988. In B. B. Shadden (Ed.), *Communication and Aging: A Sourcebook for Clinicians* (p. 367). Baltimore: Williams & Wilkins. Copyright 1988. Adapted with permission.

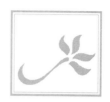

Author Index

Subject Index

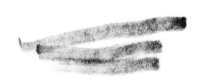

aek 8012

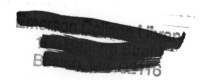